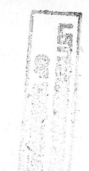
# Counselling in HIV Infection and AIDS

## EDITORS

### John Green

*Chief Clinical Psychologist*
*Department of Clinical Psychology*
*St Mary's Hospital*
*London W2*

*Honorary Lecturer in Behavioural Sciences,*
*St Mary's Hospital Medical School*

### Alana McCreaner

*Head: National AIDS Counselling Training Unit*
*St Mary's Hospital*
*London W2*

Blackwell Scientific Publications

OXFORD LONDON EDINBURGH

BOSTON MELBOURNE

Copyright © John Green and Alana McCreaner 1989

Blackwell Scientific Publications
Editorial Offices:
Osney Mead, Oxford OX2 0EL
25 John Street, London WC1N 2BL
23 Ainslie Place, Edinburgh EH3 6AJ
3 Cambridge Center, Suite 208,
  Cambridge, Massachusetts 02142, USA
54 University Street, Carlton
  Victoria 3053, Australia

First published 1989
Reprinted 1989, 1990

Set by Setrite, Hong Kong
Printed and bound in Great Britain by
Billing & Sons Ltd, Worcester

British Library
Cataloguing in Publication Data

Counselling HIV infection and AIDS.
  1. AIDS patients. Counselling
  I. Green, John   II. McCreaner, Alana
362.1'9697

ISBN 0—632—01924—7

DISTRIBUTORS
Marston Book Services Ltd
PO Box 87
Oxford OX2 0DT
(Orders: Tel: 0865 791155
        Fax: 0865 791927
        Telex: 837515)
USA
Year Book Medical Publishers
200 North LaSalle Street
Chicago, Illinois 60601
(Orders: Tel. (312) 726—9733)

Canada
The C.V. Mosby Company
5240 Finch Avenue East,
Scarborough, Ontario
(Orders: Tel. (416) 298—1588)

Australia
Blackwell Scientific Publications
  (Australia) Pty Ltd
54 University Street
Carlton, Victoria 3053
(Orders: Tel. (03) 347—0300)

Library of Congress
Cataloging-in-Publication Data

Green, John, clinical psychologist.
  Counselling in HIV infection and
  AIDS/John Green, Alana McCreaner.
    p.     cm.
  Includes bibliographies and index.
  ISBN 0—632—01924—7 (pbk.)
Counselling of.      2. AIDS (Disease)—
Psychological aspects.
1. McCreaner, Alana.      II.     Title.
  [DNLM: 1. Acquired
Immunodeficiency Syndrome—
psychology.      2. Counselling.
WD 308 G796c]
RC607. A26G64 1988
362.1'9697'92—dc 19
DNLM/DLC
for Library of Congress

# Contents

Acknowledgements                                                    vii

Introduction                                                        ix

1 The Facts About AIDS                                              1
  *John Green, Psychology Dept, St Mary's Hospital, London*
2 Laboratory Tests for HIV                                          12
  *D J Jeffries, Division of Virology, Dept of Medical Microbiology,*
  *St Mary's Hospital Medical School, London*
3 Pre-test Counselling                                              21
  *Alana McCreaner, National AIDS Counselling Training Unit,*
  *St Mary's Hospital, London*
4 Post-test Counselling                                             28
  *John Green, Psychology Dept, St Mary's Hospital, London*
5 Counselling People with AIDS, Their Lovers, Friends and
  Relations                                                        69
  *Heather George, Psychology Dept, St Mary's Hospital, London*
6 Counselling Those with AIDS Dementia                             88
  *Agnes Kocsis, Clinical Psychology Dept, St Mary's Hospital, London*
7 The Counselling of HIV Antibody Positive Haemophiliacs           108
  *Peter Jones, Newcastle Haemophilia Reference Centre, Newcastle*
  *upon Tyne*
8 Drug Abuse and HIV                                               121
  *Geraldine Mulleady, Drug Dependency Unit, St Mary's Hospital,*
  *London*
9 Counselling and Pregnancy                                        141
  *John Green, Psychology Dept, St Mary's Hospital, London*
10 Paediatric HIV Infection                                        157
  *Jacqueline Mok, Infectious Diseases Unit, City Hospital, Edinburgh*

11  The Worried Well                                                    167
    *John Green, Psychology Dept, St Mary's Hospital, London*
12  Dealing With Anxiety and Depression                                 174
    *John Green, Psychology Dept, St Mary's Hospital, London*
13  Problem Solving                                                     198
    *John Green, Psychology Dept, St Mary's Hospital, London*
14  Dying, Bereavement and Loss                                         207
    *John Green and Lorraine Sherr, Psychology Dept, St Mary's
    Hospital, London*
15  Male Homosexual Sexual Behaviour                                    224
    *Tom McManus, The Alexander Clinic, St Giles' Hospital, London*
16  AIDS in the Community                                               233
    *Terry Cotton, Social Services Dept, London Borough
    of Hammersmith & Fulham*
17  The Role of Voluntary Groups in the Community                       238
    *Janet Green, Terrence Higgins Trust, London*
18  Counselling in Developing Countries                                 248
    *John Green, Psychology Dept, St Mary's Hospital, London*
19  Training Models                                                     276
    *Alana McCreaner, National AIDS Counselling Training Unit,
    St Mary's Hospital, London*
20  Legal Aspects                                                       285
    *Diana Kloss, Faculty of Law, The University of Manchester*
21  Ethical Questions                                                   301
    *Reverend Dr Kenneth Boyd, Institute of Medical Ethics, Edinburgh*
*Appendix A*:  Relaxation                                               314
    *Agnes Kocsis, Clinical Psychology Dept, St Mary's
    Hospital, London*
*Appendix B*:  Suggested Reading List                                   325
    *Simon Vearnals, National AIDS Counselling Training
    Unit, St Mary's Hospital, London*
*Index*                                                                 329

*Helen Higgins*

# Acknowledgements

It is impossible for us to thank everyone who has helped us with our thinking about this book without making it look like a telephone directory. However, we would like to specially thank Patricia O'Connell, Simon Vearnals and Dr Susan Forster for helping us with the editing of some of the chapters.

We would also like to thank all the many friends and colleagues from statutory and voluntary agencies who have helped us to think through the issues surrounding the counselling of those with HIV infection and AIDS. We are particularly grateful to those in developing countries with whom we have worked for helping us to widen our appreciation of the issues surrounding counselling in its international context.

We would also like to thank the many course participants who have attended the National AIDS Counselling Training Unit courses over the past three years and have helped us to challenge and extend our understanding.

Special thanks go to the authors of chapters who have extended busy days into busy nights to get their chapters to us. We would like to thank our publisher Richard Miles for his unfailing good humour and support.

Finally we would like to thank our patients who have helped us more than anyone else.

John Green
Alana McCreaner

# Introduction

There is currently no vaccine which can prevent the spread of HIV infection. Only changes in behaviour by those at risk can halt its spread. The counselling of those infected with the virus can help them to make those changes in order to avoid infection or to prevent the infection of others.

However, HIV and AIDS counselling is not just about preventing the spread of infection. It is about promoting and maintaining the physical and mental well-being of all those whose lives are touched directly or indirectly by the HIV virus — people with AIDS, those with HIV infection, those at risk, their lovers, family and other carers.

The term 'counselling' is one which is applied to this sort of work worldwide. Unfortunately, different people mean different things by the term 'counselling'. It is used variously to mean supporting others, offering information so that people can make decisions, helping people practically, helping people to assert control over their lives, helping people to change their behaviour, helping people to adjust to their difficulties, and helping people to come to important decisions about their lives. As we have used the term it includes all these things and more.

However, one thing that the term 'counselling' as we have used it does *not* imply is adherence to a specific 'school' or approach to helping people. Counselling in the context in which it is used in this book is not something which *only* trained counsellors can do, it is something which anyone who is working, in whatever capacity, with people affected directly or indirectly by HIV and AIDS not only can do but *must* do.

The good HIV counsellor needs good interpersonal skills, an understanding of the social, moral, and ethical context of AIDS and the ways in which this affects peoples' lives, an awareness of the issues which confront those whose lives are touched by HIV, an understanding of the ways in which people can be helped, and an awareness of the ways in which they can be hindered by the counsellor. A good background knowledge of AIDS and HIV is also indispensable to the counsellor.

In this book we have tried to assemble material which will be of *practical* help to counsellors in their day-to-day work. We have also tried to give counsellors an appreciation of the many facets of HIV and AIDS counselling. The book does not, however, set out to provide a literature review on counselling or on AIDS. We have asked authors to explain how they go about their counselling work with patients and to provide references only where these will be of direct help to the counsellor.

We have tried to keep overlap between chapters to a minimum but, since there are common considerations in many chapters, some overlap is inevitable and indeed, we hope, helpful. We have intended that each chapter can be read as part of the overall book, but also that it will stand alone in its own right. Patients themselves do not fall into neat 'pigeonholes' for the convenience of the book editor.

We have also tried not just to convey information about the process of counselling but also about what counselling is like; in the many training courses we run each year the most common questions concern this issue: 'What do people say?', 'What sort of problems do people bring?', 'What shall I say next?', 'How shall I say it?'

We hope that, through the use of case studies and examples of counsellor-patient discussions we can go some way towards answering these questions. In doing so we hope that we will give people reading the book confidence to extend the way in which they currently work.

The book opens with brief factual information about HIV and AIDS. This is not intended as a comprehensive review of the field but as a starting point for further reading for those who are new to the field. Chapters 3 and 4 cover pre- and post-test counselling — issues which are central to all the other areas covered in the book. For instance a counsellor dealing with a person with AIDS will need to cover all the issues in post-test counselling as well as the issues covered in the chapter on AIDS (Chapter 5).

The book then looks at people who are affected in different ways by HIV, those with AIDS and those with AIDS-related encephalopathy (Chapters 5 and 6). Subsequent chapters look at individuals with particular characteristics, drug abusers, haemophiliacs, pregnant women and those contemplating pregnancy, and children, as well as the 'worried well' (Chapters 7—11).

Chapters 12–14 cover particular approaches to specific problems – anxiety, depression, helping people through problem solving, and helping with death, bereavement and loss. Chapter 15 provides a brief introduction to aspects of gay sexuality for those who may not be familiar with this. Chapters 16 and 17 go on to look at the key role of community agencies and voluntary agencies.

Chapter 18 looks at some of the differences and similarities between counselling in Western countries and developing countries, and at how models of counselling need to be changed to fit local circumstances. It also covers some of the issues which might need to be taken into account in setting up a service.

Chapter 19 suggests ways of approaching the problem of setting up a training course of key workers and managers.

Chapters 20 and 21 cover legal issues from a UK perspective and general ethical issues. Reading the two chapters together highlights the extent to which the two issues are inextricably intertwined.

Appendix A provides advice on the important issue of helping patients to reduce stress and to relax. In Appendix B we have selected a very few books which we have found helpful and stimulating from the many excellent books which are available in this area.

Finally, we would like to mention the vexed issue of language. Different authors in the book use different words to refer to those whose lives are touched by HIV. Some people refer to them as 'patients', others as 'clients', others in other ways. The important thing, ultimately, is that they are all different ways of describing *people*, individuals with their own fears and hopes, their own problems and their own strengths in facing up to the difficulties which HIV can bring into their lives.

We have used the convention of 'he' meaning the patient or doctor as opposed to he/she, for the sake of simplicity.

# Chapter 1

# The Facts About AIDS

JOHN GREEN

## AIDS: The background to the disease

This chapter is intended only to give a brief introductory overview of the field of AIDS as a basis for further reading. It is important that anyone working in this area should read widely in the field and ensure that they have adequate background knowledge. Without it they cannot hope to offer sensible advice to their patients, who may themselves be particularly well-informed about the field.

The first cases of AIDS were recognised in the United States in 1981. It is clear that there had been sporadic cases in different areas of the world in the late 1970s, and possibly before that time, but that the disease was rare virtually everywhere before the 1980s. Since that time AIDS has become a major pandemic.

AIDS is an acronym standing for 'Acquired Immune Deficiency Syndrome'. It is caused by a virus of the retrovirus family, the Human Immunodeficiency Virus (HIV). While HIV is the agreed name today, it is still sometimes referred to under names used in the past – HTLV-III, LAV and ARV.

The HIV virus invades cells which bear the necessary viral receptor site on their surfaces. This site is called the CD-4 antigen. Chief amongst these cells are white blood cells, the T4 or T-helper cells. T-helper cells act to switch on the immune system when the body is under attack by infectious agents. They also play a key role in the body's defences against cancer by mobilising immune system processes which act to kill cancer cells.

In AIDS many of the T-helper cells are invaded by the virus and killed and others are impaired in their functioning even though they are not infected. The result of this is that the immune system, the body's defences against disease, does not switch on properly in response to invasion by infectious agents and the response to cancer cells is impaired. Not all aspects of the immune system are heavily impaired since not all aspects rely on the action of T-helper cells, but the damage is extensive. The consequence is that the person with AIDS becomes vulnerable to infections and tumours which a person with a normal immune system is usually able to fight off without difficulty. These infections and tumours are called 'opportunistic' because they take the opportunity of the suppression of the body's defences against disease to take a hold.

### The virus

The HIV virus is one of a family of viruses, the retroviruses, which occur in many different species of mammal. There are at least three other retroviruses found in man, two leukaemia viruses (HTLV-I and HTLV-II), and what is probably a second AIDS virus, HIV-2. HIV-2 appears to be very similar in its effects to HIV. Currently it is thought to be rather rare outside West Africa, although there is evidence that it is spreading geographically. Whatever is said about HIV in this book appears to apply equally to HIV-2. The geographical and biological origins of HIV remain uncertain.

Because of the existence of HIV-2 some workers call HIV 'HIV-1'. For convenience in this book we refer to HIV-1 as, simply, HIV. However, counsellors should be aware of the alternative nomenclature.

The virus particle itself consists of a core of genetic material, the blueprint for the virus to reproduce itself. This core is in the form of a double strand of RNA. Attached to the RNA is a special enzyme unique to this group of viruses called reverse transcriptase. Around the core are two concentric cases of protein and then outside them a layer of lipid, essentially fat. This lipid layer must be intact for the virus to be able to survive outside a host cell. A large number of things can damage this lipid membrane or envelope, including heating, washing-up liquid, bleach and a whole range of disinfectants. Studding the membrane are molecules of glycoprotein which is one of the chief substances which the body recognises as foreign.

Figure 1.1 shows the way in which the virus invades a cell. As noted above, it invades cells which carry the CD-4 antigen on their surface. A number of cells of the immune system carry CD-4 but the greatest concentration of CD-4 appears on T-helper cells.

The virus first fuses with the CD-4 receptor site. It is then pulled

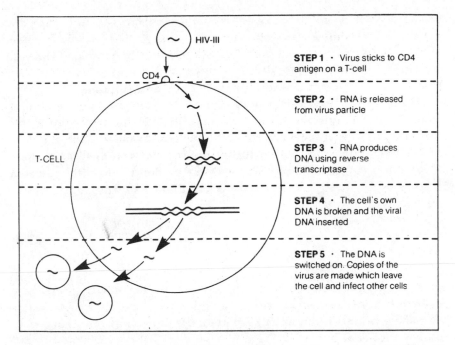

*Fig. 1.1* The infection of a T-cell by HIV (Source: Green, J. and Miller, D. (1986) *AIDS The Story of a Disease.* Grafton Publications.)

inside the cell. The outside of the virus particle is stripped off and the viral RNA with its attached reverse transcriptase is released into the cell. Once free, the RNA makes a copy of itself in DNA, the material from which human chromosomes — the genetic material of the cell itself — are made. In nature DNA makes RNA and RNA makes the chemicals the cell needs to maintain itself and carry out its functions. In the cells of animals RNA copies of DNA are used as a template for the production of proteins which the cell needs. DNA copies can only be made from RNA with the help of a special enzyme, reverse transcriptase, which the virus particle contains.

Once the virus has made a copy of itself in DNA it breaks the DNA in the cell's own chromosomes and then builds itself into the break. Once a person is infected with this virus, the virus becomes a part of the make-up of the cells of that person. It is for this reason that it is likely that someone infected with this virus will stay infected for life. When the cell's own DNA becomes active the viral DNA carried within it is also activated. As the cell's DNA is replicated the viral DNA contained within it is also replicated and can be used to produce viral proteins. These then leave the infected cell, stealing part of the cell wall as they go to make their membrane, thus completing new virus particles. These can go on to infect other cells and other people. Eventually the infected cell will die as a result of its viral load through a number of different possible processes and the infected individual has one less T-helper cell to fight infections and tumours.

The routes of transmission of this virus are covered in detail in Chapter 4. It is important to stress here that, in the everyday world, the virus has only been known to be passed on by sex, by blood-to-blood contact, by the mother to her unborn child *in utero* and, probably, through breast milk. There is no evidence, despite extensive studies of the families of those infected, that this virus can be passed on by casual contact.

## After infection

Most people infected with this virus do not even know that they have been infected, at least for some considerable time after infection. A few show a mild influenza-like illness after infection but many show no symptoms at all.

During the first few weeks after infection the virus begins to multiply in the body. The body recognises that the virus is foreign and tries to mount a defence against it. As it does so it produces antibodies in response to viral proteins on the surface of the virus and virus-infected cells. Antibodies are Y-shaped chemicals which stick onto foreign chemicals including some of the chemicals which make up invading organisms. The chemicals which antibodies stick to are called *antigens*.

Antibodies allow various cells to attack invading organisms as well as initiating certain chemical processes aimed at destroying the invader. Each antibody is specific for only one antigen, in other words antibodies aimed at HIV are quite different from those aimed at measles or salmonella. Because each virus or bacterium causes the body to produce very specific antibodies against it, it is possible to detect the fact that someone has been infected with HIV by looking for antibodies against the virus (this issue is covered in more detail in Chapter 2).

After infection it takes at least 8–12 weeks for a detectable antibody to appear in the blood. During the period between infection with the virus and the appearance of antibodies against it, routine antibody tests will be negative. However viral antigens are present in the blood and the virus may be cultured from body fluid. The individual at this stage is potentially highly infectious *even though he has a negative blood test* for antibody.

At the time that antibodies against the virus appear in the blood, detectable viral antigens disappear from the circulation and do not reappear for an indefinite period of time. The subsequent reappearance of these antigens in the blood suggests increased viral replication and is associated with a deterioration in the clinical state of the patient.

At about the time when antibodies appear in the blood some people experience a glandular-fever-like illness, usually mild but sometimes quite severe. This is the so-called 'seroconversion illness'. The illness eventually disappears, sometimes in a matter of days but sometimes only after many weeks, and the patient becomes well again.

After the appearance of antibodies in the blood most people who are infected with the virus then experience no evidence of being infected. They are said to be 'asymptomatic seropositives' because they test positive for antibodies against the virus but they have no symptoms of infection — although they are able to pass on the virus to others. Most asymptomatic individuals are quite well by all objective measures, although some do show immune system abnormalities even though they feel well.

A proportion of patients show persistent generalized lymphadenopathy (PGL). This just means persistently swollen lymph glands throughout the body. Lymph glands tend to swell when someone has an infection or malignancy which causes the immune system to become activated. HIV is a persistent infection. However, there has been debate in the AIDS field as to whether someone with PGL actually has a worse prognosis than someone who is asymptomatic. In fact there is now good evidence that someone with PGL, but with no other symptoms of infection, has the same prognosis in terms of risk of going on to develop AIDS as someone who is asymptomatic. The presence of actual symptoms in an HIV seropositive person leads to a worsened prognosis regardless of whether they show PGL or not.

Patients may continue to stay in the asymptomatic or PGL stage for years after infection, in good health. However, a proportion of patients will progress. In many patients who progress there is the appearance of fevers, of 'night sweats', and of loss of weight. A general feeling of malaise and of lack of energy often appears. They may show signs that they are not fighting off infections as they should, but do not develop any of the diseases which are diagnostic of AIDS. Patents in this stage are described as having ARC (AIDS-related complex).

Examination of the blood of those with ARC shows a pattern of the gradual reduction in the number of T-helper cells in their blood. At the same time antibody levels against the virus, especially those aimed at the core of the virus, start to fall. As they fall the level of virus in the blood and other body fluids starts to rise. It is thought likely that as individuals start to become ill they again become even more infectious to others. It is thus possible that someone infected with HIV may be most infectious just before antibodies appear and after he develops symptoms, although he may well be infectious in between these times.

There is undoubtedly an overlap between having AIDS and having ARC, with some people with ARC having worse immune functioning than some of those with AIDS. They may just not yet have developed an infection or tumour which would allow a diagnosis of AIDS to be made. The distinction between AIDS and ARC is, thus, a rather artificial one and some workers have preferred to avoid the use of the term ARC, preferring instead to look at the broad spectrum of HIV as a continuum of immune system damage without sharp artificial dividing lines. While this probably fits the facts rather better, the distinction between AIDS and ARC is a very real one in the minds of many patients and so the distinction between AIDS and ARC continues to be made.

## AIDS

An individual is diagnosed as having AIDS on one of three criteria: opportunistic infections, opportunistic tumours, or AIDS-related encephalopathy (sometimes called AIDS-dementia).

### Opportunistic infections

Opportunistic infections tend to be infections which a normal person is easily able to fight off. A person with AIDS becomes prone to disease caused by organisms which are all around us in the environment but which do not normally make us ill. Many of these infections can be treated by antibiotics and other drugs. Unfortunately, drugs which work very well in someone whose immune system is intact often work rather less well in someone who is unable to mount much of an immune system response. Nonetheless many opportunistic infections are potentially treatable and episodes of opportunistic infections can often be successfully treated. It often happens, however, that a person with AIDS will succumb to an opportunistic infection and die.

The opportunistic infections that individuals get depend on what organisms they are exposed to. Consequently the infections seen in a man in London, in a temperate zone, will differ from those seen in a man in the tropics. Exposure to infections may also vary with life style; genital herpes which fails to heal is not uncommon in gay men with AIDS but is rare in, say, haemophiliacs. Different levels of exposure to different organisms also probably explains why Kaposi's sarcoma (see below) is common in gay men but rare in intravenous drug abusers.

In Europe and the United States the most common opportunistic infections include:

- *Pneumocystis carinii pneumonia*, a protozoal lung infection causing fever, shortness of breath and a dry cough.
- *Tuberculosis*, a mycobacterial infection which attacks not just the lungs but other major organs as well. In people with AIDS it is often caused by atypical mycobacteria rather than the common mycobacterium tuberculosis.
- *Cryptosporidiosis*, caused by a protozoan, causes a profuse and persistent diarrhoea.
- *Cryptococcal meningitis*, an inflammation of the covering of the brain caused by a yeast-type fungus.
- *Toxoplasmosis*, caused by a protozoan, a common infection in the general population acquired from eating raw meat or from cat faeces; in people with AIDS it can cause extensive lesions in the brain.
- *Cytomegalovirus*, caused by a virus common in the general population; it produces damage to the brain and eyes, including progressive blindness as well as gastrointestinal and lung disease.
- *Herpes simplex (HSV)*. This extremely common, normally self-limiting, infection can cause long-lasting sores which do not heal.
- *Oral and/or oesophageal candidiasis*. This common yeast, usually known as 'thrush', can show extensive growth in the mouth and alimentary tract of people with AIDS.

Some problems are recognised as occurring much more frequently in HIV infection although they do not form part of the definition of AIDS itself. These include seborrhoeic eczema and folliculitis of the skin, recurrent shingles, certain bacterial infections of the chest, sinuses and skin and severe wart infections.

Most of these infections are common in healthy people but they take on a different aspect in someone who is immunocompromised (has immune system damage). For instance cytomegalovirus does not normally cause blindness and, while warts are virtually universal, in a person with immune system damage they are more extensive and respond less well to treatment. These changes in the pattern of common infections are caused by a failure of the immune system to control the disease-causing organism and restrict its scope.

### Opportunistic tumours

Opportunistic tumours behave in much the same way as opportunistic infections: they take advantage of the immune system being damaged to get a hold. In some cases opportunistic tumours are themselves the result of oncogenic (cancer-causing) viruses. It is possible, for instance, that Kaposi's sarcoma is the product of cytomegalovirus infection in an immunocompromised host. Amongst the most common tumours are:

- *Kaposi's sarcoma (KS)*. A bluish or reddish cell overgrowth which arises in the endothelial cells lining the blood vessels and which appears with equal frequency throughout the body. For obvious reasons it is usually noticed on the skin or in other accessible sites such as in the mouth. It is very rare except in individuals with AIDS or other causes of immune deficiency. Unusually it causes death when it is extensive in internal organs, but more usually the KS patient dies of some other AIDS disease.
- *Non-Hodgkin lymphomas*. Tumours of the lymphoid cells, usually B-cells.
- *Ano-rectal carcinoma*. Tumours of the anus and rectum. Since they are more common in gay men it is possible that an infectious agent is responsible.

Of these tumours KS accounts for the overwhelming majority of opportunistic tumours found in AIDS.

### AIDS dementia

Some individuals with AIDS show evidence of central nervous system impairment caused by direct infection of cells of the central nervous system by the HIV virus itself. This area is covered in more detail in Chapter 6.

### The natural history of AIDS

Once infected with the HIV virus some individuals will progress rapidly to AIDS, although the majority will not develop AIDS for some years. Even amongst individuals infected in the early 80s, most have not so far gone on to develop AIDS. On the other hand there is no sign that the risk of developing AIDS reduces over time, i.e. the risk in the eighth year is not necessarily any lower than that in the fifth year — roughly 4–6 per cent per annum of most populations studied. We do not know what proportion of individuals infected with HIV will eventually go on to develop AIDS. In part this will be affected, of course, by the future development of effective treatments aimed at preventing viral replication. There is no evidence currently to suggest that everyone infected with the HIV virus will necessarily go on to develop AIDS.

The fact that some individuals progress rapidly to AIDS while others remain essentially well for many years is something for which there is, as yet, no complete explanation. One factor may be the extent to which individuals who progress have co-factors, things which increase the probability of progression. One set of co-factors of particular interest are other infectious diseases. Infectious agents may promote viral replication either by causing activation of T-cells (which makes uninfected cells more susceptible to infection and makes virus production more likely in infected cells), or by themselves suppressing immune functioning to some extent or, possibly in the case of some viruses, by acting to promote the activity of HIV viral genes within an infected cell. There may be other co-factors for the development of AIDS but these are, as yet, not clearly defined.

There may be other reasons why some individuals are more likely to develop AIDS early on. What these might be remains unclear.

AIDS is usually thought of as a universally fatal disease. In fact, the picture is more complicated than this: there are a number of long-term survivors from the early days of the epidemic. By and large, these are individuals who have KS only. They are in the minority of those who develop KS, but they do exist. It is possible that a number of people with AIDS can 'get stuck' at a particular level of immune system damage and, while they do not actually get better, they do not get worse over long periods of time.

The reason why long-term survivors tend to be those with KS is that KS can develop at a stage where individuals have less immune system damage than is usual in individuals who develop, say, pneumocystis. Therefore *on average* those with KS only, tend to have less immune system damage than those with opportunistic infections. Some opportunistic infections tend to develop at lower levels of immune system damage than others. Individuals who have oral candida as their only opportunistic infection tend, like those with KS only, to have less immune system damage than those with pneumocystis or cryptosporidiosis.

Overall then, there is a spectrum of disease in AIDS, with some people diagnosed as having AIDS having less immune system damage than others.

As the treatments available for opportunistic infections have improved, the average survival time for those developing opportunistic infections has increased, simply because they are less likely to die during any bout of opportunistic infection. This trend is likely to continue and it is probable that survival time for all those with AIDS will gradually lengthen for this reason alone.

## Epidemiology of AIDS

Different countries have a different pattern of spread of AIDS. In America and in Europe the two single largest categories of individuals infected currently are homosexual men and intravenous drug abusers. Haemophiliacs and a number of individuals receiving blood transfusions have also been infected in the past, although the use of heat-treated factor VIII concentrate and the screening of blood, combined with voluntary abstention from donating by those at risk, should ensure that infections in these categories will be rare in the future. A small number of health professionals have also been infected by exposure to infected blood, for instance through needle-stick injuries, but this is an extremely rare event.

In Africa and some other areas of the world heterosexuals are the main risk category. It remains unclear to what extent heterosexuals outside other risk categories will become infected in the West. There have already been many cases but in percentage terms the incidence amongst heterosexuals remains low. It is now clear that the virus is transmitted by normal vaginal intercourse and is not necessarily related to the presence of damage to the vaginal tract, although such damage may conceivably aid transmission.

It is often argued that the virus is more easily spread through anal intercourse than through vaginal intercourse. There is no clear evidence to support this viewpoint; different studies on heterosexual spread to the partners of those known to be infected have produced widely differing estimations of risk. Similarly it is not clear whether male to female transmission is more efficient than female to male transmission. In part these differences between the results of different studies are probably the result of small sample sizes; in part they may reflect differences in the stage of illness of the partners.

What remains clear is that the number of cases of infection world-wide is likely to continue to increase until there is a change in risk-behaviours amongst those at risk or there is an effective, cheap vaccine available. There is, at the time of writing, no sign of an effective vaccine and even were a suitable vaccine to be produced it would take time before it could be tested and made widely available.

As the number of infections continues to rise, so the number of cases of AIDS will continue to rise and people will continue to die unless an effective treatment can be developed. It is likely that over the next few years a number of new drugs will become available. Already one drug, AZT (Zidovudine), is in wide use in the West and early results are promising in terms of keeping patients alive. It does not appear to constitute a cure, that is it does not eliminate the virus, it only keeps it under control.

In order to halt the deaths worldwide a drug not only needs to be effective, it needs to be cheap in itself and it needs to be free from side-effects which either require high-technology medicine to control or extensive laboratory facilities to monitor or which are expensive to treat in themselves. A drug without these features may be useful in the West but is unlikely to make much impact on the disease on a global scale.

Until the vaccines and drugs appear, counselling and health education are the only tools available to us to prevent transmission, and, as far as possible, to keep well those who are already infected. In the last analysis, also, counselling is important as a key part of maintaining the quality of life of those who already have the disease. If we cannot cure people, we can at least do that for them.

# Chapter 2

# Laboratory Tests for HIV

D J JEFFRIES BSC MB BS MRC PATH

## Introduction

Following the recognition of the AIDS epidemic in 1981, there was a period of over two years before it became generally accepted that the causative agent was a retrovirus. If the epidemic had started 10 years earlier it is most unlikely that we would have isolated and identified HIV-1 by the end of the decade. We would certainly not have reached the present stage of developing specific and sensitive diagnostic tests, prototype vaccines and specific antiviral drugs. The reasons for the rapid expansion of our knowledge of HIV lie in a series of major milestones in the sciences of virology and molecular biology.

The understanding of retroviral replication came with the description of the viral enzyme reverse transcriptase by Baltimore, Temin and Mizutani in 1970. Detection of the activity of this enzyme allowed the identification of HIV when it was first cultured by Barré-Sinoussi and her colleagues at the Pasteur Institute in Paris (1983). Another important development was the identification and purification of T-cell growth factor (interleukin 2) by Morgan *et al.* in 1976. This natural substance permits the continuous culture of lymphocytes in the laboratory and it was this key ingredient in the medium which led to the isolation of the first human retrovirus, human T-cell leukaemia virus type I (HTLV-I) in 1980, and HIV-1 in 1983. In 1984, Popovic *et al.* reported the adaptation of HIV-1 to cell lines which constantly shed virus without being destroyed and this allowed the preparation of concentrated and purified preparations of the virus which were then available for genetic analysis, and for the manufacture of the first generation antibody tests.

Cloning of gene fragments has led to the availability of totally pure antigens, and techniques for purification of antibodies together with monoclonal antibody production have refined serological tests to the present levels of accuracy. Nucleotide sequence analysis of many different isolates of HIV-1 has revealed a high degree of mutation over a relatively short time period. These mutational events are restricted to certain sections of the genome and the changes have not, as yet, been reflected by changes in sensitivity of laboratory tests. However, the discovery of a new AIDS retrovirus in West Africa (HIV-2) and recognition of this virus in certain European cities means that new diagnostic tests, currently being developed, must soon be introduced.

## Virus culture

HIV can be grown from the blood (and occasionally other body fluids) of people with AIDS and those with a positive antibody test. The technique is very expensive in reagents and time and is not a routine investigation at present or in the foreseeable future. Virus culture is mainly reserved for research work and for investigating patients with immune deficiency states which are not obviously due to HIV-1 or HIV-2. Another situation in which virus culture is of critical importance is the assessment of infection in the newborn baby. Three-quarters of the babies born to HIV-1 antibody positive women lose their antibody by the end of the first year of life; this does not, however, indicate that they are uninfected, as virus can sometimes be grown from their blood cells.

## HIV-1 antibody tests

### (a) Significance of positivity

Antibody tests were introduced for the diagnosis of HIV-1 infection in 1985. They remain by far the most important way of detecting asymptomatic carriage of the virus and, if necessary, for confirming the aetiology of AIDS-related symptoms. At first, caution was exercised in interpreting the finding of a confirmed positive antibody test and many individuals were told that it only indicated 'exposure at some time in the past' to HIV-1, implying that they may have developed antibody and eliminated the virus. We now know enough about the infection to realise that this event is most unlikely to occur, if ever. It must be realised, and conveyed to the individual concerned, that a confirmed positive in the antibody test means that infection with the virus persists and is almost certain to be present for life. In addition to this, the lack of neutralising capacity by the immune system of those infected means that, unless protective measures are taken, there is likely to be a continuing risk of infection to sexual partners. Most other viral infections result in complete recovery with the development of solid neutralising antibody which protects against reinfection. There are however some other infections (e.g. the carrier state of hepatitis B) in which the virus persists and neutralising antibody is not produced.

There is little prospect that drugs will be developed to eliminate HIV-1 from its integrated state in the chromosomes. There is a high probability, however, that long term suppression of the virus will be achieved by advances in the preparation of safer anti-retroviral agents. Apart from countering the damage caused by the virus in the immune system and the nervous system antiviral therapy may also reduce infectivity.

### (b) Seroconversion

The development of increasingly sensitive immunoassays used as screening tests for HIV-1 antibody has allowed the clear definition of antibody responses following infection. Studies of seroconversion in individuals in whom the time of infection is known indicate that most have developed detectable antibody within two months and virtually all by three months. The finding of a positive screening test is often preceded by the influenza-like acute illness now associated with HIV-1 infection. Once a confirmed positive test result has been obtained, it will remain positive despite progression to the stage of full-blown AIDS. In some of the studies based on less sensitive assays, some individuals were reported as antibody negative for long periods before seroconversion was detected and some patients with AIDS were found to revert to antibody negativity. It must be remembered, however, that no serological test can be expected to be perfect and there is still a possibility that, on rare occasions, seroconversion may be delayed for longer than three months. The loss of antibody in infected infants was referred to above and there have been isolated reports of isolation of HIV-1 from seronegative adults (Groopman *et al.*, 1985; Mayer *et al.*, 1986). In a recent study of patients with persistent generalised lymphadenopathy (Forster *et al.*, 1987), 9/84 (12 per cent) were antibody negative on enrolment and seven of these seroconverted within periods of up to 36 months. It is possible, however, that their lymphadenopathy was caused by agents other than HIV-1 and that they became infected from further exposures during the course of the study. Further work will clarify the incidence of delayed seroconversion following infection. In the meantime, a negative antibody test six months after known (or suspected) exposure to HIV-1 will provide a reasonable basis for reassurance. Follow-up testing, if considered necessary, will increase the confidence of the counsellor (and the individual concerned) that infection has been avoided.

### (c) Screening tests

It is not the purpose of this chapter to describe the laboratory techniques used in HIV testing. These have been reviewed recently by Mortimer and Clewley (1987). The first antibody screening tests were hurriedly produced to screen blood donors in the interests of the transfusion recipient. These crude assays which incorporated an impure extract of the virus erred on the safe side as far as the recipient was concerned and consequently yielded an unacceptably high rate of false positives (approx. 1 per cent). The majority of these repeatedly positive reactions could be shown to be false by confirmatory tests but with the need to introduce antibody testing for other reasons more specific tests were urgently required. These are now in general use and are either based on much cleaner preparations of virus grown in cell culture or incorporate totally specific antigens prepared by recombinant DNA technology. With the currently available screening tests (most of which are enzyme-linked immunosorbent assays, or ELISAs) the incidence of repeatable false positives is less than 0.1 per cent. This means that the likelihood of a positive screening result being a false positive in an individual who has been engaged in high risk activity is low, although it must of course be repeated and confirmed before conveying the information. On the other hand, before embarking on extensive screening of people at very low risk of infection, the problem of the anxiety generated by the finding of repeatable positives must be seriously considered, particularly as the confirmatory tests are sometimes equivocal. An example of where routine screening, if introduced, could cause major problems as a result of false positivity is in the antenatal clinics in the UK.

### (d) Confirmatory tests

Once an individual has been found to be positive on two samples of blood it is then essential to carry out confirmatory testing before conveying the information and counselling. The first test to be widely introduced for this purpose was the immunoblotting technique (or western blot). This test, which demonstrates differential antibodies in the serum against a range of different viral proteins, is still widely used and, if a clear-cut result can be obtained, provides reliable evidence of true infection. Some serum samples produce equivocal results, however, with antibody reaction against only one of the proteins, (p24)p, and these reactions may be non-specific. Discriminating ELISA tests have been developed which detect antibody to the core (p24 antigen) or surface (gp41 antigen) of the virus and these provide a very satisfactory method of confirming antibody positivity. Other techniques based on immunofluorescence are less commonly used now than when antibody testing was first introduced. In nearly every case it is now possible to confirm or refute the finding of positivity in the screening tests. On very rare occasions the results of different confirmatory tests are found to be conflicting and if this occurs a further sample of blood should be tested and if necessary the results should be sent to other laboratories for independent assessments.

**Prognostic tests**

It has become clear recently that detailed serological evaluation of individuals who are antibody positive will lead to the possibility of assessing the likelihood of development of HIV-1-related diseases. The combination of specific tests for HIV-1 antigen and core (p24) antibody, together with measurement of CD-4 lymphocyte numbers, the CD-4/CD-8 ratio and possibly beta-2 microglobulin levels, provides a package of predictive tests. It must be strongly emphasised, however, that such an assessment is based on a statistical probability of progression and cannot be applied to give a judgement of the expected future course in an individual case. Indeed, individuals have been observed to remain asymptomatic for years despite the finding of abnormal blood tests which have been strongly correlated with disease progression.

*(a) Antigen testing*

The introduction of sensitive ELISA tests which are able to detect HIV-1 antigen in serum at certain times in the course of infection has made a major contribution to the serological assessment of those exposed to infection. Many individuals have been found to have a phase of antigenaemia in the period before they develop a positive antibody screening test. (Allain *et al.*, 1986). In theory this provides the opportunity for diagnosis of HIV-1 infection early after exposure and before the antibody screening tests become positive. This test has not, as yet, become routine as the expense and time involved renders it unsuitable as an additional screening system. It has not been introduced as a routine for blood donor testing partly for logistic reasons but also because after voluntary exclusion of donors the rate of antibody positivity, in most countries, is so low as to make its use unnecessary at present.

The antigen test has another, and potentially very important, application as a predictive index in asymptomatic HIV-1 antibody positive people. A return of antigenaemia, together with a decline in core (p24) antibody (see below) correlates strongly with progression to AIDS. If an asymptomatic carrier develops a positive antigen test there is a greater than 50 per cent chance of progressing to AIDS within a few months. This (together with the other predictive factors) should provide a logical way of selecting individuals for trials of anti-retroviral drugs as they become available. In addition to this, experience with the early use of Zidovudine (AZT) has shown that a decline of antigen levels in the blood occurs during treatment. Thus, antigen measurements should provide an effective way of indicating efficacy of drugs *in vivo*.

The sequence of antigen and antibody responses following infection with HIV-1 is illllustrated in Fig. 2.1.

Other possible uses of the antigen test currently under evaluation are its possible value in assessing infection in infants born to HIV-1 antibody positive mothers and in the investigation of central nervous system disease by measuring antigen responses in the cerebrospinal fluid.

## (b) Core (p24) antibody testing

As indicated previously this test, made possible by the preparation of pure antigens by genetic engineering, allows the quantitation of antibodies to the major core protein of the virus. It has been shown in several studies (Lange *et al.*, 1986; Weber *et al.*, 1987) that the decline of core antibody is another important predictor of disease and, in fact, is seen to fall before the return of antigenaemia. This reduction of antibody to a major viral protein may indicate imminent collapse of the immune system or, conversely, may be due to consumption of circulating antibody molecules by an increase in antigen production. Whatever the mechanism, it is to be hoped that effective treatment of the infection will be followed by an increase in the level of core antibodies but this has not yet been seen in patients receiving Zidovudine.

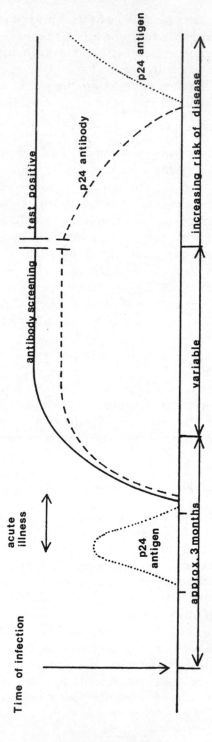

*Fig. 2.1* Diagram to illustrate the serological changes in blood following infection with HIV–1.

## Conclusions

Remarkable progress has been made in the development of diagnostic tests for HIV-1. Similar tests are becoming available for HIV-2 and, if necessary, they will be introduced as part of the screening package. It must be remembered that serological tests can never be a perfect way of diagnosing infection. This has been observed over many years with long established tests for common infections such as rubella and hepatitis B. The reason for this lack of total accuracy results from individual variation in immune responses and the danger of cross-reaction with antibodies to other antigens. Nevertheless the HIV-1 tests now available are at least as good as any of the laboratory tests for other viruses. Health care workers have been right to apply caution and to tread slowly before introducing widespread and indiscriminate antibody screening. The predictable prejudices imposed by society, enhanced by irresponsible approaches from the media, have understandably made those at risk hesitant about being tested. Indeed, at the present time many would argue that there are few benefits to the individual in being tested and found to be HIV positive. This situation is likely to change, and possibly very soon, with the introduction of non-toxic and effective prophylactic drugs. There will then be a need not only to identify antibody positives but also to carry out the predictive tests with a view to therapy.

## References

Allain, J-P., Laurien, Y., Paul, D.A. and Senn, D. (1986) 'Serological markers in early stages of human immunodeficiency virus infection in haemophiliacs' *Lancet*, **ii** p. 1233.

Barré-Sinoussi, F., Chermann, J.C., Rey, F., *et al.* (1983) 'Isolation of a T lymphotropic retrovirus from a patient at risk of acquired immune deficiency syndrome' *Science*, **220** p. 868.

Forster, S.M., Osborne, L.M., Cheingsong-Popov, R., *et al.* (1987) 'Decline of anti-p24 antibody precedes antigenaemia as correlate of prognosis in HIV-1 infection' *AIDS*, **1** p. 235.

Groopman, J.E., Hartzband, P.I. and Schulman, L. (1985) 'Antibody seronegative human lymphotropic virus type III (HTLV III) infected patients with AIDS or related disease' *Blood*, **66** p. 742.

Lange, J.M., Paul, D.A., Huisman, H.G., *et al.* (1986) 'Persistent HIV antigenaemia and decline of HIV core antibodies associated with transition to AIDS' *British Medical Journal*, **293** p. 1459.

Mayer, K.H., Stodddard, A.M., McCluskey, J., *et al.* (1986) 'Human T lymphotropic virus type III in high-risk antibody negative homosexual men' *Ann. Int. Med.*, **104** p. 194.

Mortimer, P.P. and Clewley, J.P. (1987) 'Serological tests for human immuno-deficiency virus' In: *Current Topics in AIDS*, Gottlieb, M.S., Jeffries, D.J., Mildvan, D., Pinching, A.J., Quinn, T.C. and Weiss, R.A., Eds. John Wiley: Chichester. p. 133.

Popovic, M., Sarngadharan, M.G., Read, E. and Gallo, R.C. (1984) 'Detection, isolation and continuous production of cytopathic retroviruses (HTLV–111) from patients with AIDS and pre-AIDS' *Science*, **224** p. 497.

Weber, J.N., Clapham, P.R., Weiss, R.A., *et al.* (1987) 'Human immuno-deficiency virus infection in two cohorts of homosexual men: neutralizing sera and association of anti-gag antibody with prognosis' *Lancet*, **i** p. 119.

# Chapter 3

# Pre-test Counselling

ALANA McCREANER

The IIIV antibody test has been freely available throughout the UK since October 1985. Most Western countries and an increasing number of developing countries either have introduced, or will shortly introduce, facilities for testing. In most countries in the world the incidence of HIV in the population has steadily risen and with it the need for expert counselling of people who are considering taking the test.

The aims of pre-test counselling are:

- To ensure that any decision to take the test is fully informed and based on an understanding of the personal, medical, legal and social implications of a positive result. At one level, this is a mere practical application of the traditional medical ethic of informed consent to a procedure.
- To provide the necessary preparation for those who will have to face the trauma of a positive result. Such preparation is vital in that patients who have been prepared for a positive result are able to face that result much more equably.
- To provide the individual, whether he eventually elects not to be tested, or elects to be tested and is found to be positive or found to be negative, with necessary risk reduction information on the basis of which he can reduce the risk of either acquiring HIV infection or passing it on to others.

It is crucial in pre-test counselling to gain the trust which is clearly essential in the discussion of the more intimate areas of the person's life. It is always advisable to provide assurances that what is discussed between the counsellor and the individual will be kept confidential. In some countries confidentiality is guaranteed by law, as it is in the

*21*

UK by the NHS (Venereal Diseases) Regulations, 1974; this regulates disclosure of any relevant information. In countries where limits are placed on the extent of confidentiality these limitations should be made explicit at the outset of counselling.

Each person will have distinctive needs and the discussion should develop towards identifying these needs. Once a session is under way an effective counsellor will remain alert to the danger of over-directing the individual and particularly of anticipating his or her decision about whether to take the test.

There are several stages in providing pre-test counselling; the order in which these will be covered will probably differ from individual to individual. However it is always important to be consistent and to ensure that, by the end of the session, all necessary areas have been covered.

### Assessing risk

The first stage is to make an assessment of the level of risk of the individual. The most important risk factors may vary somewhat from country to country and sometimes from area to area within a country. An awareness of the most common types of passage of infection in an area is vital to the counsellor carrying out pre-test counselling.

However, in pre-test counselling it is always necessary to guard against being 'blinded by statistics' and pre-judging the risk factors of any person on the basis of superficial questioning. The counsellor should also be aware of the fact that the importance of different risk factors may change over time, and his assessment of what is and what is not an important risk in a particular area will also have to change. Moreover, inevitably, some individuals who appear to have relatively low levels of risk will turn out to be infected. For instance, in areas where heterosexual spread is uncommon occasional cases will occur. While some individuals are 'low risk' far fewer will be 'no risk'.

It is therefore essential to carry out a comprehensive sexual and life style history. This should cover:

- The sexual behaviour of the individual and, where known to the individual, the sexual behaviour of any partners.
- Any history of injecting drug abuse.
- Past blood transfusions prior to the introduction of screening of donations.
- Use of blood products for the treatment of haemophilia prior to the introduction of screening and/or heat treatment.

- Invasive procedures carried out under non-sterile conditions such as cosmetic procedures, ritual scarification and circumcision. This will also include repeated injections carried out with inadequate sterilisation procedures, as they are by unqualified healers in some countries.

On the basis of such an assessment it is helpful to give the individual an estimation of likely risk. Where the risk appears minimal the person should be told so. On the other hand no actual risk, however slight, should be dismissed out of hand.

## Discussing the test

Confusion over what the test can actually tell us is very common. It is essential to be able to explain, in jargon-free language, exactly what the test measures. Visual material illustrating the process involved is most helpful.

A clear account of the limitations of the test should include the problems of false negatives and false positives. In particular it is important to discuss the length of time which it can take before measurable antibodies appear. These issues are considered in more detail in Chapter 2. Clearly a man who has had risky sex the day before cannot rely on a negative test result on sera collected that day to show him that he is not infected. This sort of consideration can be unsettling for those who look to the test to resolve their anxieties once and for all, but it must be stressed that the test brings with it no guarantees.

Another matter which often needs clarification is the difference between having HIV infection and having AIDS. Many people coming for the test still believe that it is a test for AIDS rather than for HIV infection.

## Thinking through possible results

People coming for the test have often thought through what a negative result would mean for them but have not thought through the repercussions of a positive result. The advantages and disadvantages of being tested for the particular individual have to be fully explored. In the end it will be that person's choice whether to be tested and the process of choosing will involve a self-assessment of his or her ability or desire to cope with knowledge of being HIV antibody positive.

## Other issues which the individual needs to consider

Some of the issues covered below are specific to the UK although they will have parallels in other countries. Counsellors need to familiarise themselves with local legal issues and with the practices of insurance companies and employers in their area.

### Possible legal and financial repercussions

Prospective employers and insurance companies have traditionally required applicants to complete medical questionnaires. Now the inclusion of specific questions about HIV is becoming more common. Particularly in the case of insurance companies, counsellors should ensure that they are familiar with current standard questionnaires.

Increasingly insurance companies, and some employers, are asking whether the individual has been *tested* for HIV infection. In some cases they are asking whether the individual has *sought advice* about HIV infection. If these questions are answered inaccurately contracts of insurance or of employment may be voided. In some cases even a negative result can lead to insurance companies asking further questions; whether this will influence the terms of insurance cover is likely to depend on the insurance company and how satisfied they are with the answers they receive.

### GPs (family doctors)

An individual who knows himself to be infected should inform his GP and dentist. The advantage of doing this is that these professionals can play a full part in the care of the individual. What they look for in their work, and how they interpret this, may be affected by knowing that a patient is infected. It is often helpful for the counsellor to contact the GP, always with the patient's agreement and without referring to the individual, to find out *in general* what that GP's attitude to, and knowledge of, the care of the seropositive person is. Clearly a patient who is unhappy about his GP or that GP's ability to deal with the consequences of HIV infection should change his GP.

One special problem which faces GPs is that they may have to fill in medical forms about a patient for insurance companies or for employers. If they are aware that a patient is seropositive they will, legally, be bound to reveal this.

### Travel

Freedom of travel may be adversely affected by a positive result. Some countries are currently requesting proof of being HIV negative before issuing a work-permit or visa. Clearly, for the high-risk individual required to travel as part of his work, this can be a considerable problem.

## Who should the individual talk to about the test?

In most countries AIDS is a heavily stigmatised disease. The stigma of being known to be seropositive can lead to loss of friends, family, and in some cases homes and employment. Even where the law protects individuals against loss of employment it is sometimes difficult to enforce such a law, particularly as the individual may be reluctant to face the even greater publicity which might be generated by a court case.

Thought needs to be given in advance to who the individual can rely upon for support and total discretion during the time when the test is being considered or the result awaited. Many people need such support from friends or family to help them to cope and it can be a very healthy thing. The counsellor can, of course, provide some support, although he will not be there at all times to talk things over with.

Prudence dictates, however, that the confidants should be kept to a minimum. In many countries there are also voluntary bodies who give confidential support and advice to those considering the test or awaiting the result. These can act as a valuable support to the individual who feels that no-one is available in his personal life to provide that support.

At the pre-test counselling stage the individual also needs to begin to think through the issue of sexual partners and which of them will need to be told and how. This issue is covered in more detail in Chapter 4.

## Advantages of the test

Being tested has a number of drawbacks for many people. However it can also have considerable advantages for some individuals and it is important to discuss these with the individual.

### *Those who have discontinued previous risk behaviours*

For a woman who has previously had risk behaviours, for instance injecting drug abuse, and now wishes to become pregnant, there can be considerable advantages in having the blood test since this may have an important influence on her decision.

Similarly, a couple who, having previously been at risk, wish to establish a monogamous relationship and who do not wish to continue with safer sexual practices, may decide to have the test.

Individuals should be aware of the limitations of the test when using it for these purposes.

### Reducing uncertainty

For some individuals having the test is an advantage simply because it reduces uncertainty.

### Helping in behaviour change

Some people feel that knowing whether they are positive or negative may help them to change their behaviour. Caution must be exercised here. Some people feel that they will change their behaviour if they know themselves to be positive *but not if they know themselves to be negative*. This needs careful exploration.

It is also worth bearing in mind that good counselling can help people change their behaviour regardless of whether they are tested or not. Working out whether knowing a result will help to change behaviour is a decision for the patient, not for the counsellor.

## Taking a decision

Written material summarising the main points covered in pre-test counselling should be available for all. It is particularly useful for those who need more time to consider before reaching a decision. It is helpful to tell the individual that they do not necessarily have to take a decision there and then. They can always return later to have the test.

## Reducing risk

Whatever the decision with regard to taking the test, everyone who has felt himself or herself to be at risk should be introduced to risk-reduction techniques in the course of counselling, and this should be done regardless of how high or low the risk is perceived to be. Individual behaviour can and does change. Someone whose behaviour is relatively low-risk at the moment may not be low-risk in the future and pre-test counselling is an important occasion for the provision of general health education about HIV.

It is important to cover the issue of safer sex (see also Chapter 4). This is a delicate area touching as it does on the most private behaviour and needs sensitive handling to overcome embarrassment. Non-sexual modes of transmission should also be identified and discussed, including injecting drug abuse, materno-foetal, non-sterile invasive procedures, etc.

While counsellors will be most concerned to cover all proven modes of transmission, they must also be prepared sympathetically to discuss fears and to reassure about the absence of domestic and social transmission, e.g. household contact, including sharing of kitchen and toilet facilities, hugging, touching, kissing, etc.

Although dealt with separately here for convenience, risk reduction education is an integral part of the counselling session and it has been shown that necessary behaviour change can be achieved by counselling alone rather than being dependent on a positive test result. Some, however, will want to take the test as an incentive to change behaviour.

Individuals who decide to be tested should be given an appointment to see both the doctor and counsellor for their result. Fridays should be avoided where possible to ensure that those who prove positive do not have to face the weekend without access to the counsellor should they need support.

# Chapter 4

# Post-test Counselling

JOHN GREEN

This chapter looks at the counselling of those who are tested and found to be infected with the HIV virus. However, the approach is much the same with those who are untested but at risk of infection or those who are seronegative but at risk of infection. It is just as important to counsel someone who is untested or negative but at risk as it is to counsel someone known to be infected.

The chapter uses a case, that of Paul — a gay man — to give a feel of what it is *like* to counsel someone about HIV, the sorts of issues they raise and the sorts of things the counsellor needs to be thinking about. It is not, of course, a script to be followed. Every counsellor will approach the issue slightly differently according to his or her personal style.

## Breaking the news

COUNSELLOR: 'Hello Paul [shaking hands with the patient], come in and sit down. You've come in for your test results?'
PAUL: 'Yes.'
COUNSELLOR: 'OK, I have the results back from the laboratory and they are positive, you have been infected with the HIV virus.'
PAUL: 'Oh, damn.'
COUNSELLOR: 'Are you surprised?'
PAUL: 'No, not really, I thought I would be, but it's still a hell of a shock.'

The exact wording of what happened doesn't matter so much as the structure. The important things are:

- To open the meeting in as friendly a fashion as possible; shaking hands and using first names helps. The tone of voice can't be conveyed on the printed page but it's important to sound as though one is pleased to see the patient and is interested in him as a person.
- To check that the patient has actually come for his results. He may have changed his mind and not want them, but still want to talk.
- To tell the patient straightforwardly, without evasion or qualification, what the results are. Many counsellors want to try to 'dress up' the results so that they are more acceptable to the patient (and easier for them to give), it doesn't work. The news *is* often unacceptable, at least initially. There is no way to make it acceptable and trying to qualify it only leaves a confused patient who is sometimes not even sure whether he is infected or not. Almost as bad, it tells the patient that the counsellor can't handle the news — and if the counsellor can't handle it, how can the patient be expected to?
- To indicate to the patient that the counsellor is ready and willing to talk by asking an appropriate question, 'Are you surprised?', 'Were you expecting it?', 'How do you feel about the news?'. What is said actually matters less to the patient than it does to the counsellor. The patient is likely to be trying to absorb the information and won't usually be listening all that carefully. It's just a way of showing the patient that one is listening.
- To listen carefully to what the patient says next; it is often an important clue to what is uppermost in his mind.

## Taking it in

The reactions of people to being told they are positive vary enormously:

'It can't be true, I only did it once.'
'It's a relief really, just to know.'
'Does that mean I have AIDS?'
'How will I tell my wife?'
'It's what I expected.'
'What am I going to do?'

The important thing is to listen to what the patient is saying and to encourage him to voice his thoughts. Some patients simply sit in silence. It's easy to think that nothing is happening; it is. The patient is thinking over the information, often his mind is racing. Getting him to verbalise what is going on helps because it is possible to pick up the key issues for that patient. On the other hand barraging him with questions sometimes simply worsens the situation by constantly interrupting his train of thought.

Responses fall into three main categories:

*Statements*     'It can't be true, I only did it once', 'It's what I expected'. These are ways into the counselling, openings to start the patient on telling the counsellor more. Possible responses might be 'You only did it once?', or 'You're not surprised?' or even 'Uh-huh'. Of course there is no perfect answer, all the counsellor has to do is to indicate that he is listening and interested in hearing more.

*Questions*     Factual questions such as, 'Does that mean I have AIDS?' should be answered factually — 'No, it doesn't because...' (assuming it is known that the patient does not have AIDS). However some questions are not factual questions at all — they are expressions of anguish; for instance, 'How will I tell my wife?' could be saying, 'Tell me how to tell my wife', but is much more likely to be a statement like, 'I'm going to have to tell my wife and the thought terrifies me'. 'What am I going to do?' falls into the same category. The answer in these cases is not to provide an answer but to start to encourage the patient to talk about the situation; 'You're worried about your wife?' or, 'Tell me about your wife' or, 'Go on', are the sort of responses that the counsellor is going to use in these circumstances.

*Reactions*     The patient might burst into tears or he might swear or just sit there glassy-eyed and silent. Nothing is more off-putting to counsellors than a reaction of this sort since they are usually geared up for a dialogue. There is a strong temptation for the counsellor to start babbling on about anything that comes into his mind. When the patient is crying most counsellors feel distinctly uncomfortable and try to reduce their discomfort by stopping the patient crying in any way possible. Mothers with crying children usually try to achieve this by distraction ('Oh, look at the fire-engine, isn't it big!'). Uncomfortable counsellors use the same tactics, sometimes by talking about irrelevancies, often (interestingly) by offering drinks — 'Let me get you some water', 'Would you like a coffee/aspirin/handkerchief?' (the tea-and-sympathy approach).

There is nothing wrong with offering coffee and handkerchiefs. Indeed I have made it a habit to keep a box of paper tissues on my desk to provide patients with a tissue if they cry. On the other hand it shouldn't replace an appropriate response.

The key is to acknowledge the patient's feelings and to give permission for him to behave in the way he is doing. Most patients feel very embarrassed if they cry, as with Paul:

COUNSELLOR: 'It's a shock even when you expect it, isn't it?'
PAUL: 'Oh God, I'm sorry, I shouldn't cry, it's stupid.'
COUNSELLOR: 'That's OK, lots of people cry when they're told, it's normal. Here, have a tissue.'
PAUL: 'I'll be all right in a moment.'
COUNSELLOR: 'Take your time, there's no hurry.'

Sometimes touching the patient, maybe putting a hand on his shoulder for a moment, helps as much as anything. It says a lot, but interestingly it takes a confident counsellor to be able to do it without feeling awkward, given the taboos against touching in Western medicine.

### Getting the discussion going

Exactly what order the counsellor and the patient discuss things in very much depends on what the patient feels is most important. It is likely to come out of what the patient brings up during the 'taking it in' stage. However there are a number of different areas which need to be addressed or at least touched on during the course of the first session and, perhaps, returned to in subsequent sessions. Here I will call them 'blocks'. The order of blocks and how much time is spent on each will entirely depend on circumstances.

In reality, of course, blocks overlap and a counselling session will be far more messy than is presented below, with the topic switching backwards and forwards. But this doesn't detract from the fact that the *counsellor* should have some sort of structure in his mind of the issues that need covering, otherwise large areas might not be covered.

### *AIDS/HIV block*

'Do I have AIDS?'
'How long have I got to live?'
'Will I die?'
'What are the chances of a cure?'
'Is it painful to die of AIDS?'
'Where did this virus come from?'

Patients usually want to know factual information about AIDS and HIV infection. A lot of the information is about aspects of the infection as it affects them. However, they often have a general curiosity about AIDS and HIV and it is likely that taking a general interest in the whole area helps some people to come to terms with being infected.

It is worth going through certain basic information, even with a well-informed patient. It's reassuring to hear from the lips of an 'expert' confirmation of what the realities of the situation are. It's also important not to assume that just because certain information has been gone through in pre-test counselling it shouldn't be covered post-test. Repetition of material can be very reassuring.

Of course it is important to be right in what is said about factual issues and to admit the limits of current knowledge or of personal knowledge about the topic. An up-to-date grasp of the current literature on AIDS is indispensable to any counsellor in this field.

Sometimes patients have gathered misleading information from things they have read or have misunderstood. This sort of issue is particularly important, since it is usually much easier to fill in gaps in people's knowledge than it is to correct information that they *think* they know, which is, in fact, incorrect. Wide reading is helpful here because patients will often have read items about AIDS and HIV in the newspapers or seen them on the television and these are quite often factually incorrect. It pays to know what is likely to come up.

Glossing over areas of difficulty in order to reassure patients and to avoid a long and technical discussion seldom works. One patient, having listened patiently to me providing a rather glib explanation of some technical point he had raised (and leaving out several important points in the process), produced a copy of an earlier book and, opening it, pointed to a paragraph and said, 'That's not what you said here . . .'.

In fact, almost any technical issue can be understood by almost any patient if the explanation is clear enough and simple enough. Paul raised one such issue:

PAUL: 'Why is the HIV virus killed by washing-up liquid?'
COUNSELLOR: 'Well, the virus itself is wrapped in a sort of coat made of something called lipid. Really this is a very thin layer of fat. If this coat is damaged then the virus dies. Now, washing-up liquid breaks up fat. Do you ever roast a joint of meat?'
PAUL: 'Yes.'
COUNSELLOR: 'Then there's a lot of fat at the bottom of the tin?'
PAUL: 'Yes, sure.'
COUNSELLOR: 'And what do you do to clean it?'

PAUL: 'I put it in hot water with washing-up liquid and that takes the fat off.'
COUNSELLOR: 'That's right, and the same thing happens to the virus. You put it in washing-up liquid and the outside of the virus is broken up and it dies.'

The common spine of what usually needs to be got across is as follows:

AIDS is not the same as HIV infection. Many people who have HIV infection are quite well. At the moment it is impossible to say who will go on to develop AIDS amongst those infected with the virus. It is not even possible to give a percentage figure for the proportion who will go on to get AIDS. Different studies come up with different rates. In part this is the result of different populations. For instance early on in the epidemic haemophiliacs had much lower rates of progression to AIDS than gay men. If one looks at studies at the moment which show rates over eight years the individuals in those studies were infected right at the start of the epidemic. It is possible that they may have had higher rates of co-factors (things which tend to increase the risk of going on to develop AIDS). For instance, men infected with a sexually transmitted disease (STD) at a time when it is relatively rare tend *on average* to have more partners and a greater risk of contracting other STDs, which may in turn be co-factors for the development of AIDS.

Within the limitations of the available data it would appear that once someone is infected they are always at risk of going on to get AIDS and there is no sign so far that this risk reduces as time goes by. However it is worth remembering that the longest period people are known to have been infected is only about ten years. Moreover there is no evidence that *everyone* infected with the virus will eventually get AIDS; they might, but there is no evidence that they definitely will.

However, for the person with HIV infection there is no need to look forward into the mists of time. Progress is being made in the treatment of AIDS, even if more slowly than one would hope. There has also been considerable progress in the treatment of opportunistic infections. Already people with AIDS live much longer than they used to. There is a very good chance, for anyone infected today, that by the time they develop AIDS there will be an effective treatment for it. Treatment here needs to be distinguished from 'cure', the elimination of the virus from the body which looks a long way off, if indeed it is possible. Moreover even without treatment not everyone dies, or at least has died so far. There are individuals alive today, with KS only, who were diagnosed in the early 80s, even, in a few cases, retrospectively diagnosed from before the time AIDS was recognised.

Of course the person infected with HIV may go on to get AIDS and may die. There is no point in avoiding this issue, the counsellor knows it and the patient knows it. In explaining about risks it is important to make it explicit rather than producing a relentlessly and possibly unrealistically optimistic message. Without mentioning it the counsellor is likely to appear to be providing an untrue view. Moreover it is always important to tell the patient the truth. Again, Paul asks about this:

PAUL: 'Will I get AIDS and die?'
COUNSELLOR: 'I don't know, no-one can tell you for sure that you won't. However, you may not get AIDS and even if you do, you may not die. Let me explain...'

Many patients don't really understand what AIDS is like. Even if they have had friends who have had it they may only have seen one or two cases and have, therefore, formed an inaccurate picture of what it is like. The counsellor can help to redress this.

Clearly the picture of a gaunt, sickly individual waiting for death in a hospital bed is not typical. Many people who have KS alone look and feel physically well. Those who have opportunistic infections are often well physically in between bouts of infection. For them the disease consists of periods of being well, during which they can lead a normal life, interspersed with bouts of acute illness. Of course during one of these bouts they may die, or they may recover and be as well as ever.

Many people with AIDS fear that they will die alone and in pain. People with AIDS and those with HIV infection often fear this more than the prospect of dying. They should be reassured that this will not happen to them. Modern pain-control methods and good clinical care should ensure that no-one dies alone and in severe pain.

It is important that the counsellor should be aware of current treatments and current research and be able to give the patient a realistic appraisal of these. The information above is current knowledge. It will inevitably change over time and it is important to keep abreast of these changes.

One question which comes up often with patients who have HIV infection is:

'Have I got AIDS?'

Those who test positive for the HIV virus should always have a medical as soon as possible after their results come back. This serves to reassure the patient that he does not have AIDS. It should be followed up with regular check-ups wherever possible, perhaps three-monthly or six-monthly. The patient should be encouraged to come into the clinic or consult his own GP if he becomes worried about his health in between appointments. Everyone who is HIV seropositive is bound to get sick from time to time, just as anyone who is HIV negative will get sick. However the seropositive person is very likely to feel that sore throats, stomach problems, chest infections, skin rashes and so on are the result of the HIV infection rather than part of the common lot of humanity. Feeling that there is always a ready source of sympathetic advice does more than anything else to reassure someone in that position.

### Transmission block

Knowing how the virus is passed on and how it is not passed on is a key issue in counselling someone about HIV infection. It is easy to give patients a list of dos and don'ts but to fail to explain where the advice comes from. Giving them reasons why the virus is transmitted in some ways and not in others helps them to remember the advice and allows them to make judgements about what the risks are in novel situations not covered by the advice.

Table 4.1 covers current understanding of transmission.

### Infection control block

'I share a house with three other people, am I putting them at risk by sharing the bathroom with them?'
'What do I do if I cut myself?'
'I want to have acupuncture, can I have it?'

The information about the routes of transmission gives a natural springboard to go on to cover practical issues about how the virus can and can't be passed on. It is important to cover what is not a risk as well as what is a risk. Table 4.2 shows the sort of advice which might be offered.

There is no evidence that HIV virus can be casually transmitted and patients should always be reassured about this. The families of those who are infected with the virus remain uninfected, except where there is sexual contact. It is important to put the message across in a way

**Table 4.1**   Transmission of the HIV virus

The HIV virus is found in and known to be transmitted through:

**Blood and blood products**. If infected blood from one person gets into the body of another person, the recipient may become infected with HIV. Infected blood transfusions (rare since the introduction of screening of blood) and blood products like factor 8 concentrate (prepared from batches of whole blood) are known to have passed on the virus. Intravenous drug abusers pass the virus by sharing syringes heavily contaminated with blood; by drawing blood back into the syringe after they have injected they contaminate the syringe particularly heavily. There is no evidence that the virus can penetrate intact skin but some evidence that under unusual conditions infected blood coming into contact with damaged skin can lead to infection.

**Tissue and organ transplants**. The considerations are as for blood and blood products.

**Semen**. Semen can contain large concentrations of virus. If infected semen gets into a person's body, for instance, via the rectal lining, vagina or cervix, the recipient can become infected. The route for this is unclear. The vaginal tract, cervix and rectal mucosa all contain cells related to T-cells and it is likely that this is one route of infection. Damage to the vagina, cervix or rectum will increase the likelihood of infection by allowing direct access of the virus to underlying tissues and blood vessels. However, there is no evidence that such damage is essential to transmission.

**Vaginal and cervical secretions**. Vaginal and cervical secretions can contain the virus. A man having vaginal intercourse with a woman infected with the virus can be infected in this way. The virus may pass across the surface of the glans either by being picked up by cells there or through lesions in the glans. There is no evidence that severe damage, if any damage at all, is required for transmission to occur.

**Breast milk**. Breast milk contains the virus and there have been a small number of cases in which babies appear to have been infected by being breast-fed by mothers acquiring the virus after birth through blood transfusions. There is no evidence to show whether an uninfected baby born to an infected mother can subsequently be infected through breast-feeding. Breast milk can be pasteurised.

**Intra-uterine infection**. Mothers can pass on the virus to their babies in the womb, and possibly during birth.

The HIV virus is found in the following but there have been no recorded cases of transmission through these routes:

**Saliva**. The virus is sometimes found in the saliva of those infected but at low titre (small concentration). There is no evidence that anyone has been infected through exposure to saliva and transmission through this route seems very unlikely.

**Tears**. The virus is found at low titre in tears of some people. There is no evidence of any transmission through this route and it is hard to imagine it being a risk.

**Table 4.1** (*contd*)

---

**Urine**. The virus is found at low titre in urine but there is no evidence of transmission and it is hard to imagine it being a risk.

**Faeces**. The virus is probably present in faeces but, again, risks appear minimal or non-existent.

**Other body fluids**. The virus is probably present in other body fluids but the risks of transmission appear extremely low.

**Overall**. The risk of infection is related to two things. The first is the amount of virus present in a body fluid or tissue — the higher the concentration, the greater the risk. The second is the fact that the virus has to get *into* the body to cause infection. There is no evidence that it is able to cross intact skin, therefore the virus must come into contact either with non-skin surfaces like the vaginal and rectal linings, or be carried through the skin, as with blood transfusions.

Very large numbers of people are infected with the virus worldwide. It is impossible to rule out very rare cases of unusual transmissions but there have been so many cases so far that it is possible to be confident about how the virus can and cannot be transmitted.

---

which encourages people to mention their fears. The danger is that they will be made to feel that they cannot mention their worries because they will look foolish. It is worth tackling this issue directly:

COUNSELLOR: 'Now we've talked about what to do and what not to do, is there anything that you think you'd feel uncomfortable about or anything which worries you particularly?'

PAUL: 'Yes. My sister comes round on a Sunday and brings the kids. I really like having them there but now I'm afraid to kiss them or even touch them.'

COUNSELLOR: 'A lot of people feel like that when they learn that they are infected. But the HIV virus can't be passed on just by touching someone or hugging them or kissing them on the cheek. A lot of people worry particularly about passing the virus on to children but there isn't any need to. The rules are no different for children than for anyone else, you would have to get your body fluids into their bodies and you can't do that by hugging them or kissing them on the cheek.'

PAUL: 'But what if they have a cut on their cheek?'

COUNSELLOR: 'The cut would have to be open and you are assuming that the virus can be passed on through saliva, and there's no evidence for that. But tell me, do you ever kiss anyone on an open cut?'

PAUL: 'No, I suppose not. I suppose if the virus was passed on that easily everyone would have it.'

**Table 4.2**   Infection control advice

Someone who is infected with the HIV virus or who thinks he might be should:

**Not** donate organs, tissues or body fluids including blood, semen and breast milk. He should not carry an organ donor card.

**Not** have any surgical or other invasive medical or cosmetic procedure carried out except under proper sterile conditions. So he should not have ear-piercing, tattooing, skin-cutting, ritual scarification, ritual circumcision or any other non-medical procedure unless he knows that the practitioner is taking proper infection-control measures. In the case of acupuncture for instance, the patient should seek assurances that appropriate sterilisation of needles is practised or disposable needles used. Otherwise there may be a risk of transmission of HIV to others or of acquisition of other infections by the patient.

**Not** share wet-shave razors or toothbrushes with others (they may be contaminated with blood).

**If** he cuts himself he should stop the bleeding and cover the cut with a clean dressing. He should mop up the blood using a paper tissue, newspaper, leaves or any absorbent material to hand and flush this down the lavatory or if this is not possible burn or bury it. Surfaces can be washed down in one part bleach to ten parts water for extra safety. If someone else cleans up the blood they should use household rubber gloves.

**Not** share syringes or needles with anyone else.

**Not** worry about transmission through casual contact, including shaking hands, kissing on the cheek, or normal social contact.

**Not** worry about others catching HIV virus from the WC, bath, or washbasin.

**Not** worry about possible transmission through cups, cutlery or crockery. None of these things is a risk.

**Remember** that the virus is not airborne, nor can it be caught from coughs and sneezes.

**Lead** a normal life.

---

COUNSELLOR: 'That's a very important point; with so many people in the world infected we would know if it could be casually transmitted, and we know it's not. You hug your sister's kids and kiss them on the cheek, it's good for you and it's probably good for them, too.'

The above dialogue highlights several important points. It is important to treat people's worries seriously, even if they seem out of proportion. It's important to explain why they are not realistic. Often people will cite some extreme set of circumstances such as 'what if they have a cut on their cheek' and it is important to either explain why this is not a risk or to try to sort out some kind of strategy to avoid it if there is a real risk. It is absolutely crucial to get people thinking about transmission using the information you have provided or things they already know. That's why the statement, 'I suppose if the virus was passed on that easily everyone would have it' is so important and why the counsellor should pick up on it and encourage the patient — 'That's a very important point'.

Getting people to apply abstract information to their own lives will give them the confidence to apply it. In thinking over the practical applications of what they have learnt they will fit the information into their own way of thinking and it will improve their chances of remembering it.

### Reducing personal transmission risks

Anyone who is engaging in high-risk behaviours needs to modify those behaviours, whether they are seropositive or seronegative. When the counsellor starts to look at changing behaviour with a patient it is important that they should cover all the risk behaviours, even if these do not apply directly to the patient's life at the moment. People's lives and their sexual and other risk behaviours may change over time.

So with gay men, the risks of vaginal intercourse and of transmission through sharing syringes and needles should be covered. Contrary to the popular view, it is not uncommon for some gay men to engage in sex with women from time to time. Similarly some heterosexual men sometimes engage in sex with other men. Moreover it is worth bearing in mind that most things which gay men do sexually, including anal sex, are quite common amongst heterosexual couples.

So for any patient it is important to cover *all* the issues surrounding sex and also the issues surrounding sharing syringes (see Chapter 8), although the amount of discussion on syringe-sharing with a middle-aged man who has never injected drugs and says he never will is likely to be a lot less than that with a young man who is currently a user or who has many friends who inject.

### Sex

For most patients sexual transmission is the way they caught the virus and the way they may pass it on to others. Sex is likely to be one of the most critical areas for counsellor and patient to discuss. However, sex is an interaction between people as well as a physical act.

COUNSELLOR: 'When you and your lover Jeff have sex, what sort of things do you do?'
PAUL: 'Anal sex mainly, sometimes mutual masturbation.'
COUNSELLOR: 'Are you both active and passive?'
PAUL: 'Yes.'
COUNSELLOR: 'Have you ever used a condom?'
PAUL: 'A few times, but we don't usually use one. I don't really like it, though Jeff likes them more. It makes sex artificial, I can't feel what I'm doing somehow. Also we've had breakages.'
COUNSELLOR: 'How often?'
PAUL: 'Maybe half the time.'
COUNSELLOR: 'That's really high, let's come back to that in a moment. What else do you do? Oral sex?'
PAUL: 'No, I don't like it. Jeff likes it more and he does it sometimes.'
COUNSELLOR: 'Jeff sucks you sometimes?'
PAUL: 'Yes, that's right.'
COUNSELLOR: 'But you never suck Jeff?'
PAUL: 'That's right.'

It's always important for the counsellor to check that he has understood the patient correctly. It's very easy to make assumptions about what people mean and store up a whole lot of confusion for later. Unless the counsellor has a particularly good memory he should take notes, if the patient doesn't mind. In the dialogue above the failure rate for condoms is much too high, it's an issue which the counsellor is going to want to come back to.

COUNSELLOR: 'Anything else you do? Rimming? Fisting?'
PAUL: 'No, I suppose we have a pretty straightforward sex life, just anal sex and playing about.'
COUNSELLOR: 'What about mutual masturbation, do you enjoy that?'
PAUL: 'Yes I do, we both do. We mainly have it when we're tired.'
COUNSELLOR: 'But it's not a replacement for anal sex?'
PAUL: 'No, anal sex is more intimate, it gets us close together in a way that mutual masturbation doesn't.'

Penetrative sex often has a different value attached to it. It is always worthwhile finding out what the patient's attitude towards various sexual activities is. To what extent is one sexual activity seen as equivalent to another? To what extent do different activities fulfill different functions in the patient's life? It is a mistake to assume that all sexual activities can be considered on one dimension — how exciting they are; things are much more complex than that.

COUNSELLOR: 'What about sexual partners other than Jeff?'
PAUL: 'Yes, I have other sexual partners from time to time, maybe three or four last year.'
COUNSELLOR: 'What did you do with them sexually?'
PAUL: 'Mainly mutual masturbation or oral sex.'
COUNSELLOR: 'They sucked you?...'
PAUL: 'Both.'
COUNSELLOR: 'I thought you didn't like it?'
PAUL: 'It avoids having to have anal sex with them?'
COUNSELLOR: 'Did you have anal sex with any of them?'
PAUL: 'Yes, I did once, I picked up a guy at a party, he was very attractive, I was very drunk and I guess that I was very unwise.'
COUNSELLOR: 'Did you use condom?'
PAUL: 'No, I didn't, and then I wished the next day that I had or, better still, that I hadn't done it at all.'
COUNSELLOR: 'Were these short-term or long-term affairs?'
PAUL: 'They were one-night stands while Jeff was away. I told him about them when he came back, we've made it a rule to tell each other about what we're doing. I didn't tell him I'd had anal sex with this guy though, we'd agreed with all this trouble about AIDS that we would stick to lower-risk activities.'
COUNSELLOR: 'You do different things with Jeff than with these other men, why is that?'
PAUL: 'It's mainly because of the risk of AIDS, anal sex is special to me because it's closer so it's important to my relationship with Jeff. The other guys were just for excitement, a part of a good evening, and really I wanted to keep sex with them safe, though I did go all the way once when I hadn't intended to. Even when we had oral sex I wouldn't let them ejaculate in my mouth and I didn't ejaculate in theirs.'

The sexual interview above is, of course, only a small part of a much more detailed discussion about Paul's sex life. However, it does show certain important features. The counsellor asks specific questions about exactly what the patient does sexually, and where the patient doesn't mention something (for instance oral sex) the counsellor specifically asks. The counsellor also tries to build up a picture not just of what Paul does but who he does it with and what meaning Paul attaches to different aspects of his sexual behaviour. Understanding the context in which sex takes place is vitally important in trying to help someone to decide the best way to make changes in his sexual behaviour.

Some terms for sexual activities may be unfamiliar to the counsellor, for instance 'rimming' (oral-anal sex) or 'fisting' (inserting the hand into the rectum). A counsellor coming across something unfamiliar in someone's sex life should simply ask what it means:

PAUL: 'Jeff and I also like water-sports.'
COUNSELLOR: 'What's "water-sports"?'
PAUL: 'Urinating on each other.'
COUNSELLOR: 'Right.'

Patients are usually only too happy to explain unfamiliar terms.


## Relationships

Finding out about relationships is just as important as finding out about sex. In Paul's case he has two sorts of sexual relationship, a steady one with Jeff, and casual relationships. It's important to explore these in detail and to work out how they are going and what sort of functions they fulfil. There will also be other non-sexual relationships in Paul's life; these are considered under 'Social support', later in this chapter.

### Primary sexual relationship

COUNSELLOR: 'How long have you known Jeff?'
PAUL: 'About eight or nine years. We met at a club one night and just took it from there.'
COUNSELLOR: 'Do you live together?'
PAUL: 'Yes, we moved in together after about three months and we've been together ever since. We rented a flat to start off with but about four years ago we bought the flat together.'
COUNSELLOR: 'How is the relationship between the two of you?'
PAUL: 'It's very good, we get on really well together.'
COUNSELLOR: 'What's Jeff like?'
PAUL: 'He's ten years older than me. He had a pretty wild time before we met but I think that he was getting to the end of that phase when we met. He was looking to settle down into something more permanent. He's a good man.'
COUNSELLOR: 'In what way?'

PAUL: 'He's very quiet, very organised and very patient. He never argues about things, if I get annoyed or upset he sits down and we talk things through. I get pretty aggressive, verbally aggressive, when I get annoyed, but he just sits it out.'

COUNSELLOR: 'How does that make you feel?'

PAUL: 'At the time it makes me feel mad, he just sits there so cool and calm and I'm really angry. After a bit I start to cool down because he doesn't rise to the bait. Then we start to talk about things.'

COUNSELLOR: 'Is the way he handles things a good one for you?'

PAUL: 'If we both started shouting that would be it, but...'

COUNSELLOR: 'But...?'

PAUL: 'Well, sometimes I wish he was a bit less cool?'

COUNSELLOR: 'When you get angry?'

PAUL: 'No, not then. Generally.'

COUNSELLOR: 'How do you mean, "generally"?'

PAUL: 'He's very quiet, sometimes I wish he was a bit more demonstrative. I know how he feels about me but I wish that he'd actually show me how he feels.'

It's important when exploring a person's relationships with him to look at the positive aspects as well as the negative. In all but the most dead relationships or in the most perfect relationships (of which I have yet to see an example) there are pros and cons about the relationship. Since most counsellors are looking for the problems a person has they tend to ignore the good things in their relationships. This produces an imbalanced and incomplete picture. Moreover, helping someone to make changes doesn't just mean getting round his problems, it also means building on the strengths in his life. If you don't know what the strengths are, it's hard to build on them.

Discussing relationships is one area where counsellor prejudices tend to show up more than in any other. Many counsellors have strong ideas about what makes good and bad relationships, often based on common sayings or ideas in their own culture. In Western cultures common ideas are:

'If one partner has an affair there must be "something fundamentally wrong with the relationship".'

'Relationships where there is little overt display of affection must be bad ones.'

'In a good relationship all sex is kept within that relationship.'

'In a good relationship people sit down and talk about their feelings.'

'A relationship in which there are a lot of rows is always a bad one.'

'A couple should always do most things together, *or* each partner needs to lead a "life of their own" if the relationship is to prosper.'

Many popular paperback books have reached the best-seller lists by advocating this sort of idea or other ideas of the same kind, generalisations about the way to build an 'ideal relationship'. In fact the key issue is what the couple themselves want out of the relationship and whether it is giving them what they want. All the above statements are true for some couples, for others none is true.

Even fairly obvious ideas about couples can be wrong. For instance, most counsellors believe that physical violence in a relationship means that it is inevitably no good. These beliefs are based on heterosexual couples where the weight/size/aggressiveness of the partners is usually uneven. However, in a few gay couples I have seen they have chosen to resolve unresolvable differences in the last analysis by fighting it out. In none of these cases does significant tissue damage seem to have occurred and the issue in hand seems to have been sorted out in the post-fight discussion rather than by sheer strength. This does not mean that this is the right way to resolve differences or that the counsellor should not explore other ways in which they might sort things out, but it does mean that such relationships are not necessarily disastrous, as might be thought superficially.

Particularly, but not exclusively, in gay relationships it is not uncommon for a couple to live together, have a warm and loving relationship, and yet seek sexual activity outside the relationship. Quite often one finds that long-established gay couples have ceased all sexual activity with each other.

What matters in a relationship is what the members of the couple think about that relationship and what's in it for them. Researchers into relationships such as Stuart (1980) and Jacobson and Margolin (1979) have stressed the issue of the rewards and costs which are inherent in relationships for the individual.

Whatever initially brings people together, their satisfaction with their relationship comes from the balance between what they get out of the relationship and what they have to put into it. Obviously the balance of rewards and costs has to be considered over a period of time; in any relationship there will be unrewarding hours, days or even weeks. However on balance a relationship which is all cost and no gain is likely to be an unhappy one. One which brings a lot of gains and relatively low costs to both partners is likely to be a happy one. Rewards in this case are emotional rewards, sexual rewards, the opening up of possibilities (even simple ones like having someone to go to the cinema with), and material rewards (like being able to share the costs of a house). Costs are likely to be emotional, sexual (like having to engage in unwanted sexual activity), the restriction of opportunities (not being able to do what one wants because of the other person) and material costs (having a lower standard of living through having to support the partner).

However, satisfaction or lack of it is not all that clearly related to whether people stay together. Studies on marriage do not show a clear relationship between how happy a relationship is and how likely it is to survive. One way to look at it is to look at what alternatives a person has. People are likely to continue in a relationship if the alternatives look worse. A man may stay in an unhappy relationship in a comfortable house if the alternative is living alone in a damp bedsit. He is likely to stay in an unhappy relationship if he feels that he is unlikely to be able to form a happier one elsewhere. Perhaps that is one reason why younger people tend to have less stable relationships: they perceive themselves as being more easily able to make a favourable change.

A lot of people stay in unhappy relationships because the short-term unhappiness of splitting up, with attendant loneliness and financial problems, outweighs for them the possibility of having a happier life in the long term. Where a relationship between people is very unhappy the patient sometimes wants to break out of that relationship and helping him to sort out the short-term problems can allow him the freedom to make a change.

For the counsellor assessing a relationship with a patient one of the key issues to look for is what the patient gets out of the relationship, what he doesn't get out of the relationship which he feels he should, and what the costs are for him from that relationship. Where a relationship is presenting problems it is important to consider with him the ways in which he can make it more rewarding and can reduce the costs to him of the relationship. It may, of course, be that what the patient really wants to do is end the relationship. It is perhaps not surprising how often the moment when a patient finds out he is HIV positive or has AIDS is the moment when he decides to take action and to end a relationship which has gradually been getting less and less happy over the years. As a number of people with AIDS have said to me in different ways, 'I may not have long to live, I want to be happy in the time I've got left and being happy means getting out of this relationship'.

In the case of Paul he has, it appears so far, a basically good relationship. It sounds as though it might be even happier if his lover were more demonstrative. Later it will probably be useful to go back over this issue and find out how important it is to Paul — is it very important to his well-being or just a minor irritation which doesn't really matter to him all that much, at least not enough to want to put the effort into doing something about it?

### Other sexual partners

COUNSELLOR: 'What about your other sexual partners, what do they give you?'

PAUL: 'How do you mean?'

COUNSELLOR: 'You've said you have a basically good sex life with Jeff but that you also have sex with other people. What do you get out of those relationships, is it novelty, excitement...?'

PAUL: 'It's a mixture of things, really. Sex is good with Jeff but it's rather comfortable, like a well-worn pair of slippers, I know exactly what we are going to do and when and where. One thing I get out of casual relationships is excitement, another thing I get is a boost to my self-esteem. These people give me positive feedback, they tell me I'm attractive in a way that Jeff usually forgets to do. Also when I have too much to drink I don't think too clearly and the heat of the moment tends to take over.'

COUNSELLOR: 'Where do you meet these other partners?'

PAUL: 'Clubs mainly; both Jeff and I used to go to the clubs pretty often and I still know a lot of the crowd; once this year I met someone at a party. In the past, people we've known as friends once or twice but not any more, too complicated.'

COUNSELLOR: 'And you tend to meet them when Jeff is away?'

PAUL: 'That's right, he travels a lot on business and when he's away I get pretty lonely on my own. Our friends are really more Jeff's friends than mine, I feel; I do go and see them when he's away but I never really feel they are *my* friends. So I tend to go out to the clubs. Jeff is, in any case, not all that keen these days to go out socially to clubs or the theatre, he likes us to have friends round or to go round to dinner with them. So while he's away I tend to do the things he doesn't like doing.'

It is important to build up a clear picture of the context in which sex takes place with partners other than the primary partner and to try to find out what role these play in the patient's life. This serves two functions, to build up a picture of the structure of the intimate relationships of the patient and to form the basis for discussion about safer sex.

**Putting safer sex into practice**

There is a lot of information about today on the subject of safer sex. The current information is contained in Table 4.3.

Gay men in particular have made tremendous changes in their sexual behaviour in the light of the spread of HIV. However, change has not been complete and not everyone has changed. Heterosexuals in the West have hardly changed their behaviour at all. The reason is straightforward: putting safer sex into practice is difficult. Moreover, safer sex is much more difficult to make fun.

In general safer sex is non-penetrative sex. Non-penetrative sex seems to differ from penetrative sex in that, to many people, it is not so intimate. Even though the orgasms from masturbation seem to be as strong or stronger than those from penetrative sex people tend to value penetrative sex more. This is particularly the case with heterosexuals. While some gay men have given up penetrative sex, very few seropositive heterosexuals I have seen have done so. This probably reflects the greater range of sexual behaviours gay men have always engaged in besides anal sex. For heterosexuals other sexual activities, with the possible exception of oral sex, have been seen as foreplay prior to intercourse rather than as means of satisfaction in themselves. Safer sex can be made fun for both gay men and heterosexuals but it takes time and imagination.

The other problem with putting safer sex into practice is sorting out all the difficulties which surround it. It's worth considering the options open to Paul in more detail and this is where the detailed questioning about his sex life comes in. For both the counsellor and the patient this sort of review of options is extremely important. They should do it together. It is often helpful for the counsellor to actually write out in front of the patient the options available. The patient may, of course, come up with other options and these can be incorporated. In Paul's case he could:

**With his primary partner:**

(1)  Choose to have non-penetrative sex only. In this case he may have to work with his partner to make this more interesting and more intimate. In their relationship anal intercourse fulfills a special function in terms of intimacy. Unless safer sex can go some way to fulfilling the same function he is likely to go back to penetrative sex at some time in the future whatever his good intentions.

**Table 4.3**   Current safer sex advice

**Vaginal intercourse**: A high risk of transmission of the virus, both male—female and female—male. Only totally safe way is to avoid completely. If this is unacceptable a condom should be used, with extra lubricant. It is possible that those gels with spermicidal agents like nonoxynol-9 may offer additional protection through some anti-viral action in case of condom breakage. Condoms should never be used with oil-based lubricants like Vaseline which may weaken the rubber. A range of lubricants made for use in sex is available. Because of occasional failures with condoms and the vital importance of avoiding pregnancy a back-up method of contraception should *always* be used — the diaphragm with spermicide (which has the additional advantage that it protects the cervix), or the pill.

**Anal intercourse**: High risk of transmission of the virus from active (insertor) to passive (insertee). The risk of transmission from passive to active is hard to assess but appears to be considerably lower although still significant. Only safe course is to avoid anal intercourse completely. Use of a condom provides protection to both partners if it remains intact; however, condoms tend to have a higher rate of failure in anal than in vaginal sex because of the greater mechanical stresses, and no generally acceptable condom appears to offer a total freedom from breakages. One which did would be likely to be so thick that there would be a major loss of sensation for the user. Extra *water-based* lubricant should always be used with condoms, never lubricants based on oil or grease which may weaken the rubber.

**Oral sex**: Very hard to assess the risk because it is difficult to find a sample of individuals who only ever have oral sex and don't engage in high-risk penetrative sex. Risk in fellatio is likely to be lower if ejaculation does not occur into the mouth. Risks from cunnilingus impossible to determine. Oral sex is probably best avoided until more is known. Fellatio can be made safe with the use of a condom, a method used by some prostitutes but usually considered unaesthetic by most people for obvious reasons.

**Sharing sex toys**: For instance sharing dildoes or other objects inserted anally or vaginally. At least one case of transmission through this route has probably been identified (in a lesbian couple, one of whom was bisexual). To be avoided.

**Water sports**: Urinating on partner or into partner's body. The latter practice is to be avoided since while the urine itself may not be a risk it is hard to carry it out without penetrating the partner.

**Inserting hand (fisting) into anus**: Almost always causes bleeding from ano-rectal area, tends to be risky because it is usually followed up with anal intercourse with recipient bleeding on active partner and having a damaged ano-rectal area. As an isolated behaviour probably small risk provided the skin on the hand of the insertor is free from lesions, but very unusual as an isolated activity.

**Oral-anal contact (rimming)**: Spread of HIV through this route, assuming there is no concurrent bleeding, seems unlikely. However the risk of the transmission of pathogens from the gut, which may be particularly virulent in the immunocompromised individual or may even act as co-factors for the

**Table 4.3** (*contd*)

---

development of AIDS, makes it best avoided. This particular activity is probably responsible for the high incidence of gastro-intestinal problems identified in populations of gay men in the 70s, the so-called 'gay bowel syndrome'.

**Mutual masturbation**: Safe, can be engaged in with as many people as an individual wishes.

**Body rubbing (frottage)**: Rubbing penis or clitoris against the intact skin of partner (not mucous membranes). As for mutual masturbation.

**Other activities**: People show enormous imagination in their sex lives and, as such, sometimes present the enquiring counsellor with unexpected activities not referred to in the literature. However, these can usually be assessed straightforwardly. Any activity which involves contact between body fluids and body surfaces which are not covered in ordinary skin (for instance the glans, vagina, eyes, lips, etc.) or with skin surfaces which are damaged, is likely to be best avoided.

---

If he chooses this option then the counsellor is going to have to help him, and possibly the two of them together, to think through how to make safer sex work for them.

Making safer sex more exciting is very important. It needs imagination and a willingness to explore. Incorporating fantasy, erotic materials like books and videos and erotic talk between the partners can all serve to boost excitement. It is well worth the counsellor exploring with the patient what he finds exciting and erotic and what he fantasises about and then encouraging the patient to build these elements into safer sex.

(2) Engage in penetrative sex, but use a condom. This is not 100 per cent safe but they may be willing to take the risk. However, there is an extra worry here: the breakage rate for condoms when they use one is staggeringly high, probably because they are misusing them in some way. This needs further investigation to find out why there are so many breakages and if it is through misuse Paul and his partner will need instruction in how to use condoms properly.

(3) They may choose to continue to have anal sex, after all they may already have passed the virus between them, indeed Jeff may have given it to Paul in the first place. Let's look at this option:

COUNSELLOR: 'Has Jeff been tested?'
PAUL: 'No, he hasn't, but we've been having anal sex for a long while, I guess he must be infected if I am.'

COUNSELLOR: 'Not necessarily, only about half the partners of gay men infected with the virus are themselves infected.'

PAUL: 'Why should that be so?'

COUNSELLOR: 'There's probably a combination of reasons. Firstly it is possible that some people are resistant to the virus, although I don't think this is something which anyone should count on. More likely is the possibility that the infectiousness of people who have the virus may vary over time. It is likely that a person is most infectious just after he himself has been infected, before antibodies have been produced which restrict the amount of virus being produced. There is probably a second peak if someone begins to become sick, as his immune system becomes weakened it is no longer able to restrict production of the virus and he may get more infectious again. However between these times it is thought possible that a person's level of infectiousness may fluctuate unpredictably. He may be hardly infectious at all one week and much more so the next. There is also probably an element of sheer bad luck in all this — enough virus coming into contact with the right cells at the right time or not. So even if the virus hasn't been passed on yet, it doesn't mean it can't be in the future.'

PAUL: 'What if Jeff has the test and turns out to be positive, will it be OK to have unprotected anal sex together?'

COUNSELLOR: 'That's more difficult. There are two possible problems. Firstly, it may be that repeated exposure to the virus may cause problems, we're not sure whether this is true but extra doses of a virus that your partner is currently controlling *might* break down that control. Moreover either or both of you might have sexually transmissible diseases which you haven't yet passed on to each other. Herpes is an obvious example of a virus which one partner can have for quite a period of time without passing it on to his partner and then suddenly it can be transmitted. But there are other viruses like that which are only produced by a person intermittently. The problem with these is that they may act as co-factors in the production of AIDS in someone infected with the virus.'

PAUL: 'So it is best not to engage in unprotected anal sex?'

COUNSELLOR: 'That's right, and there is another reason. Even if both of you are infected you may not have caught it from the same person. There's a lot of variation in the virus so it might be that you have two different strains of the virus which you could pass to each other. We don't know what the effect of that would be. It may be that when you are infected with one strain you won't get another but the evidence is unclear at the moment.'

PAUL: 'A different strain might be more aggressive in causing disease?'

COUNSELLOR: 'We just don't know. At the moment I think it is safest to avoid unprotected sex, even between two people who are infected.'

**With other partners**:

Paul has options here:

(1) He could restrict his sexual activity to his primary partner. He has other partners because:
   (a) His sex life with Jeff is a bit hum-drum, the sexual excitement has gone out of it. If he's going to cut out outside sexual activity he is going to have to build up the excitement of his sex life with Jeff.
   (b) His partners make him feel attractive, Jeff doesn't. This goes back to the issue of Jeff not conveying his feelings in the way Paul wants. It needs careful going into to try to find ways of getting Jeff to provide more feedback to Paul.
   (c) Sex is part of the social scene he is involved in. This is tied into two other factors: (i) He likes going to clubs and has to go without Jeff because Jeff doesn't want to go, and (ii) When Jeff is away he gets lonely and the clubs are a place where he can get social contact. On the other hand it frequently leads to sex with others. He could therefore: (i) Go, but avoid situations in which he is likely to end up having sex, or (ii) Persuade Jeff to go with him when he goes to clubs, or (iii) Not go to clubs at all. In the case of (ii) or (iii) he is going to have to find some other social outlet when Jeff is away.

(2) He could still have other partners but only have safe sex with them. This seems to break down when he has been drinking despite good intentions, suggesting that if he is going to carry it through he is going to have to ensure that he doesn't get drunk *and* get himself into a position where he is likely to have sex at the same time.

This sort of option analysis is very useful. Setting out the options and going through them with the patient is a very good way of structuring decision making for the patient. It takes time but it often helps very much to actually put down what the possibilities are and go through the pros and cons in logical order. It also helps to decide what steps the patient needs to take if one or other option is to be adopted.

I would cover, at least verbally, all the information contained in the above option appraisal. I would encourage the patient to do it jointly with me and to correct any errors and to add any information or options he felt I had left out. It should be our *joint* appraisal of the options in which my part is largely to help him to structure the picture.

## Telling sexual partners

### Current sexual partners

Virtually every patient wants to tell their current sexual partner. There is usually little debate on the subject. There are good reasons why they should. The partner may not be infected and may be able to take steps to ensure that he does not become infected. In the case of heterosexual couples if the partner is female she may need to take steps to avoid pregnancy. If the partner is having relationships outside the couple they may have to take steps to protect or inform those partners. The partner needs to take steps to protect his own health if he is infected.

Occasionally one comes across a patient who does not wish to tell his partner. This is exceptionally rare, apart from in one set of circumstances: it is not uncommon to find the partner of a person with AIDS saying that he does not want to tell his partner that he too is infected because it would only add to his partner's worries. This is an understandable reaction; whether it is the right reaction will entirely depend on the couple. However, it does no-one any harm.

The rarest case of all is the individual who does not wish to tell his sexual partner even though the partner has been at risk *and doesn't know it*. One occasion on which this occurred was in the case of a gay man who had agreed with his sexual partner early on in the HIV epidemic that in view of AIDS they would not have sex outside their relationship. He had broken this agreement and had a brief affair with another man and had become infected. He was stricken with guilt. In another case a man who was bisexual (but whose wife knew nothing of his activities) had become infected. Again, he was unwilling to tell his wife what had happened. Both were quite prepared not to have sex again with their partner, but were reluctant to tell.

This is in my personal view a situation in which the counsellor should try as hard as possible to persuade the patient to tell his partner. There is no point in being censorious and giving the individual concerned a lecture on the subject of 'responsibility', or whatever. The first step is to try to find out *why* he will not tell his partner and to try to come up with a strategy to overcome the problems he has. Then it is important to rehearse with the patient the reasons why it is important for him to tell his partner.

In both these cases there was a combination of two factors — shame at deceiving the partner and fear of being rejected by the partner. In the case of the bisexual man he had to make a double disclosure, that he was infected and that he was bisexual. Both were also uncertain about how to actually go about the task of telling the partner.

After discussion, both saw that to have deceived the partner in the first place might be shameful, but it was minor compared with the shame of knowing that one had in fact become infected and not passing that news on. Neither, in the last analysis, could face living with that particular shame, and decided to tell. In both cases the resolution of the worries about being abandoned was for the two members of the couple to come to see the counsellor and to talk the issues through with the counsellor acting as 'referee'. In practice it worked very well, both relationships survived the experience, although it was hardly comfortable for either.

But suppose that, ultimately, one has a patient who just will not tell his partner. What should the counsellor do then? Should he tell the partner against the patient's wishes? There are legal issues here (see Chapter 20). The precise issues concerned in terms of law depend on the country the counsellor is working in.

However, there is also a moral dilemma for the counsellor which can't be avoided. Unfortunately for the counsellor it is a moral issue where the 'right' answer is very hard to discern. It is clearly a matter of balancing the rights of the patient against the rights of the partner mixed in with considerations about the 'privileged' relationship between the patient and the counsellor. Different people who have looked at the issue have come up with different answers largely because they have tended to start from different premises. Initial prejudices tend to lead to the eventual answer people come up with. This is profoundly unhelpful for the counsellor who, unlike most of those discussing the issue, actually has to take a decision and put it into action.

There is, however, one practical consideration, which tends to get lost in the ethical debate. If a patient feels that he or she cannot tell the counsellor the truth and be sure that that information will not be passed on to others, that patient will be deterred from seeking counselling in the first place. If he doesn't come for counselling, how can he be persuaded to tell his partner? A guarantee of confidentiality serves one very critical purpose: it allows people to come forward and reveal information about themselves which they would not otherwise be able to reveal. In this set of circumstances it is the reason why I personally would not pass on information against a patient's will, however uncomfortable that decision might sometimes be.

For the counsellor who cannot operate on these terms there is an alternative. If he feels that he cannot under all circumstances keep information confidential he can make the limits of confidentiality clear to the patient at the outset of the counselling. If the patient is not agreeable to this arrangement it should be made clear to the patient that he can be passed on to another counsellor.

## Past sexual partners

For the patient who is infected there may also be a question as to whether he should tell his past partners, and if so, how far into the past he should go. This issue, assuming the patient doesn't know when he was infected, can be a difficult one. There is, probably, a case for telling very immediate past partners, for instance someone the patient has just split up with. Going further back into the past tends to present problems. Patients may well have lost touch with past sexual partners and many of those past sexual partners may view the re-appearance of the patient in their lives with a distinct lack of enthusiasm, especially if they have formed new liaisons.

Going back into the past is a matter of common sense, a matter of what is practical and reasonable. For a gay man in London today there is little point in going into the distant past because levels of infection amongst gay men are high. Anyone that they had sex with in the distant past will quite probably have been exposed to other infected people since having sex with the patient. Moreover gay men in London are well aware of the risk of getting HIV infection and anyone who has been at risk will be alerted to the fact.

## Future sexual partners

Whether future sexual partners are to be told by the patient is a matter of what the patient will do with them sexually. Where only no-risk safer sexual activity such as mutual masturbation and body rubbing is to be engaged in there is, strictly, no need to tell future partners. However, many patients do, from time to time, go rather further than they would like sexually. If a patient intends not to tell future sexual partners, he has to be aware of the extent to which he must remain entirely in control of what he is doing sexually. If he cannot be sure of remaining in control, he has no option but to discuss the issue with future partners.

For Paul, who tends to go rather further than he would like when he has had a few drinks, an obvious step would be that if he did want to have sex without telling his partner he should severely limit his drinking in situations where he might end up having sex.

For some people, both gay men and heterosexuals, not telling future partners is not really an option at all. As mentioned earlier, amongst heterosexuals no-risk safer sexual activities tend to be a prelude to penetrative sex rather than an alternative to it. The young seropositive heterosexual haemophiliac boy just starting to take girls out is not going to have to tell the girls that he is infected if he is only going to take them out or to engage in petting. Eventually, if he finds a girl he wants to form a long-term relationship with he is going to have to tell her at some point. When he does so he is quite likely to end up with a rejection. He may minimise this risk as far as possible by forming as strong a relationship as possible with the girl before telling her. However there is no way in which he can avoid a very strong probability of rejection. Also, by telling her, he is exposing a personal and socially stigmatising fact about himself. He must be sure that, whatever her reaction, she will not tell that fact to others without his agreement. Guiding him through this sort of problem is not likely to be easy.

## How to tell others

Telling sexual partners that one is infected with HIV is very stressful. It needs careful attention from both counsellor and patient. Sometimes it is very straightforward, the patient is confident that he can handle the telling. For other patients it is a very difficult issue and needs careful thought.

Where a patient has difficulties there are several things which the counsellor can do.

### *Helping the patient to pick a time and occasion*

When telling a partner it is helpful to choose a time when the partner is relaxed and when there is time to discuss the issues through. The counsellor and patient can work together to select or work out how to achieve such a time. It is clearly a mistake for the patient to tell his partner just before the partner leaves for an important business meeting, for instance. On the other hand there is seldom likely to be a perfect time to tell.

### Practising telling

It is extremely valuable for the patient and the counsellor to practise together how to tell the other person and what to say. This can be done in the form of role-plays. The counsellor needs to get a clear picture of what the partner is like and how he usually reacts to difficult news. The patient should be able to provide this information. The counsellor can then take on the role of the partner and the patient can practise telling him. In this way the patient can gain confidence in telling, practise different ways of telling to see which is the best, and the counsellor can help with suggestions as to how the patient can handle the situation better. It also helps if the counsellor and patient occasionally exchange roles so that the patient can feel what various approaches are like for the person being told.

Where a patient intends to tell a partner it is always wise to ensure that he has fully understood the facts about HIV since the conversation may well turn to issues of fact at some point.

### Being available for the partner

The counsellor should always make it clear to the seropositive person that he would be only too happy to see or get a telephone call from the partner after he has been told. The partner will himself often have things he wants to talk through and he has a right to do so with the counsellor. In this sort of situation the discussion with the partner sometimes turns to issues surrounding the patient. The relationship between counsellor and patient and between partner and patient are both confidential ones. It is important to establish with, say, the patient, what aspects of his discussions with the counsellor he is or is not willing to have discussed with the partner.

### Seeing the couple together

When a patient has told his partner it is often helpful for the counsellor to see them together as a couple if they wish this. Particularly where there are relationship stresses or where putting safer sex into practice is an issue for them it can be helpful to deal with the issues jointly, but making it clear that each has the right to see the counsellor individually as well.

### Telling the partner for the patient

Rarely, patients do not wish to tell the partner but would like the counsellor to do it for them, although it is usually much better if they tell the partner themselves. Sometimes this is because they feel unable to discuss the issues clearly enough; not everyone is verbally very adept. Under these circumstances the patient can bring the partner in and the counsellor can tell him or help the patient to tell him.

## Social support

Virtually everyone needs a social support network of some sort. Such a support network is particularly important when someone is in trouble. As the saying goes, 'That's what friends are for'. There is a large body of psychiatric research which shows that those who have little in the way of social support are more prone to just about any form of psychological and psychiatric disturbance, particularly depression and anxiety.

It would therefore be expected that those people who find themselves infected who have a good network of sympathetic friends to rely on should do better than those who have no-one. Clinical experience suggests that this is correct.

As always, however, things are not straightforward. Virtually any counsellor who has seen many people with HIV or AIDS is able to produce a list of those who have met with rejection, abuse, even physical aggression from 'friends' who have found out their status. They can also usually produce a list of patients who have experienced no problems at all. One patient of mine told, he calculated, over a hundred other people and said that everyone was sympathetic. This is, however, rather unusual.

In most cases, it is important for the patient to balance the need to obtain social support against the need to avoid unpleasant experiences. In doing this, the patient will have to consider not just the likely reactions of friends but also how discreet they are. Friends cannot always be trusted not to pass on the information to others who may be unsympathetic. Particularly with friends at work, this can be a major problem: we have had examples of people being ostracised at work after telling indiscreet 'friends'.

Support with less risk of rejection can, of course, be obtained from various support groups and voluntary agencies. These are a vital part of the support-system of many people with HIV infection and every seropositive individual should be told about the opportunities in their area and encouraged at least to try their local support group. On the other hand not everyone wants to go to a support group or finds them helpful and many people still need support over and above what such groups can give.

Some seropositives want to tell friends of their status not just in order to get their support but also because they feel that if they do not pass on the information they will be creating an undesirable block between themselves and their friends.

So it is a matter which needs to be talked through in detail between counsellor and patient. Who can the patient trust: Will that individual be discreet? How sure can the patient be of that individual's reaction?

The person newly identified as HIV seropositive will usually be well advised to tread carefully early on. There is often a tremendous need in people to share the news they have had. However, people can always be told in the future; once told they can never be un-told. The counsellor can play a very important role in reviewing with the patient who they might tell. Sometimes it is a vital role.

### Telling one's family

Many people who are seropositive want their family to know. Families can provide a great deal of social support, sometimes even more so than friends can. In general they are rather less likely to reject someone simply because they are infected. On the other hand such a rejection is far from unknown:

> Sean's father was dead. His mother, who had strong religious views, had never accepted his homosexuality. After he came to London they met seldom and she was always somewhat cool towards him. He learnt that he was infected and developed ARC. He felt sure that he was going to go on to develop AIDS very soon and wanted to tell his mother and be reconciled. After discussing it with his sister he went to see his mother. After listening to what he had to say she told him it was a judgement on his sinful life style and begged him to repent before it was too late. He left feeling much worse than when he went.

For many people who find themselves seropositive, admitting that they are infected means making a double disclosure. They have to admit that they are infected and they have to admit that they are gay, or that they have injected drugs or that they have caught the virus heterosexually through sexual activity that their family may not approve of.

Where the likely reaction of a family member is uncertain, for instance the reactions of a mother, it is sometimes helpful for the seropositive person to enlist the help of a brother or sister or other family member who is sympathetic. One patient told his grandmother, who had always been fond of him, and the grandmother told his father who was initially far from sympathetic to the idea that his son might be gay. However, the grandmother was able to sort out the situation very well.

It is also important to remember that families themselves sometimes require advice and support. This tends to be most common in people with AIDS, where the family may need a great deal of support. However it does also happen from time to time that a family member of someone who has revealed that they are seropositive seeks advice and information about HIV either in terms of worries about infection or, more usually, in terms of worries about the seropositive person.

## Telling other people

Few seropositives will have any reason at all to tell their employer. Existing employers do not usually question their workers about what they have caught since joining the firm. If employers are told they may take a very sympathetic stance; however, I have seen far too many people lose their jobs or be 'eased out' of companies when found to be seropositive to feel that that is something which can be relied upon. Telling friends at work is one issue here: if they are not absolutely discreet then there is a good chance that the news that someone is seropositive will go all the way round the company in a very short time, including to the management. It is not unknown for sympathetic employers to be faced with highly *un*sympathetic workers demanding the removal of a seropositive colleague.

There can be some difficulties, however. Some countries are asking for negative HIV test certificates before allowing foreign nationals to settle in their country. The difficulty this presents to the seropositive individual who is going to be posted to a country requiring a certificate is obvious. The only options are for the seropositive person to try to find some way out of the posting, or to tell his employer why he can't be posted to that country. Alternatively he could resign. It is a difficult situation.

## Informing GPs and dentists

Anyone who is seropositive should inform his General Practitioner (family doctor, GP) of the fact that he is infected. It is potentially very difficult for the GP to treat the seropositive patient sensibly if he does not know a potentially crucial part of that patient's medical history. Common symptoms such as a chest infection or diarrhoea may have a particular significance in someone known to be HIV seropositive.

There can be disadvantages in telling the GP. As noted in Chapter 3, the seropositive person may be asked to get his or her GP to fill out a health questionnaire for employers or insurance. Also not all GPs are very well informed about HIV and AIDS. There are even, shamefully, occasional cases in many countries, including the UK, where doctors have refused to treat someone who is HIV seropositive.

The first step in dealing with the GP is to find out whether the patient likes his current GP. A surprisingly large number of patients dislike their GP. Under these circumstances they should change to a different one.

Some patients will elect to be looked after by a clinic and will not be making use of their GP. They may, therefore, elect not to tell the GP until such time as they need to consult him.

The situation with respect to hospital medical specialists is much the same. Anyone going into hospital for, say, an operation should tell the surgeon that they are infected (or that they are at high risk). Sadly, there have been cases of seropositive individuals being refused 'non-essential' operations in the UK and in many other countries. It is always possible for the counsellor to contact the surgeon a patient will by seeing to sound him out in principle, without mentioning the patient, about his attitude towards operations on those with HIV infection. Where a patient does experience problems the counsellor is often in a good position to follow up those difficulties with the doctor concerned, or help him to find another surgeon, and should do so.

It is helpful for any counsellor to establish a personal list of sympathetic doctors, both specialists and GPs, to whom patients can be referred.

Similar considerations apply to dentistry. Some dentists are unhappy about dealing with individuals who are seropositive. There are good grounds for suspecting that gum disease is rather more common than usual in seropositive individuals. This makes dental problems more likely. The counsellor can check, in principle, what attitude a patient's dentist has to those who are seropositive. It is always wise to keep a list of sympathetic dentists in case of difficulty.

## Keeping well/positive health boosting

There is currently little that can be done medically for someone with HIV infection to affect the course of any possible deterioration in health. However it is likely that there are things that patients can do to help themselves, which will possibly reduce their risk of going on to get AIDS, or at least slow down the progress. These can be considered under two headings, Keeping well, and Health boosting.

### Keeping well

There is a theoretical risk that other infections acquired after being infected with HIV may have an adverse effect on health. There is also good evidence supporting the reality of that risk.

The most common serious infections in adults, other than respiratory tract infections, are sexually transmitted diseases (STDs). There is evidence that STD infections can provoke a worsening in health in someone who is seropositive. They act as co-factors in the development of disease. There are three reasons why this might be so: some infections are themselves to some extent immunosuppressive; the activation of T-cells in response to the new infection may increase HIV production; and some viruses may possibly act directly to stimulate HIV viral DNA. In the immunocompromised individual any serious infection should, in any case, be avoided.

It is not clear whether some STDs are more of a danger than others. It appears possible that some viruses, possibly Epstein-Barr, herpes simplex and cytomegalovirus, may be particularly active in this respect. On the other hand non viral infections may also cause problems.

Safer sex not only protects the HIV seropositive individual from passing on the virus, it also protects against acquiring infections from others. Thus it is probably helpful to an individual *even though he is already infected with HIV*. Patients should be made aware of this.

Other possible sources of infection should also be avoided. This does not apply to colds or other minor ailments. There is no way in which these can be avoided and no evidence that common minor upper respiratory tract infections are a problem in this respect. However it is helpful to ensure, for instance, that meat is well cooked and food hygiene is good to avoid possible infection with organisms causing food poisoning.

One other issue relates to vaccination. Vaccines come in two types, killed vaccines (which should present no problem) and live vaccines. Live vaccines are what they sound, live pathogens which have been weakened so that they cannot cause disease. Common live vaccines include yellow fever, polio and measles vaccines. Because they are live there is the risk that they will cause greater immune activation than killed vaccines and hence act as co-factors. It is also possible that a vaccine which cannot cause disease in a person with an intact immune system might cause disease in someone with an impaired one.

There is a small amount of evidence suggesting that live vaccines can cause a problem, with particular uncertainty surrounding BCG. On the other hand there are a number of studies looking at various live vaccines which show no problems. Against the theoretical risks from vaccines must be set the very real risk of catching the disease which the vaccine protects against. There is little point in *not* being vaccinated for yellow fever because of risks surrounding HIV, and then catching yellow fever.

The best evidence at the moment suggests that the advice should be that live vaccines should be avoided if they are not necessary. If there is a real risk of catching the wild-type organisms then it is better to be vaccinated. Sometimes there are killed versions of live vaccines and, where possible, these should be used in preference.

### Health boosting

In contrast to the information on keeping well there is, currently, little hard evidence that taking active steps to improve general health will also improve prognosis. However there have been few studies aimed at trying to show that such an approach does work, so the lack of evidence does not mean that it is *not* possible to make a useful impact.

Encouraging patients to improve their general health might be expected to have a favourable effect on commonsense grounds alone. If nothing else it can only do the patient good and will have no side-effects, a somewhat unique feature in medicine.

It is also clear that encouraging people to look after their health has a very important influence on mental well-being. Taking control of one's own health can act as an important corrective to feelings that one has lost control and is the passive 'victim' of a malevolent virus.

In fact it is relatively easy to come up with a programme designed to promote good health. Most counsellors will know what they *should* be doing to stay well themselves, even if they are not actually doing it! There are several things which the seropositive person might aim to do.

### Eating a balanced diet
This simply means what it says: eating a good range of fresh foods and not living out of packets or tins or on 'junk' food. It does not mean eating a quirky diet nor does it mean that nothing should ever be eaten out of a packet. There is *no* special 'AIDS diet' and a quirky diet is likely to do more harm than good. Sometimes quite reasonable dietary changes can have unexpected results:

Peter, a seropositive man, came in to say that he had been suffering from what he considered to be excessive frequency of bowel movements for three weeks. He felt sure that he had got an opportunistic infection. Close questioning revealed that he, a lifelong carnivore and junk food enthusiast, had shifted over to a high fibre vegetarian diet in the last three weeks. He had not made the connection between the two events.

## Getting a reasonable amount of exercise

This is self-explanatory. However, it is important that the exercise is *reasonable*. It would not be sensible for a man who has not taken exercise for thirty years to suddenly embark on ten-mile runs or hard games of squash. Swimming or walking might be better.

## Reducing stress

Stress is not always a bad thing. A little stress is unavoidable in any life. Nice things like birthdays, parties and weddings can be just as stressful as bad things. However, someone who is excessively stressed should take steps to reduce his level of stress. The counsellor can help simply by going through with the patient on a piece of paper those things which the patient finds particularly stressful and looking for ways of reducing the stress (see also Chapter 13, on problem solving).

## Relaxation

Getting adequate relaxation is also very worthwhile. This can be in the form of carrying out some of the relaxation exercises covered in Appendix A; or it can mean setting aside an hour a day to lie down and listen to some music or read; or it can mean going for a walk in the park every day with the dog. Whichever way it is handled it is beneficial to have at least an hour a day set aside for personal relaxation.

## Reducing excessive use of recreational drugs including alcohol

A drink or two in an evening is unlikely to cause any problems, so someone who is seropositive need not become teetotal. However, excessive use of alcohol by a patient needs to be looked at carefully. Alcohol in excess can not only impair physical health but can also be a severe hindrance to psychological adjustment to HIV. The use of recreational drugs should also be either eliminated or kept within sensible limits, depending on which drug is being used and its harmfulness. There is no evidence currently, for instance, that the occasional use of cannabis will cause particular problems for the seropositive person. However, used in excess it can also make it difficult for people to sort out their problems.

### Heterosexuals

Although the example chosen, the case of Paul, is a case involving a gay man, a case involving a heterosexual man or woman could equally well have been chosen and there would have been very little difference in approach. Anyone who knows how to counsel a seropositive gay man also knows how to counsel a seropositive heterosexual.

There are, however some specific difficulties for heterosexuals.

Firstly, there are the issues surrounding pregnancy. These are covered in Chapters 9 and 10. Where the heterosexual is an injecting drug abuser there are the problems specific to this group (Chapter 8).

Secondly, the availability of what *patients* consider as appropriate voluntary support groups is lower. Most support groups and organisations currently are aimed mainly at gay men. Such organisations are usually only too happy to support heterosexuals. However, the patient may feel that he has less in common with the members of such organisations and therefore they sometimes feel that such groups are 'not for them'. This is changing as new support groups aimed at heterosexuals and injecting drug users are set up by existing organisations or new organisations. However, currently it still remains a problem in many places, particularly in view of the relatively few non-injecting heterosexuals infected at the moment in most Western countries.

Thirdly, there is often an extra feeling of isolation for the heterosexual man or woman infected sexually. Most gay men will know other men who are infected. They will also find that being seropositive does not cut them off from the possibility of sexual expression since many gay men are relaxed with the idea of having safer sex with someone who may be infected. However, the infected heterosexual may find himself one of only a very few heterosexuals infected in his area and few potential sexual partners are likely to be prepared for the idea of safer sex with someone infected with HIV.

The counsellor may have to spend a lot of time with the heterosexual dealing with these issues. Because there is a greater tendency for heterosexuals to feel isolated it has been our experience that they need far more in the way of support than most gay men and tend to face repeated difficulties. Therefore maintaining continuing contact with such patients is of vital importance.

## Dealing with carers

This chapter has dealt mainly with the issues concerning the seropositive person. It is well worth remembering that others may be affected, directly or indirectly, by the patient's being seropositive.

The sexual partner of someone who finds that he is infected may himself (or herself) be afraid that he is infected. He may need help in making necessary changes in sexual behaviour or other risk activities. He may also be very anxious about the patient and about the implications for the patient of being seropositive.

If the patient and partner are willing then it often helps to see them together on a few occasions, particularly where issues surrounding their personal and sexual relationship need to be resolved. However both may also need time alone with the counsellor in addition to joint time.

Not everyone affected by the patient's being seropositive will be a sexual partner. Family and friends may be extremely anxious and worried about what will become of the patient.

Some of our own research (Kocsis *et al.*, 1988) has shown that carers and family are not uncommonly more anxious and disturbed than the patient by the issue of the patient's seropositivity.

A counsellor who sets out to provide a service to seropositive people or those at high risk will need to provide a service also to carers. Again, where carers are coming to see the counsellor because of worries about the patient's well-being it is important to explore first with the patient what he has and has not discussed with the carer. It is also important to establish what he is and is not willing for the counsellor to discuss of what patient and counsellor have talked about.

The counsellor should make clear the issue of the confidential patient–counsellor relationship early on, and also establish that the carer–counsellor relationship is a confidential one.

## Organising practical help

However good the counsellor is, his efforts will be seriously undermined unless the patient has adequate housing, enough to eat, can keep warm and has adequate access to medical and other services. The good counsellor will find himself acting to ensure that patients get the services to which they are entitled.

Organising this sort of practical help is a vital part of the work of the counsellor. Often the counsellor will be more familiar with the services available than the patient and will need to guide the patient through any difficulties involved.

The counsellor also needs to ensure that the patient has access to other hospital or clinic facilities, understands the system and how to make the most successful use of what is available. By liaising with other services, if the patient wishes, the counsellor can often play a key role in ensuring that the patient is able to get the maximum benefit from them.

## Organising the counselling

People will vary enormously in the pattern of counselling that they require. However, there are several general considerations which are well worth bearing in mind:

- It is important that counselling should be available at the time that the test results come back. Patients should never have to get their results and then come back the next day for the counselling.
- It is often impossible to get through the whole of the counselling of an individual in a single session. The counselling may have to be split over two or more sessions.
- When people have been given bad news they are often shocked and may not take in information as well as they normally would. It is important, especially when going through factual information, to keep checking that the patient has, in fact, understood and taken in what has been said.
- A patient who has had bad news may be unable to take everything in. A counsellor should never be afraid to review what was gone over in the last session before starting on the next one.
- Good counselling also implies good medical back-up. It is important that a patient who has had a positive result should be able to have a medical as soon as possible to reassure him that he is physically well or to uncover any possible health difficulties.
- It is extremely helpful to have at least two sessions with a patient, the second seven to fourteen days after the first. This allows the patient time to try out some of the things he must do and to let the information sink in and to come up with any questions he may need answering. It also allows the initial shock to wear off; the counsellor and patient will then have a better idea of how the patient is taking it and it will be possible to see if the patient is anxious or depressed, which is rather difficult to assess in someone who is shocked.

**Table 4.4** Issues which need to be covered by the counsellor

---

**Breaking the news** in a clear and sympathetic way
**Listening** carefully to the patient's response and helping him to talk through what it means to him
**Providing** facts about HIV and AIDS
**Providing** facts about transmission
**Providing** information about infection control issues
**Finding out** about the patient's sex life
**Finding out** about his relationships
**Finding out** about any other risk factors, e.g. injecting drug use
**Helping** him to implement safer sex
**Helping** him to reduce other risk factors
**Helping** him to inform sexual partners
**Helping** him to deal with relationship issues
**Helping** him to arrange a social support network or to make the best use of the one he has
**Informing** him about what hospital and voluntary services are available to help him, and how to access them
**Helping** him to decide who else he wishes to tell
**Encouraging** him to take positive steps to maintain and improve general health
**Organising** further appointments with the counsellor, and with other health workers
**Making sure** that he has adequate medical support and services
**Helping** him with practical problems such as housing, welfare benefits etc.
**Making sure** that he knows how to reach the counsellor in case of difficulty and knows he is welcome to seek help from the counsellor

---

- At the second session the counsellor and the patient can review the situation and decide how much extra time they need to spend together and either book further sessions or agree to stop at that point.
- A follow-up at three months should always be arranged to see how things are going.
- Regular medical follow-up should be arranged.
- The patient should be encouraged to get in touch if there are any problems. It is important to make patients feel that they would be *welcome* to ring up or to come back at any time. Giving the patient a telephone number to ring is most important because often patients have quite simple questions or need a little reassurance and being able to ring up means that they can have their questions answered rapidly, without having to make an appointment or come in. This reduces their distress and saves them and the counsellor time.

- Some people coming for the test need relatively little in the way of counselling. They have thought through the implications of the test in detail before coming forward to seek it. Even so, it is important at least to ensure that they have thought about all the issues covered in this chapter. It is not unusual for someone to handle the test result well at the time but later have difficulties. Even for someone who needs little counselling at the time, the booking of a follow-up and making it clear that he is very welcome to come back if he has any difficulties is very important.

## References

Jacobson, N.S. and Margolin, G. (1979) *Marital Therapy* New York: Brunner/Mazel.
Stuart, R.B. (1980) *Helping Couples Change* New York: Guilford Press.

# Chapter 5

# Counselling People with AIDS, Their Lovers, Friends and Relations

HEATHER GEORGE

The diagnosis of AIDS, or AIDS-related complex (ARC), represents a crisis for affected patients and their 'significant others' — lovers, friends, and relations. Although there are parallels with patients suffering from other life-threatening illnesses, practical and emotional problems are likely to be more complicated for people with AIDS (referred to as PWAs) for several reasons.

Public awareness of AIDS is very different, with ignorance or faulty beliefs frequently generating fear or hostility towards individuals or groups of PWAs who disclose their diagnosis. Scientific understanding of AIDS and HIV is constantly changing, so that in addition to myths and misinformation from lay sources PWAs are continually faced with new findings or guidelines from health care professionals (e.g. revision of advice about safer sex, or introduction of new treatments). Media coverage of AIDS is much greater than for other diseases, and may be misleading through oversimplification, or by distortion of details in articles which may be designed to entertain and sensationalise rather than educate. AIDS, more than any other illness, challenges our most basic beliefs about health, infection, death and dying; dependency, disability and disfigurement; sexual behaviour and orientation. Against such a background emotional support of PWAs deserves particular attention.

## Emotional reactions of PWAs

A diagnosis of AIDS or ARC represents different crises for different individuals. A range of reactions has been observed in people adjusting to their diagnosis; although these reactions and their management have been most fully observed for gay men, they are fairly general responses to loss and would seem to apply to everyone faced with a new, life-threatening illness.

It should be stressed that the most usually observed responses are given here; there is no evidence to indicate that individuals necessarily experience all those listed, nor is there any particular order of presentation suggesting universal 'stages' which everyone must 'work through' to achieve positive adjustment.

Uncertainty and beliefs about AIDS are important concepts underlying the reactions. Unlike some other terminal conditions, the course of illness varies greatly from person to person, depending on the tumours or opportunistic infections suffered and the individual's response in both physical and psychological terms. Hence for PWAs there is uncertainty about when the next tumour or opportunistic infection will occur; how long periods of relative health may be enjoyed; how much time they have left to live; and how, when and where they will die. There is the question of whether treatments or a cure will be developed 'in time' for them. In addition there is the uncertainty of reactions of others (lovers, partners, friends, family, colleagues, employers, health care staff, the media and society).

As time has passed since the first cases, underlying beliefs about AIDS become more complex and important in structuring an affected person's reactions. If images of physical pain, social isolation and intellectual decline are held as the inevitable outcome for someone diagnosed as having AIDS, these beliefs will create much mental distress as the individual considers his future. Some people have ideas about how a PWA 'should' cope, and feel guilty or a sense of failure if they experience distress.

(1)  *Shock* may occur on diagnosis, and may be manifested in a very obvious, overt way with agitation, verbal anger, thoughts and expression of disbelief, and crying. Some people may appear calm and controlled, whilst feeling emotionally numb, physically drained and generally cut off from people and events around them. Some people may feel 'too well' to have AIDS, e.g. for a PWA with one mild episode of *pneumocystis carinii* pneumonia (PCP) which responds well to treatment, or for someone with one small KS lesion it can be extremely difficult to believe there is something seriously wrong with his immune system. Despite this, denial and avoidance are uncommon where the diagnosis is communicated sensitively and clearly, and where further emotional support is offered.

(2)   *Relief* may be experienced by people who have known themselves to be HIV antibody positive, or more commonly by people
with ARC, who may suffer greater distress from repeated hospital
admissions and investigations which turn out to be negative
than from a clear diagnosis — having lived with a feeling of
impending doom, the reality can be much more manageable.

(3)   *Anger* may be generated over being infected, by frustration that
there is no cure, by the involuntary restrictions and limited
opportunities imposed on life, or by hostile or prejudiced reactions of others who fail to understand or are unable to empathise
or imagine the impact of AIDS on anyone. Some patients may
'shoot the messenger' and express anger towards the person who
breaks the news of the diagnosis, although again this is rare
with sensitive handling. Less common still is the angry reaction
of attempting revenge by spreading the virus to others — most
PWAs are over-concerned about infection to others.

(4)   *Guilt* may result from worries about infecting other people or
being a burden to others. When individuals feel stigmatised
through others blaming them for becoming infected with HIV,
they may feel guilty over a life style or behaviour which led to
exposure to the virus, or over other events or attributes unrelated to AIDS which they feel are personal faults.

(5)   *Decreased self esteem* is common since, although there has been
some increase in understanding about HIV, AIDS remains a
stigmatising and unglamorous illness which continues to elicit
hostility from some sections of the public. Some people feel
contaminated and unclean, applying the cliché of 'social leper'
when recounting their experiences of real, or anticipated, rejection. Personal events such as loss of employment and subsequent loss of income, or public ones such as media coverage
terming HIV-infected babies 'innocent victims' (implying that
adults with AIDS deserve their illness) may be seen as a confirmation of unworthiness. Alterations in appearance may be
construed as disfiguring, e.g. weight loss or skin disorders, whilst
if there are neuropsychological impairments such as word fluency
problems, the PWA may have insight into these effects of the
virus on his abilities, and feel embarrassed or inferior to the
good conversationalist or witty intellectual he used to be.

(6)   *Loss of identity* is experienced by people who feel completely
different in appearance, personality or life style from what they
were before they had AIDS, or they may feel they are different
from other people without AIDS. It is quite common for PWAs

to feel socially and sexually unacceptable, that any form of sexual activity is unavailable, and that close relationships will be impossible to establish or maintain. These feelings may be compounded by actual events that lead to a loss of role, e.g. the ending of a sexual relationship because of a partner's fear of infection; living on invalidity benefit after sick leave from employment, so that both work and income are lost; dependence on parents and/or health care workers to help in physical or daily living care so that privacy and time alone are reduced or unavailable.

(7) *Loss of a sense of security* is felt by PWAs who feel threatened by actual or anticipated changes in their lives as a result of illness. Most people take their health and independence for granted, at least when they are young, but they are likely to experience losses or changes throughout their lives as a function of ageing, e.g. greater dependence on others because of physical weakness or illness; retirement or redundancy from work with perhaps loss of income which leads to changes in accommodation; a reduced social network due to friends moving away or dying. It may be difficult for people in their middle years or old age to cope with such factors, but generally they are able to adjust because these changes may be anticipated, and they usually occur slowly, over a period of some years. However, for PWAs there may be equally disruptive changes in their lives, which could not be predicted and which occur very rapidly after diagnosis. Furthermore, knowledge and 'truth' about HIV and AIDS are constantly changing, and are complicated by myths and rumour, adding to the confusion and to the feeling that the world is no longer safe and predictable.

(8) *Loss of personal control* results when people feel that everything they do is dictated by AIDS. Work, social and personal routine may be disrupted by hospital admissions and appointments with health care workers who are continually probing and prodding for information to help in treatment and research. Individuals' life styles come under inspection by counsellors and by the public as the impact of AIDS in society is examined by social scientists and in the media.

(9) *Fear* of what may happen in future and of inability to cope may haunt a PWA. Physical symptoms of anxiety and worrisome thoughts which disrupt attention, memory and concentration may generate or exacerbate the feeling of losing control and confidence. Avoiding feared situations may lead to the development of phobias.

(10) *Sadness and depressed mood* are normal responses to adverse circumstances. Repeated episodes of illness and/or experience of
losses lead to helplessness and hopelessness about overcoming
or changing situations.

(11) *Obsessions and compulsions*, which may occur with or without
anxiety and depression, are fairly uncommon among PWAs
(although characteristic of 'worried well' people who believe
they have AIDS in the absence of any supporting evidence for
HIV infection). Obsessional pre-occupation may take the form of
disturbing, repetitive thoughts about illness, death and failure.
Possible compulsive behaviours are relentless searching for new
treatments, therapists or clinics; 'body checking' for the appearance of new symptoms; and faddism over health and diets.

(12) *Positive adjustment* occurs in some people with little intervention
from professionals. All people with AIDS or ARC should receive
support and advice about their illness on and soon after diagnosis, and be given information about professionals and agencies
offering further help with emotional problems. Some PWAs are
able to minimise and adapt to changes, concentrating on living
with AIDS rather than on dying. Others respond by making
AIDS and HIV central to a new identity, by being active in self-
help groups. Some health care workers may regard such responses as pathological avoidance or denial, but this may be
more to do with the defensiveness of the workers who are faced
with confronting their own mortality when dealing with PWAs.
Some people show remarkable adjustment to impending death,
although much is dependent on external factors and individual
situations, e.g. how other people respond when told the diagnosis, or the type and severity of physical illness.

## Support and advice on diagnosis of AIDS or ARC

People diagnosed as having AIDS or ARC are normal people in an
abnormal (crisis) situation. Although all patients diagnosed with any
serious illness may benefit from the approach given below, PWAs
should be offered particular help because of the unique way AIDS is
viewed by society. PWAs are part of society, and so are subject to
misconceptions and false information; they need orientation to the
reality of their situation. Hence overly pessimistic beliefs about their
future may be corrected, and help and understanding may be offered
when actual aspects of their illness are distressing.

*Minimising uncertainty*

Sensitive and straightforward confirmation of the diagnosis when test results become available is important. There is no easy way to break bad news, but hedging or vagueness do not protect the patient, they just add to confusion. Patients have a right to know about their physical health status, and attempting to withold information only leads to a loss of trust and confidence in the health care team when the true diagnosis is eventually learnt. Since PWAs are faced with many uncertainties, as much detail as possible about what *is* known should be given: e.g. an explanation of the symptoms of the opportunistic infection or tumour; an account of treatment(s) and side-effects, plus any tests or investigations; an idea of how long the hospital stay will be, if possible; and reassurance about follow-up care: e.g. names and status of people in the care team, support services outside hospital, including voluntary services in the area, and locations and appointment systems of outpatient clinics. Such information is important because it builds up a picture of what actually happens, and orientates the person to life continuing outside hospital.

Some people are distressed about admission to hospital *per se* — they may never have been in hospital before, or they or their friends or family may have had bad experiences — and they will need comfort, company and understanding, e.g. reassurance about how it is difficult to adapt to the ward routine, or that it is normal to feel disorientated and lose a sense of the outside world.

Initially, only a small amount of information is likely to be taken in, and the aim should be to relieve distress. There should be plenty of opportunity on subsequent occasions for emotional expression and for asking questions.

## Checking what has been understood and correcting misconceptions

After breaking the news, what is understood from being told of a diagnosis of AIDS or ARC will vary according to underlying beliefs and preparedness. Basic post-HIV antibody test issues (transmission of the virus, safer sex, increasing chances of staying healthy) need to be introduced to PWAs who did not know they had HIV, and checked for comprehension in those who did. Some PWAs may take some time to think through the implications, and be unable to discuss very much of the future; this may be a healthy defence, when people know they are not ready to examine things beyond the hospital environment. With gentle prompting and questioning any misconceptions may be corrected.

## Telling others of the diagnosis

Reassurance should be given about confidentiality — patients should know who within the hospital or clinic knows their diagnosis and has access to their notes, and what will appear on sickness certificates.

Outside the health care team, patients may wish only to inform a partner or one friend or relative. Direct help may be given where patients like a member of staff to be present when a significant other is told, or they may prefer staff to do the telling. It is useful to discuss whom else might be told, and, for those who are not told, what might be said to them: e.g. if a patient does not want to tell an employer or colleagues the true diagnosis, rehearsal or role-play of how to deal with probing or intrusive questions avoids future difficulties and fears about being 'found out'. Generally, patients eventually inform all significant others, but on diagnosis and/or when they are debilitated they may feel unable to cope with others' responses. Wishes about whom patients want to know and whom they want to see whilst in hospital are important aspects of control and should be respected.

## Examining personal resources

Emotional and practical resources outside hospital should be investigated, so that plans may be made; this is a good way of giving patients a sense of the future and of life continuing. There are no rules about how people should cope, but patients may be encouraged to look at what options are available in terms of how they will spend their time and who will offer emotional support outside hospital so that severe problems are avoided. For example, patients may wish to 'protect' their family from their diagnosis, but if relatives are the people to whom they have turned in past times of crisis it may be better to look at how to break the news to them, so that their support may be received; when patients are unwilling to burden partners or family with their worries, they should know what voluntary and professional counselling help is available; if their work is an important part of their lives and structures most of their time, they need not leave their jobs immediately if they are likely to be sufficiently fit to return after convalescence, but they may be encouraged to consider possibilities of limiting working hours and creating aims unrelated to work. Since any practical problems will interact with and compound emotional strain, enquiries about housing, employment and finance, with plans for how to sort out difficulties, will help prevent later distress.

## Discussing death and dying

People should not be forced to talk about death. Gentle enquiries are enough to ensure that they understand the significance of their diagnosis and that they are likely to die at a much younger age than formerly expected. For some people this, with plans for sorting out practical affairs such as making a will, is sufficient. For many others, talking about death with a member of staff or trained volunteer is a relief because they feel unable to do so with significant others. Patients may want to know the 'nuts and bolts': e.g. what happens to their body after death; whether partners or family may touch them when they are dead; what to do about funeral arrangements. These matters may sound somewhat distasteful, and indeed need to be discussed with sensitivity, but they may cause great worries for PWAs who have heard accounts of health care workers or funeral directors 'refusing' to handle bodies of people who have died from AIDS-related illness. Some PWAs will want to make sure that certain people are contacted and able to be there with them when they are seriously ill.

PWAs may want to examine their beliefs and feelings about death. Most people are more fearful about the process of dying than of death itself, although some have very strong emotions about life after death. Returning to a former religion, or a stronger involvement with the Church, are fairly common, and it is important that hospitals and clinics make links with clergy and religious groups who are informed and aware of AIDS-related issues so that pastoral care may be given. Frequently people who do not see themselves as religious but are wary of professional 'counsellors' will feel comforted by seeing a hospital chaplain because they perceive him as the appropriate person with whom to discuss feelings and beliefs about death.

Checking for suicidal ideas should form part of routine counselling for PWAs, since it may reflect severe depression. Thoughts about suicide are almost universal, and when they occur in the absence of other symptoms of depression should not be taken as indicative of psychological disturbance. Many people are relieved to express their suicidal feelings, and are reassured to find that they are 'normal' among PWAs. Plans and intentions to carry out suicidal acts are uncommon, but should be taken seriously with referral to other agencies for psychological or psychiatric support as necessary. For most PWAs with destructive ideas it is useful to make contracts and plans for what they should do when they feel particularly negative. They should know telephone numbers of emergency supports within and outside hospital, including 24-hour services, and be aware of the fact that they may present at any accident and emergency department to see nursing staff and/or a duty doctor for psychological as well as physical problems.

Taking things at the patient's pace is particularly important when dealing with ideas and feelings about death and dying. Approaching the area too quickly may lead to a failure to engage a patient, who feels threatened and hurt by pressure to discuss matters he feels are personal and painful. Very often PWAs work out their own timing, preferring to deal with other problems, e.g. practical aspects of their illness, or to develop a relationship with a member of staff or trained volunteer before they are ready to disclose their feelings about death.

## Developing a sense of purpose

At the time of diagnosis, or when PWAs have subsequent physical problems and hospital admissions, they may feel that life is already over and positive experiences are no longer available to them. They may need help to find the motivation to carry on, particularly when a series of changes and losses has led to helplessness and despair.

Denying the difficulties and limitations imposed by having AIDS or ARC only leads to the patient feeling alienated and alone, and that others cannot appreciate his point of view. It is important to empathise with feelings of hopelessness whilst giving reassurance about how things can change. For example, it is worth pointing out that many people in hospital feel frustrated by being 'looked after' by others, yet come to depend on staff to meet their needs and feel quite frightened of facing the outside world again. Under such circumstances it is normal to feel daunted by the prospect of leaving hospital, and to feel strange on discharge, but generally old feelings of competence and safety return quickly, very often in a matter of days.

Some people feel they have lost all that was important about themselves. Continuity with the past can be examined, to clarify roles, achievements and activities that are no longer available and those attributes and aspects of the person's life and situation which are enduring. Ambitions may be examined to sort out whether these may still be fulfilled, or to generate alternatives. Contact with another PWA can help in providing a model for coping, and in self-help groups a focus may be provided for future effort. Whether through being involved in self-help or other outlets, PWAs may be encouraged to take on new roles and master new skills — the crisis of AIDS and prospect of death enable some people to sort out what is really important in life. The aim is to maximise the quality of life in a realistic way. Building false hope is counterproductive, but by encouraging a positive attitude, 'fighting spirit' and clear idea of a sense of self-help, PWAs feel they have had and continue to have a worthwhile life.

### Emphasising individual choice and dignity

The primary concern for many PWAs is that they should not have to face a dependent and undignified existence. Worries of being left alone, of being used as an experimental guinea pig, of suffering extreme physical pain, and of being 'kept alive' are very real, usually generated by images in the media. Most people respond well to emphasising that they have choices in their future, e.g. that they would not be kept on active treatment against their will, or that they only participate in drug trials with their permission. It is important that provision is made for choice in their counselling too, with as many options as possible being presented.

### Setting 'boundaries' and providing 'safety nets'

Many PWAs will have had little or no past experience of contact with health care workers in hospital and social services, and will need to know the various roles of people involved in their care. The amount of contact will depend on how well services for PWAs have been developed, and upon the preferences of the individual workers. There are no rules about what constitutes 'emotional overinvolvement' of workers with patients, but in order to provide a feeling of security PWAs need to know who to call upon and how they may do this. Health care workers and volunteers should clarify how they may help, so that PWAs feel entitled to emotional support and worthy of receiving it, and never feel they have to face problems alone. It is important to avoid over-helping and patient over-dependence, and a continuous review of needs helps illustrate that adjustment is a matter of a patient's control as well as a counsellor's opinion.

## Longer-term support for specific problems

Studies of counselling, psychotherapy and other forms of psychological support have shown that a small number of factors are important in terms of what patients perceive as helpful. These factors have been identified as: receiving advice or specialist knowledge; the understanding given by the counsellor; and the availability of time to talk about self and problems e.g. see Murphy *et al.*, 1984; Whalen, 1987.

Such factors are certainly relevant in giving support to people after a diagnosis of AIDS or ARC.

Much emotional support may be given to PWAs by staff in primary contact — normally nurses, health advisers and physicians. A problem is that these health care workers may not have sufficient time to listen to the particular difficulties of all patients, nor may they have experience or confidence in dealing with psychological problems. When this is the case, referral to another agency may be necessary, e.g. to a clinical psychologist, psychiatrist, social worker, community psychiatric nurse, or other 'professional counsellor'.

One difficulty is that patients may be reluctant to see another person, particularly if they have already developed a good relationship with a member of staff, or if they feel uncomfortable about receiving help specifically for emotional problems. The referring agency and the counsellor can help to engage reluctant patients by explaining why the referral is being made, the form that the counselling will take, and what patients may expect from it. Anyone offering counselling to PWAs should have a sound knowledge of the basic facts about management of AIDS and HIV infection, in addition to training in counselling skills.

Depending on the experience and resources of the primary health care workers, referral for additional support may take place at or soon after diagnosis with the aim of covering the issues outlined in the last section, or may occur when a PWA requests or seems to require longer-term support.

## Helping PWAs to understand their responses

Some patients with AIDS or ARC experience more extreme emotions than they have ever had in the past, which can be very frightening and make them feel as if they are losing control or 'going mad'. Allowing time for expression of these feelings and fears, and accepting them as 'normal' and appropriate given the crisis of AIDS, can be an important part of helping with the adjustment reaction. Patients should not feel guilty about having 'negative' emotions at times, and benefit from having an opportunity to discuss these feelings with someone who will not chastise them for being morose, but acknowledge the difficulties in their situation.

Some people require a forum where they can feel understood by simple reflection of their feelings by the counsellor. Others are helped by discussing why these emotions arise.

**Structuring problems and eliciting solutions**

Many PWAs feel overwhelmed by the complexity of their situation. Reflective listening can be useful as a first step in identifying problem areas. For some patients it is useful to write a list or problem-solving chart with the possible actions they could take written alongside. It is important to identify priority areas for attention; the initial aim is to lessen distress which in turn establishes a feeling of control. The counsellor may point out that not all problems need be tackled at once, and that some things may change quite rapidly. Solutions include actions by the counsellor and by the patient (e.g. if an immediate concern was that the PWA felt very alone and isolated, the counsellor's action might be to contact agencies for times of various self-help activities, and the patient's action to attend and report back what happened); they should be elicited or negotiated rather than simply presented by the counsellor.

The model of checking beliefs and feelings, allowing description or expression of emotions, and generating solutions to problems may be established as the model for subsequent sessions.

**Anxiety management**

Experiencing symptoms of anxiety can be extremely distressing for PWAs. Since opportunistic infections or tumours may occur in the gut, lungs, skin or nervous system, PWAs may become sensitised to any changes in these systems and so misinterpret normal fluctuations in arousal levels as signs of organic pathology. If they become worried about their health, this generates more symptoms of anxiety and hence confirms their fear that they are becoming ill.

Anxiety management techniques help to avoid this spiral. It is useful to give an account of how anxiety has physical and mental concomitants, and how these overlap with the symptoms and signs of HIV-related illness — for example, that nausea and diarrhoea, breathing difficulties, hot flushes and rashes, and attention difficulties should certainly be reported to a physician if they persist, but that these symptoms may be caused by psychological distress. Patients may experience considerable relief from simply being aware of this interaction of mind and body, but generally they need further reassurance that they will be able to control anxiety symptoms by learning specific techniques.

Deep-breathing exercises, progressive muscle relaxation and guided imagery may be used alone or in conjunction, initially by the counsellor giving instructions or guidelines within a counselling session, to be followed up by exercises which the patient may practise alone. Simply providing a cassette tape with instructions for the patients to follow in routine practice is an effective and elegant way of enabling PWAs to experience regular relaxation, and to learn control of anxiety and panicky symptoms. Alternative techniques such as autogenic training or biofeedback may also be discussed and used — ideally, personalised instructions may be created, using elements which individuals find particularly effective.

Relaxation and imagery techniques may help boost confidence and build ideas of mastery, and to settle sleep if patients have difficulty falling to sleep or experience distressing dreams and nightmares.

Where panicky feelings are accompanied by distressing thoughts, imagery may be used in distraction and thought-stopping techniques where the counsellor and later the patient interrupts the chain of obsessive thoughts and focuses on some prearranged image or idea. Self-monitoring and response-limiting may help if there are compulsive behaviours — e.g. where patients feel the urge repeatedly to check symptoms and present to doctors for physical examinations, they can learn to rate the severity of their own symptoms and limit symptom-checking according to a schedule arranged with the counsellor, hence increasing their awareness of symptoms which are serious and actually require medical intervention.

One problem with anxiety management techniques is that they take some time to learn. In the short term tranquillisers and night medication are extremely useful in calming many patients, although ideally they should be used in conjunction with, or with a view to, counselling. In the long term psychological approaches are more likely to establish feelings of control and confidence.

## Combatting depression

It is normal for PWAs to feel depressed at times, in response to loss. For some, this may develop into a more severe disorder of mood, where the individual feels extremely pessimistic about himself, his situation and the future. This may be as a consequence of untreated long-standing anxiety, or where limitations and losses imposed by HIV-related illness have not been accompanied by development of a new life style and the individual has essentially withdrawn from everyday life.

Since depressed people frequently feel they are bound to fail, it is important that unrealistic goals are not set by themselves or others. Intervention in counselling can begin from assessment — initially when asking about self, mood and activities, the counsellor may challenge reports of absolute depression and failure (i.e. that the patient 'always' fails, feels low, or does not enjoy things), by focusing attention on any success, times when he feels less depressed, or anything that has been enjoyable. This must be balanced by the patients' need to feel that the counsellor understands the degree of their distress, and should be given time to express negative feelings; they are often relieved to have their reports of guilt, low self worth, crying, poor concentration, loss of interest and reduced activity diagnosed as depression which is treatable.

In subsequent sessions the counsellor can gradually orientate a PWA to more optimistic views of self and future. The aim is for the patient to feel less helpless, less hopeless and more in control. Initially the counsellor may have to assume control and be directive in generating less pessimistic and more realistic alternatives to the patient's views. For example, the counsellor can suggest that the PWA writes or thinks of a self description, plus an account of the ideal image. These may be used as material to examine whether the person has a style of expecting too much, of setting goals too highly and so setting up situations that are bound to fail. Activities also may be planned in a structured way to avoid failure and maximise the likelihood of changing mood by manipulating the situation. If there is a time of day when a patient feels less depressed, this time may be used to engage in certain 'tasks' set by the counsellor via negotiation with the patient. For example, if a PWA is depressed by feelings of fatigue, a simple structured exercise programme may be followed with the aim of building some stamina; if the problem is withdrawal from social activities the PWA can gradually build up contacts within his existing network or develop new ones via self-help groups; if physical illness or disability curtails many previous activities, attention may be focused on what is still available, e.g. enjoying company and conversation, or being able to give advice to friends. The counsellor can encourage patients to 'reality test' pessimistic predictions of future activities; almost invariably patients find they have distorted things, and the reality is that they are able to cope and may even enjoy situations. Even PWAs with suicidal thoughts may be helped by an intervention which allows emotional expression, examines ideas of self, and generates courses of action.

Antidepressant medication can be useful, particularly when there is marked sleep and/or appetite disturbance (early morning wakening, anorexia and weight loss) or where there are obsessive thoughts with depression. Psychiatric admission is rarely required, even when patients are suicidal, since destructive thoughts are often contained by regular counselling sessions which build feelings of security and safety.

## Dealing with relationship and sexual difficulties

Frequently PWAs anticipate problems in relationships, and although in many instances they will wish significant others to be involved in counselling, some PWAs may wish to keep the counsellor as a confidant. If so, or if others are not willing to attend, much can be gained from discussion of difficulties in individual sessions.

Many PWAs welcome the opportunity to express their feelings about others, and are helped by an examination of the problems by the counsellor who may be able to 'take the attitude of the other' (i.e. give an idea of how a PWA's reactions may seem to a partner, friend or relative), or structure problems more easily as an observer of the relationship. If PWAs feel that there are ideas or feelings they wish to express to others, these may be rehearsed or role-played with the counsellor.

Communication difficulties sometimes lead: to sexual problems, particularly if PWAs experience a loss of libido related to guilt over having been infected by someone other than a regular or long-term partner; to depression and low self-esteem which make them feel unattractive or unworthy of sexual attention; or to fears of infecting their partner with HIV. They may also find it difficult to establish how partners feel about sexual activity. In such circumstances, sessions with the PWA alone can help in examining how feelings may be conveyed to partners or elicited from them. Where sexual problems are long-standing or involve more than a loss of interest, both partners need to attend for therapy.

## Counselling significant others

Partners, friends and relatives are helped by the same basic interventions as PWAs, i.e. advice and information about the illness, reassurance about how to cope with changing situations and intense emotions, opportunities to express these feelings, and methods of managing stress. Caring for and coping with someone with AIDS can lead to emotional reactions which are similar to those experienced by PWAs themselves.

Significant others caring for PWAs frequently worry about breaking down or failing to cope. Observing changes in someone with AIDS can be very distressing. Physical changes in appearance are often easier to cope with than changes in personality and behaviour. Even acute confusional states caused by infections such as toxoplasmosis or by metabolic imbalance, which clear with treatment and time, are very disturbing to witness — it can seem that the PWA is no longer the person they used to know. The adjustment reaction for significant others continues after a PWA dies, hence provision for follow-up and bereavement counselling is important.

### Supporting a partner, lover or spouse

For partners who are current or past lovers of a PWA, news of the illness may generate many worries about their own health status as well as concern for the diagnosed person. It can be difficult to show care for the PWA when experiencing nagging fears about whether they too have been infected, and they may overtly or internally feel anger at being put at risk of infection, a sense of betrayal if they were unaware of other sexual contacts or drug use by the PWA, or see themselves as failures because the PWA 'went outside' their relationship for stimulation. Partners may feel these emotions so strongly that they initially reject the PWA, although complete or long-term rejection is very uncommon — they need to acknowledge feelings of resentment or hostility, sometimes with a counsellor, but in general even partners who have been put at risk of HIV infection by the PWA are primarily concerned about that person's welfare, and how they will each cope with the illness.

Changes of role within the relationship are inevitable. The PWA may be the one who has been more practical, assertive or in control — i.e. in some way construed as the carer of the other — and it may be very difficult for the couple to adjust to a role reversal when the PWA needs to receive the care.

Frequently both partners will know they have been HIV antibody positive, will have faced issues about who infected whom, and have prepared to some extent for one of them to develop AIDS. The situation becomes very complex if both partners have AIDS, since the roles of giving or receiving care may fluctuate and so continue to reverse; each is aware that it is impossible to know who will survive the other.

If sexual contact is to continue between a PWA and partner, it is important that each feels comfortable with any activity in which they engage. Sometimes couples feel tense and at a loss about how to deal with sex. Counselling can help in allowing time and opportunity for each to express what is desired, and the counsellor can help by reflecting back these needs and wants and by giving guidance on what would seem to satisfy both parties so that sex becomes enjoyable and relaxed again. When the partner is untested or HIV antibody negative, the couple may decide to continue with sexual contact which risks HIV transmission. Often it is the partner who desires the closeness of sex with the PWA, since it is a pleasure and intimacy which will cease when the person dies. The PWA may be extremely worried about infecting the partner and fail to enjoy sex as in the past, so again joint counselling sessions can help in reaching a compromise to suit both parties. Although such a couple may be encouraged to limit activities to safe or safer sex, it is imperative that the counsellor recognises the needs of some PWAs and partners for close and sometimes 'unsafe' intimacy.

Changes in health of PWAs are likely to involve changes in the practical situation for partners too. Partners may require more psychological support than PWAs, possibly needing to adjust to loss of joint income, accommodation and activities in addition to loss of the person they used to know. They may attempt to meet all the needs of the PWA, and feel unwilling to allow professional and voluntary carers or family and friends into the relationship. Counselling is important to acknowledge the temptation of 'giving all' to the PWA whilst giving 'permission' to allow others to take on responsibility for some of the care. The partner needs to preserve some independent identity, so that resentment is avoided, the PWA can enjoy the pleasure of others' company and caring, and the partner can begin to examine how life may be after the PWA's death. Partners can be encouraged to pay attention to themselves by pointing out that their care for the PWA will only be maintained if they look after their own health and lessen their stress levels. Furthermore, completely to 'look after' someone with AIDS is rather patronising − the PWA needs to be able to give as well as receive in the relationship.

When partners are the closest to the PWA − even if not the 'official' next of kin − counsellors and other staff should show their understanding of the significance of the relationship. Offering bereavement counselling − preferably involving some contact with staff who have cared for the PWA − can help make a partner feel involved. Support may be required many months after the death, since often by then family and friends withdraw their support, feeling that the partner should be 'getting over' the trauma. Some partners may feel they adjust too quickly, but often they grieve in advance of the death as they react and adjust to a decline in the PWA's health. They may need reassurance about developing new relationships and creating a new life without feeling guilt for being 'unfaithful'.

### Support for families

Support for families may begin when a PWA informs relatives of the diagnosis. For gay PWAs this may be the first time they have disclosed their sexual orientation to parents, siblings or extended family members. Some families may feel shocked by this in addition to the shock of news of the illness. They may find it easier to talk of their feelings about their son's sexuality with a counsellor than with the PWA himself. They may feel they have 'failed' as parents by raising a gay son, and so need help to see that a homosexual life style is non-pathological and 'normal'.

Such support may be offered, although explicit discussion may not be necessary since often parents have a tacit understanding of their gay son's life style.

Almost all families have many questions about the infection risks, illness, treatment and management of AIDS, which they may find difficult to ask the PWA himself. They may need reassurance about the care given by staff and friends, particularly if they live some distance from the PWA's home. They may ask about how they should behave, and need to be encouraged to make the PWA feel part of everyday family life and not try to overprotect. Parents and older siblings may find it very difficult to accept that the PWA is likely to die before them, and may search desperately for information on treatments to give hope of a cure; they can be helped to focus on the quality of life for the PWA being more important than longevity.

By mutual agreement a PWA may move back to the family home, or parents move in to help provide care. This may lead to problems of adjustment where the 'adult child' returns to being a dependant, and parents may need help in coping with the PWA's frustration and other strong emotions which can be evoked by such a situation.

After the death of a PWA, relatives can feel very isolated, particularly if they have no contact with the PWA's friends and are unable to discuss the death with their own friends. Group support is invaluable in helping families feel less alone, but where this is not possible or desired individual follow-up, even by telephone, can help families to adjust to the loss.

*Supporting friends*

Some PWAs feel closer to friends than to family. Friends can feel helpless or inadequate when someone has AIDS, and may not maintain contact, feeling they are intruding on intimate or family relationships. Sometimes friends reject a PWA because of their own fears of hospitals, illness and death. Occasionally gay friends may attempt to deny the implications of AIDS for their own lives by staying away from a friend with AIDS; others may have difficulty coping with feelings of guilt about remaining free from HIV infection if they have lost many of their friends through AIDS-related illness.

Friends can be helped by reassuring them that they have a role to play with someone with AIDS. Merely maintaining contact can help a PWA feel 'normal', so that just by 'being there' a friend is offering support, even if the diagnosis is never mentioned. Friends may wish to help with difficult situations or problems generated by AIDS, by offering practical help or by being the confidant with whom the PWA can discuss fears and worries. As with partners and families, friends have their own needs and feelings; for all significant others counselling can help by finding the balance between meeting the needs of the PWA and their own, an equilibrium which is difficult to find when painful and extreme emotions make a PWA and carers lose sight of how distress can most successfully be relieved.

## References

Murphy, P. M., Cramer, D. and Lillie, F. J. (1984) 'The relationship between curative factors perceived by patients in their psychotherapy and treatment outcome: An exploratory study' *British Journal of Medical Psychology*, **57**, pp. 187–192.

Whale, G. (1987) 'Distinctive contributions from clinical psychologists?' *Clinical Psychology Forum*, **8**, pp. 11–14.

# Chapter 6

# Counselling Those with AIDS Dementia

AGNES KOCSIS

It seems that the world is now threatened with dramatic change in the incidence of dementia in the young adult population. As the virus which causes AIDS manifests itself in an exponentially increasing number of individuals, we seem to be faced with patients who are suffering not only physical but also mental effects — or are we? It is currently accepted that a large number of AIDS patients have indications that the virus is in their central nervous system and a smaller proportion of them have clinically apparent dementia, unrelated to opportunistic infections, in the late stages of their illness. It is also the case that a small number of individuals present with neurological signs (e.g. motor weakness, loss of sensation, confusion) as the first symptom of HIV infection. However, at the time of writing, it is not at all clear when signs of central nervous system infection first become apparent in otherwise asymptomatic individuals. Nor is there certainty about the proportion of asymptomatic seropositives who might be suffering mild cognitive impairment.

This uncertainty in a sensitive and anxiety-provoking area of HIV symptomatology has several vital implications for the HIV counsellor. Primarily, seropositives as well as PWAs will be in need of information and reassurance. However, in addition to the opportunity for discussion, the counsellor may well be in the position of having to partake in a decision-making process which will influence clinical management. This is because patients themselves, or their intimate carers, may present with or describe symptoms of, say, slowness, tiredness, anxiety and confusion. The counsellor may then have to try to assess whether the symptoms are likely to be due to some organic process, or whether they are purely functional — a set of psychological responses, perhaps, to being seriously ill. The outcome of such decisions will lead to alternative interventions for the patient. The counsellor must therefore be alert to the various possibilities and must be well-informed. This chapter seeks to present some of the issues that must be considered and where possible to offer some approaches to the problems. It is divided into two parts the first giving the background theorising and facts as we know them; the second making practical suggestions for counselling with sketches of role-plays you might do to help think about the issues.

## PART I: BACKGROUND

### History of our knowledge of central nervous system involvement of HIV

Navia and Price in New York were the first to detail symptoms in their patients that pointed to the possibility of the virus directly affecting the brain (Navia and Price, 1986). The symptoms they reported as affecting AIDS patients fall into what they refer to as a triad of cognitive, motor and behavioural dysfunction which together they baptised the AIDS Dementia Complex. Cognitive symptoms related to four areas: memory, concentration, speed of thought, and confusion. Behavioural symptoms were either gross withdrawal and apathy or high agitation, hallucinations and confusion. Motor symptoms divided into weakness, unsteadiness, poor coordination and tremor.

Their assessment of dementia was at the time based on their informal, that is to say not objectively charted, observation of patients over time, together with results of the mental status examination and neurological examination. During the mental status examination the clinician will, for example, ask a patient to count backwards from 100 in jumps of 7 and in the neurological exam will ask him, for instance, to perform a variety of motor tasks such as rapidly touching fingers to thumb in sequence. Observation of difficulties in such tasks, as well as of general presentation of patients, thus led to questioning of whether HIV could be affecting the brain. There was initially some doubt as to whether this could be so, since PWAs often suffer from opportunistic infections which may themselves affect the brain. Was HIV having a *direct* effect — or was it only *indirectly* responsible? A great deal of evidence has since accumulated that the virus *does* directly invade the brain and other parts of the nervous system. Its presence in the central nervous system in PWAs is indicated by the facts that it is possible to culture HIV from cerebrospinal fluid and to isolate the virus from the brains of PWAs.

### How the virus can affect the brain

The virus is likely to be acting directly on the brain cells and is not simply present incidentally, since it is found in those cells present in the central nervous system which carry the CD-4 receptor. As discussed in Chapter 1, it seems that in order for an HIV virus to attach itself to a cell in the human body, the cell must carry this CD-4 molecule. The molecule is on the surface not only of cells in the cellular immune system, such as T-helper lymphocyte cells, but also on cells of the humoral immune system. Instances include the antibody producing B lymphocytes and another group of immunologically active cells called monocytes or macrophages. These bone-marrow derived macrophages are widely dispersed in the tissues of the body. However, they are also present in the central nervous system, as microglial cells. Microglial cells are one of the group of cells that make up the glial ('glue') cells of the brain. All brain cells are either neurons or glial cells. Neurons are the nerve cells themselves and appear to be the main cells involved in our thought processes; glia, which outnumber neurons by about 10:1, are their satellites. It is mainly the cells of macrophage or lymphocyte origin which are infected in the brain. However, a minority of other cells have also been shown to be infected, notably some oligodendro-cytes, which form the myelin sheath around axons and thus contribute to the speedy conduction of messages in the nerve network. This may be potentially relevant to our understanding of symptoms observed in AIDS dementia, such as psychomotor slowing, which may be due to demyelination − the deterioration of this myelin 'fast-conductor'.

### When and how the virus is active in the central nervous system

Little is known at the time of writing about the exact effects of the virus on the workings of the central nervous system. However, it seems possible that there are at least two distinct manifestations of central nervous system involvement which may have different bases. On the one hand it has been noted that at the time of seroconversion (when antibodies to HIV are first produced) patients may have a mononucleosis (glandular fever) type of illness with fever and malaise, sometimes accompanied by signs of central nervous system involvement such as headache, dizziness and confusion; these symptoms tend to disappear along with the other physical signs and individuals can feel well and alert for a long period subsequently. When people develop AIDS, however, some will experience slowing and overall problems in thinking and motor coordination which appear to persist. The latter set of symptoms are probably related to changes in brain cells, perhaps associated with demyelination in some areas, whereas the early changes may be due to a more general and transient immunological response.

Little is known, too, about the factors which might influence the rate of progression of central nervous system involvement. Clinicians, especially in the United States, have perceived that progression is usually slow and steady — but these reports are so far based only on observation and not on objective testing of cognitive functioning. The fact that there may be early and then again much later manifestations of central nervous system invasion as mentioned above, should not of course lead us to conclude that there is a steady progression from one to the other.

There are also quite frequent reports of late onset of clinically apparent cognitive deterioration with very rapid decline shortly before death. It has been suggested (Pinching and Parkin, 1987) that it is possible for severe opportunistic infection in PWAs to concurrently stimulate replication of virus in the brain through the immunological response of latently infected brain cells, thus leading to rapid progression of encephalopathy.

## Problems with assessing the direct impact of HIV on the brain

There are three kinds of problem with assessing the extent of HIV impact on the brain. The first concerns the complexities of assessing whether someone is cognitively impaired (thinking and performing less well than they should be or used to). The second is in deciding whether any apparent deterioration is due to damage to the brain (organic impairment) or to, say, anxiety (functional impairment). These two issues are discussed further below.

If you have succeeded in solving the first two problems, and conclude that a seropositive individual or a PWA is indeed suffering cognitive impairment due to organic causes, the third problem still remains, of determining whether, for that individual, it is the HIV virus which is actually to blame. For it is of course not at all the case that signs of cognitive impairment in seropositives or PWAs are always due to direct effects of HIV. This is because some of the opportunistic infections which take advantage of the immune system's weakened defences also themselves attack the brain. These may be infections caused by other viruses, usually the viruses which carry DNA in their genome. These include most commonly cytomegalovirus, but also the herpes viruses such as varicella-zoster and herpes simplex. Progressive multifocal leukoencephalopathy can also be caused by opportunistic infection by the JC papovavirus. Lymphomas can occur through opportunistic viral infection – the Epstein-Barr virus, for example, leads to the development of Burkitt-type lymphoma, and Kaposi's sarcoma is an opportunistic tumour probably caused by a viral pathogen (Weber, 1988). Cerebral toxoplasmosis, caused by a parasite, is also common. More rarely, bacterial infections can occur. In addition, patients sometimes suffer epileptic fits or vascular accidents such as haemorrhage.

Any of these infections could cause symptoms of confusion, headache, motor impairment, dizziness, memory loss and personality changes, however transient. Counsellors should be aware of the range of possible reasons for these presenting symptoms for they may well have the most contact with the patient and be in the best position to make a medical referral for investigations to be carried out. This could be crucial since the above infections are mainly responsive to treatment.

Finally, any infection may affect cognitive functioning. Anyone who has had a bout of 'flu knows that it is difficult if not impossible to work at full rate or as accurately as usual. In fact, investigators have shown that just having a cold can lower one's effectiveness by reducing hand–eye coordination, as can influenza by slowing reaction times (Smith *et al.*, 1986).

## The assessment of cognitive impairment

It is helpful for the HIV counsellor to be familiar with some of the commonly used testing procedures and the information we have gleaned from them, partly so that their own understanding of a patient's presentation can be enhanced and partly so that they can be informed – and in turn inform the patient – of investigations that may be available and in which the patient may be asked to participate.

The assessment of possible cognitive deterioration has not been considered to be so crucial from a practical point of view with, say, the elderly dementing. Pensioners are not usually in situations, for example, where they are handling dangerous machinery or performing complex tasks vital to the community. They are *expected*, perhaps exaggeratedly so, to be less capable than when young. The possibility of HIV-related cognitive deterioration, however, has something of the status of a hidden disease. This person is young and looks well – but could he be seropositive? Could he be dementing? Can he fly this plane?

Apart from the demands of the public and employers to know what the effects of HIV are likely to be on an individual's work skills, there are other important functions for assessment of cognitive functioning to fulfil. As far as clinical management goes, a judgement that a sero-positive individual has an affected central nervous system is currently likely to lead clinicians to prescribe a centrally acting drug (Zidovudine (AZT) is at present the most widely on trial). The evaluation of the effectiveness of this drug as far as the central nervous system goes also requires cognitive assessment. One would predict that if HIV affects the brain and Zidovudine prevents replication of the virus, cognitive functioning should also improve.

There are also questions to be answered about the overall *nature* of the virus' effect. One of the theoretical questions of interest is whether dementia in those with AIDS resembles one of the dementias we are familiar with. Is it, for example, more similar to Parkinsonian-type problems or to dementia of the Alzheimer's type? Does it resemble an ageing process or does it look like impairment resulting from insult to a particular part of the brain's neuronal network? Comparisons may be worthwhile in that we can then make some informed guesses about how the virus may be causing the damage to the brain. Additionally, such understanding could lead to hypotheses about the effectiveness of various drugs, including anti-psychotic agents, and about the kind of psychiatric manifestations we might be expecting to see.

Our present uncertainty about the extent, nature and natural history of central nervous system involvement is essentially due to the limitations of the methods currently available. Although, as discussed, we know the virus exists in the spinal fluid of some asymptomatic sero-positives and PWAs and we know retrospectively from post-mortem examination that there was virus in the brains of people who died of AIDS, these methods do not allow us to chart the *progress* of infection or to assess the actual *impact* on the individual's thinking, memory, concentrations, etc. Other methods, such as computerised tomography (CAT scans) and nuclear magnetic resonance imaging (NMR), produce images of the brain which, although potentially useful in showing areas of brain involvement and especially in detecting the presence of opportunistic infection such as toxoplasmosis, are insufficiently sensitive to allow us to glean the information we need. Clinicians — and indeed probably most people who know a patient well — can tell when dementia is gross. That is why it is called 'clinically apparent' dementia. But it is assumed that dementia is the tip of the iceberg. Subtle early signs of central nervous system involvement and hence the impending dementia need to be looked for with sensitive instruments.

The most effective method of charting invasion of the brain is probably to look at the effects on brain 'output' — i.e. thinking — directly. This is done by using neuropsychological tests — a range of tasks which have been developed as ways of testing the efficiency and power of an individual's thought processes. These all come under the heading of 'cognition'. Understanding and remembering what you read, learning your way about a new town, memorising a telephone number and doing the crossword are all typical examples of 'cognitive functioning'.

## Some points about neuropsychological tests

There is no one magic test which will allow you to diagnose AIDS-related cognitive impairment with certainty in a few minutes. This is not surprising given the complexity of the questions involved: 'What is intelligence?'; 'How do we think?'. When looking for impairment in thought processes we are looking for patterns: patterns which are similar in people at the same stage of disease or with the same signs of central nervous system involvement, such as viral particles in the spinal fluid; patterns within individuals which point to a particular kind of impairment or which show change over time. On any one reaction time test, a patient may be thinking of dinner, or not trying very hard. Over several tests one can get an average measure which gives a more accurate picture. Testing again in some months will give an indication of change.

Cognitive testing is also sometimes criticised on the grounds that individuals may not do well simply because they are under stress, or feeling miserable. This is true, though in most trials currently being carried out, patients are concurrently assessed for psychiatric symptomatology. Where this is done, it is possible to look at the effect on test performance of, say, merely being anxious, by correlating levels of anxiety in the whole group with the actual scores on the testing. From the overall correlation therefore, one can predict for a particular individual, given his anxiety, or lack of it, how he is likely to perform. His actual score can therefore be adjusted to take anxiety level into account and only a performance significantly worse than expected on this basis would give rise to concern.

### Results from neuropsychological testing

What has such testing told us? There are now several trials under way internationally, comparing the performance of PWAs in tests with that of asymptomatic seropositives and those without the virus. Early studies are not consistent in that they do not agree on the proportion within each of these groups who seem to show cognitive impairment. For example, one US study cited 87 per cent of their AIDS patients and 44 per cent of asymptomatic seropositives as showing cognitive deficits (Grant *et al.*, 1987). Our own research points to a much lower rate of impairment — certainly under 50 per cent of AIDS patients and not more than 15 per cent of seropositives. Evidence for these lower rates has also been found by other workers in the United States. The reason for the discrepancy is probably the criteria used for judging someone to be impaired — and also whether one takes account of anxiety levels as well as factors like how intelligent an individuals is. In our own study, for example, we found that there was a significant difference in anxiety levels between the seropositives (asymptomatics — AAPs — and those with persistent generalised lymphadenopathy — PGLs), the PWA group and the seronegatives (see Fig. 6.1). Understandably, amongst those with AIDS especially, there were more individuals experiencing moderate to severe anxiety.

It is very interesting to note also people's subjective perceptions of changes in themselves. The only two areas in which seropositives and PWAs differed significantly from controls was in their perception of deterioration in their own memory and concentration. This is shown in Figs 6.2 and 6.3. It is clear that the AIDS group and to a lesser extent the asymptomatics are concerned about memory and concentration. But does this indicate that they are experiencing HIV-related cognitive impairment?

The answer here is not simple. As far as concentration goes, their ratings of impairment were very significantly correlated with their *anxiety* scores but not with their impairment score on the neuropsychological tests. In other words there seemed to be no organic impairment, but anxiety could have been contributing to difficulties in concentration. However, subjective perception of *memory* impairment was correlated both with anxiety and with impairment scores overall.

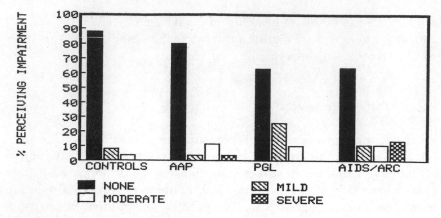

*Fig. 6.1*   Memory change by group

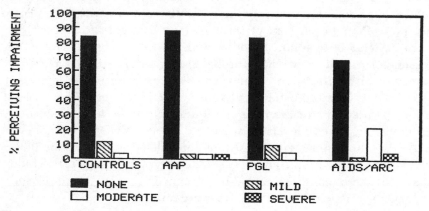

*Fig. 6.2*   Concentration change by group

Some people, therefore, are noticing real problems with their memory and this in itself might make them anxious. However, those people who reported only absent-mindedness − forgetting what they came into the room for or forgetting to register someone's name, for example − tended to be anxious only and not suffering objective impairment. More serious signs are probably concerned with difficulties in memorising when trying to learn complicated material.

If a patient reports concentration problems alone, therefore, he is perhaps only anxious. If he thinks he has memory problems this could be due to anxiety or else to real impairment. It depends somewhat on the type of problem he is experiencing.

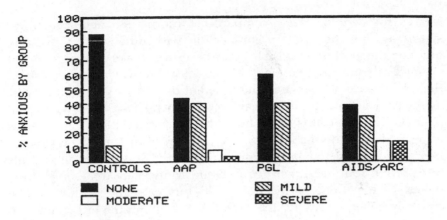

*Fig. 6.3*   Anxiety scores by group

Our own research shows that those PWAs who are clearly suffering from central nervous system effects do not generally become less accurate. They tend, however, to slow down in their responses. Tasks which involve attention and some physical activity simultaneously are difficult for them and the ability to perform more than one task at a time is lessened.

Various trials are now being conducted on the effectiveness of Zidovudine in reversing cognitive deterioration. No firm evidence has yet emerged. Our own evaluation indicates that some individuals on Zidovudine therapy appear to improve — at least for a time. The kinds of tests which show improvement are those which are measures of speed of varying kinds. Current work appears to indicate that the improvements are not always maintained, or not maintained in all patients. At present patients can only be advised that the drug is experimental and nothing can be guaranteed about its consequences. However there is a possibility that even the extent of decline referred to may be reversible and it can encourage patients to know this. Hopefully, as research moves forward, the likelihood of our being able to tackle this aspect of AIDS will also increase.

**Monitoring the patient**

Ideally, as a part of proper clinical management, all seropositives as well as PWAs should undergo cognitive testing when their diagnosis is known and then at six-monthly intervals, or with any shift in their clinical state. The advantage of such monitoring is that each patient acts as his own basis for comparison. Information about cognitive state may then be used in conjunction with other clinical signs to monitor the individual's state over time and make decisions – for example, about drug treatment. Moreover, as knowledge accrues about the significance of change in the different diagnostic groups it may be extremely valuable in future years to have such background data about patients. However, it is understood that in many settings this counsel of perfection cannot be followed for a variety of reasons. If no psychological testing is available on site, or if there is no time for all patients to be tested routinely, then requests for testing may come only at the behest of a patient or his doctor. In this case the testing can be clinically meaningful with the caveat that although the test results can be matched to an estimate of premorbid intelligence, there is less certainty in a given case that the patient is performing worse than he should be. So long as psychiatric aspects are taken into consideration, however, 'one-off' testing can be extremely valuable.

## PART II: PRACTICAL ISSUES IN DEALING WITH PATIENTS

### Should one discuss the possibility of dementia with patients?

The issue of possible cognitive impairment is unlikely to be relevant in pre-test or immediate post-test counselling. Issues to be dealt with in these sessions are covered in Chapters 3 and 4. However, as public awareness of possible AIDS dementia increases, patients may start to ask, 'Am I going to go senile?'. At this point, as with other sensitive issues in the counselling of HIV, it is most helpful to be direct and factual yet without giving more information than the patient is asking for. Thus, it is unnecessary to pour out details of how cognitive performance may be assessed or of the number of diseases which might cause cognitive impairment if the patient is just asking about the likelihood of experiencing problems. Again, as always, the giving of information as far as we know it must be done in the context of careful listening and openness to discussing the feelings underlying the question. Sometimes patients have experience of elderly relatives with Alzheimer's and are therefore particularly frightened by the possibility of senility. They may feel their identity threatened by their recent diagnosis – What does it mean to now be labelled HIV sero-positive? – Am I going to lose my mind as well as my body? Again, however, it is irrelevant and intrusive to pursue such lines of discussion unless the seropositive individual indicates that this issue is of particular concern.

In similar vein, the essential idea behind subsequent counselling is active listening and awareness from all the professionals involved. One PWA told me what a relief it had been when friends finally mentioned how slow and clumsy he had been recently and allowed him to talk about his fear of losing his mind instead of pretending to ignore his difficulties. In this case, none of his doctors had given him the opportunity to ask questions about it either. The professional counsellor or clinician may therefore be the only one who is willing to discuss the patient's fears about dementia and to give advice when the concerns are based on real decline as well as when they are the product of needless anxiety.

## Talking about it with the carers — lovers and friends

Counsellors, Buddies, Frontliners and other professional and voluntary workers may have to deal not only with the patient, but with his lover, friends and family. They may also need to ask questions and mention anxieties about the possibility of dementia even when they are not noticing any problems in the patient as yet. They need the same factual information and reassurance as the seropositive individual. If he is indeed suffering from memory and concentration difficulties, then the carers may need a considerable amount of advice and practical help as well as the opportunity to discuss their feelings. Some suggestions for counselling the carers are given below.

As a general point about 'whether or not to talk about it' it may be helpful to consider that while talking may provide enormous relief, it is not necessarily so for everyone; and for those who do indicate the need, the time and the listener must be appropriate. We do not discuss all aspects of our lives with everyone — for good reason. A patient may be able to talk about physical aspects of his health with some people and aspects of cognitive impairment with others. For some, professionals provide a cooler, less emotionally charged atmosphere which is reassuring. For others only intimates are experienced as being helpful rather than intrusive. Moreover, these preferences may change according to mood and state of health. The counsellor should always be willing to talk and to be frank — but it is rarely necessary to force the topic. If, for example, it is clear that a patient is regularly forgetting to take medication or is taking a double dose, a word with the carer to get an automatic pill-box may be more effective than confronting the patient.

### Distinguishing HIV-related cognitive impairment from psychiatric manifestations

What if the issue is suddenly brought up by a seropositive without any clinical symptoms some time after infection? For example, he may present with anxiety about deteriorating memory or difficulty with reading, following the script of television programmes or remembering appointments. The probability of a seropositive without symptoms having objective impairment is low. In this category he is not suffering from any opportunistic infection that might be affecting his thoughts. It is just possible that he is one of the small number who present with neurological complaints as a first symptom of HIV infection, or he is showing signs of an opportunistic brain infection. However, there are a number of other alternatives:

(1)   he is anxious;
(2)   he is depressed;
(3)   he has heard about AIDS dementia and is starting to imagine that his memory and concentration are getting worse;
(4)   any combination of the above.

How can one decide between these alternatives? There is, of course, no way of being absolutely certain. The important thing is to ask questions related to each alternative so that none is ignored. Then a decision can be made as to whether a referral is necessary or whether the counsellor and the patient can sort the difficulty out together. Here, then, is a short check-list of questions relating to the above alternatives. They are not comprehensive and can only act as indicators of the areas to be explored. Ongoing consultation and information exchange with professional colleagues expert in the various areas is obviously necessary.

#### A short check-list for possible neurological involvement

* Any weakness or numbness in arms or legs?
* Any sensory loss — diminution of sense of smell, taste or touch?
* Any tremor not caused by anxiety? For example, when reaching to put sugar in coffee, combing hair, writing?
* Recurrent or persistent headache not associated with stress?

- Dizziness unrelated to panic attacks?
- Unusual slowness, clumsiness when performing routine tasks?

Any positive findings would indicate that a referral for a neurological check-up would be appropriate.

### A short check-list for anxiety

Where memory and concentration problems are presented by the patient it is worth bearing in mind the findings reported above, i.e. that perception of problems in these two areas is highly correlated with anxiety although organic impairment is not ruled out.

- Do you feel tense and worried?
- When you have problems concentrating, what do you find yourself thinking about? Is it about your illness or other worries, or about how to escape from these worries?
- Can you give examples of your memory problems? Are they more than just episodes of absent-mindedness? Are you forgetting things you are actually trying to memorise more quickly than you used to?
- Do you wake early or have problems getting to sleep?
- Are you finding it difficult to eat or are you overeating compulsively?
- Do you find yourself more aware than usual of your bodily responses: e.g. whether your heart is racing or misses beats, whether your breathing feels uncomfortable, the amount you are sweating, pain in your chest, dryness in your mouth?
- Are you more aware than usual of how people are responding to you, questioning whether you are liked and successful?

Positive answers to any of these questions suggests anxiety, although one would normally expect to see several components together. Some individuals, however, are not aware of anxious feelings apart from their physical symptoms. As a standardised measure of anxiety it might be helpful to use the Spielberger State and Trait Inventory (STAIS and STAIT). Alternatively, the Hospital Anxiety and Depression Scale is a quick screen for both anxiety and depression. For ways of dealing with anxiety see Chapter 12 on anxiety and depression.

### A short check-list for depression

If you notice any difficulties with his speech or he reports slowing and appears lethargic, is constantly overwhelmingly sleepy for no good reason or is very confused, he should be referred for cognitive assessment. But you should also enquire about depression.

- Has his level of enjoyment in everyday activities decreased?
- Does he feel himself to be less likeable and successful than he used to?
- Is he especially sensitive to people's remarks about him?
- Does he feel guilt about present or past behaviour and think about this a great deal?
- Has he stopped looking forward to anything?
- Does he consider suicide? If so, has he formed a plan and does he have the means?

If the answer to any of these questions is positive then it might be helpful to use a standardised psychiatric questionnaire to assess the extent to which this person might be depressed and might require medication as well as counselling. The Beck Depression Inventory is commonly used.

### A short check-list for AD self-observers

It is possible that, having heard of the AIDS dementia, he has been observing himself. It is surprising how many errors of memory and absent-mindedness we can find in ourselves if we start counting! Therefore check on the following:

- Is there any special reason why these things might be worrying you? Have you perhaps wondered whether being seropositive is going to affect things like your memory?
- Are you worrying about your health overall? Does your lack of concentration relate to worrying?

If none of the above questions in any of the check-lists is relevant, then either cognitive testing should be carried out for the first time or the data from ongoing testing should be examined.

For a PWA the above alternatives still need to be taken into consideration, since it is likely that less than half will have objective impairment. Nevertheless, the probability is higher and while counselling may be most valuable in reducing difficulties and anxieties, cognitive monitoring as an adjunct is always advisable.

No mention has been made of patients presenting with psychotic symptoms — paranoia, mania, violent uncharacteristic aggressive outbursts, hallucinations and delusions. There is some evidence that some of these symptoms may occasionally occur in PWAs, possibly related to organic brain changes. If a patient appears to be behaving very oddly and especially if he is very unwilling or unable to discuss possible reasons, psychiatric referral is essential.

## Suggested workshop exercise

In counselling it is often helpful to role-play with colleagues to help prepare oneself for the kind of issues which may arise. The advantage of role-plays is that often one is able to experience some of the feelings which go along with the real-life situation in a safe environment when one can take time to think and discuss. It helps to bridge that enormous gap between having an idea of what to do in theory and having to actually do it in practice. To help with setting the scene for role-plays, or at least thinking through some examples, some sketches are presented below which have been used by Andrew MacCallum and the author. They are meant to be springboards for thought and the comments below them are just suggestions based on our own experience. These sketches can be given to small groups and pairs asked to act out what might go on in the interaction. In this way ideas can be pooled.

(1) Bob is 25 and has been living with Vincent for four years. Vincent, a few years older, has AIDS. Over the last four months he has become slow, clumsy, withdrawn and forgetful and can do very little for himself. Bob feels that Vincent is quite unlike his old self and finds it hard to know how to deal with him. Vincent's doctor says there are no signs of the dementia being due to opportunistic infection. Bob feels very guilty because some days he wishes Vincent would just die. He also finds it difficult to look after him as he has a demanding job and during work finds himself worrying about how Vincent is getting on. Bob has finally been persuaded to come and see you. How would you counsel him?

If Vincent has begun to show clinically apparent signs of AIDS dementia he is not, given our current inability to treat, likely to live for much longer than a year. Thus Bob may not have much longer with him. We know that, paradoxically, bereavement is easier to bear where there has been a good relationship with little ambivalence. At the moment, when Vincent dies, Bob is set to feel guilty that he did not do enough for him and did not make the most of their time together. He therefore needs to be able to accommodate the negative feelings, probably by talking and perhaps some problem solving. How necessary is it to him and to Vincent that he should spend all possible time with him? How can he prioritise his time so as to fit in with Vincent's actual rather than imagined wishes? Sometimes it may be helpful to go over the history of the relationship, remembering the good times so as to help make sense of the effort that Bob is currently putting in.

Where death is imminently anticipated, feelings of loss may precede actual death. Where personality changes are involved *actual* loss may also start before death. This experience needs to be acknowledged. However, in addition to listening to the feelings it may also be helpful to work with the carer on finding an alternative framework for the new relationship. For example, if a patient is not as lucid as he was, it does not necessarily mean that it is impossible to 'get through'. Part of the sense of loss may arise from the fact that the partner no longer offers the *same* pleasures and 'rewards' as before. Sex may not be practicable, but touch and massage will still usually be pleasurable. The person may be finding it hard to read, but music can be enjoyed together. Long talking sessions may be tiring, but short ones are not ruled out.

There are two essentials to find out from Bob during the session:

(a) *Communication*    Do they talk about the symptoms of HIV together and the way AIDS is affecting their relationship? Our research on the effects on intimate carers indicates that in relationships where there is communication about these issues the carers are less anxious and depressed overall. Sometimes of course anxiety makes it difficult to talk, partly because the problems lose all perspective. Communication is not ruled out by slowing or withdrawal in the patient, but again Bob might find it helpful to question his own expectations from such communication as well as the style of conducting the conversation. Lovers may be in the habit of conducting quite complex protracted discussions about their relationship and things that matter to them. This may no longer be possible where one of them is finding it hard to concentrate and is more easily confused and therefore frustrated. It can therefore be helpful to rehearse simple, straightforward messages, 'I love you, I'm worried about you. Would you like me to spend more time with you or can you manage alone?', and so on.

(b) *Social support*    Who else is around to be with Vincent during the day? What social support is, or might be, available if mobilised? Voluntary agencies can be very helpful in providing a supportive network; friends, too, though sometimes people have to be prompted to remember actually to ask friends and not just wait.

Finally, it seems that Bob has come to see a counsellor with some reluctance. Maybe, as a work-orientated individual with high standards for himself, he sees counselling as an admission of weakness which

would suggest he cannot deal with Vincent's needs. It might be helpful to remind him of something we were told by a carer whose lover
died a few years ago. He said: 'At no time during the year between his
diagnosis and death, nor indeed in the long months before his diagnosis, did I ever receive any advice, counselling or support. I regret
this not so much because of the benefit I would have got, but more
because of the help I might have been able to give my lover. Looking
back I feel I should have gone out and looked for help but at the time I
was just overwhelmed by the situation.' The carer who asks for help
when necessary will in turn be able to help his lover.

(2)   Hal is a writer. He is HIV positive. Friends who know he is HIV positive have
noticed that he forgets appointments with them or turns up very late with some
unbelievable excuse. Once at a dinner party they noticed that he took medication
twice, forgetting that he had already taken it. When driving a friend to his home he
took the wrong turning along a very familiar route, and his flat was full of unposted
letters and manuscripts. One of these friends rings you for advice. Would you advise
him to confront Hal with these bouts of apparent absent-mindedness, and how would
you explain what was happening to him?

Our research has shown that being absent-minded is in itself not a
sign of cognitive impairment. Absent-mindedness is more of a personality trait: any increases in its incidence are far more likely to be a
result of anxiety. Any signs of absent-mindedness therefore need to be
taken in the context of the individual's overall personality. Perhaps
Hal was always like that and his friends had overlooked it — perhaps
because of how writers are expected to behave. What seems normal in
a writer may look suspicious in a seropositive if one is on the lookout.
  If there is an actual change, however, it is possible that Hal is feeling
under stress. It would therefore be much more appropriate for friends
to explore this possibility than to raise his anxiety by suggesting that
he might be heading towards dementia.

(3)   Brian has been in hospital for two months. His condition has deteriorated. He is
now bed-fast, can hardly talk and is sometimes incontinent. He now also needs to be
fed. Although when he was well he was very popular, he is now a strain to be with.
The staff on the ward are distressed that Brian's friends are not visiting more. They
mention this to you when you are visiting the ward. What suggestions would you
advise them to make to these friends?

To some extent the comments made on the first example, relating to
lover rather than friend, also apply here. The aim is to make sure
expectations are realistic and to try to make interaction as rewarding

as possible within the situation. This usually means rewarding in a different way from before. When friends visit hospital they may feel that they should talk with the patient. Therefore if they cannot do so, they feel useless and frustrated. They can however be given other roles. For example, feeding the patient can be comforting for both. So can sitting quietly together, perhaps with the television on in the background or some music. It is very helpful if staff convey these suggestions explicitly and show understanding of the visitors' difficulties. Friends can be encouraged to feel that it is enough, and indeed the most sensible, to pop in for just a few minutes on a regular basis. In our experience it is also very helpful if staff can take a minute to chat to friends. This often makes problems and unrealistic expectations apparent. They can be discussed, and frequently solved with a simple practical suggestion.

> (4)   Robin has just been diagnosed as having AIDS. Apart from the fear of dying he is fearful of becoming demented. He is contemplating suicide because he saw his grandfather go senile and he would rather die than be like that. What would you say to him?

It is useful here to explore, to acknowledge and to inform. All three activities are crucial, as in all aspects of HIV and AIDS counselling. Feelings and facts both need to be considered. Exploration of Robin's associations with dementia will allow the counsellor to understand Robin's personal view. Acknowledgment of the fears will allow him to feel that he is understood. However, he can be reminded of the fact that the probability of his escaping without dementia is high. Moreover, mild forgetfulness, distractibility or slowness can, with planning, be compensated for and can restore the all-important sense of control. One of our patients early on started keeping a diary, 'to get into the habit — in case I do become forgetful'. It is possible to arrange one's environment so that interruptions are few, to choose to work or read when less tired, to break up tasks into smaller elements, to ask to be reminded, to rely on mechanical aids — calculators, watch alarms, tape-recorders, automatic pill boxes. The essential message to convey is that control is possible and that adjustments, if necessary, may not be so hard to make. Sometimes individuals will focus their anxieties on one aspect of the illness or symptomatology to the point of rumination, and fear of dementia may be one of these. If this kind of rumination is apparent, it may be wise to consider the overall pattern of the patient's life. Is there too much time to think and too little distracting, pleasurable activity, for example? In that case, focusing on improving the quality of his life overall may immediately banish ruminations about future dementia.

## Two conclusions

We have to live with uncertainty in this, as in many other aspects of our understanding about the virus. These points, however, are certain:

- Some people with AIDS who do not have clinically apparent dementia nevertheless do show some memory decrement and slowed reaction times on some neuropsychological tests, especially where attention and motor performance are both needed together. However, currently it is only the minority of people with AIDS who suffer from clinically apparent dementia. If you die from AIDS you are most likely *not* to experience gross confusion, muteness, withdrawal or motor effects.

- Whether or not someone is experiencing difficulty through organic impairment, the counsellor's main task is to support and look for ways of dealing with the problems that arise. Even if anxiety and low mood are not the primary reasons for a person's cognitive difficulties, he will be immeasurably assisted in maintaining self-respect and a sense of control by being reminded of what he can do for himself to mitigate the everyday effects.

## References

Grant, I., Atkinson, J.H., Hesselink, J.R., Kennedy, C.J., Richman, D.D., Spector, S.A., and McCutchan, J.A. (1987) 'Evidence for central nervous system involvement in the Acquired Immune Deficiency Syndrome (AIDS) and other human immunodeficiency virus (HIV) infections.' *Annals of Internal Medicine*, **107**, 828–836.

Navia, B.A., and Price, R.W. (1986) 'Central and peripheral nervous system complications of AIDS' In A.J. Pinching (Ed), *AIDS and HIV Infection. Clinics in Immunology and Allergy*, **6**(3) 543–558.

Pinching, A.J., and Parkin, J.M. (1987) 'Clinical snippets' **1** 247–260. In M.S. Gottlieb *et al.* (Ed), *Current Topics in AIDS* Chichester: John Wiley and Sons Ltd.

Smith, A.P., Tyrrell, D.A.J., Coyle, K., and Willman, J.S. (1986) Selective effects of minor Illnesses on human performance. *Br. J Psychol*, **78**, 183–88.

Weber, J., (1988) 'The biology of HIV' in L. Paine (Ed), *AIDS: Psychiatric and Psychosocial Perspectives*. London: Croom Helm.

# Chapter 7

# The Counselling of HIV Antibody Positive Haemophiliacs

PETER JONES MD FRCP DCH

The full extent of HIV infection in the haemophilic population of industrialised countries only became apparent in 1985. In that year it became clear that the majority of people treated with multidonor clotting factor VIII concentrates within the preceding five years had been infected with the AIDS-related virus. Paradoxically, most people with haemophilia living in developing countries without recourse to modern therapy had escaped this iatrogenic infection. What was not known in 1985, and is only now becoming clearer, was the likely extent of overt disease in those testing positive for HIV antibody. As time into the epidemic passes early optimism that the majority of those infected would remain well has had to be tempered. The increasingly gloomy prognosis for anyone infected has meant that the foundation of helpful counselling, reliant as it is on factual information, has shifted. Most people can accept and adapt to bad news quickly and remarkably well, but failure to come to terms with adversity increases with uncertainty. Difficulties in being able to give a realistic prognosis, ill-founded arguments about casual spread, and disagreements about testing and management within the health care professions made public by unprecedented media hyperbole, add to that uncertainty. In consequence, effective counselling of individuals, their partners and their families has to be continually adapted to the changing picture of the epidemic.

In this respect infected people with haemophilia are no different from others carrying the virus. In other respects there are differences, often profound, which should be recognised if haemophilic families are to be given adequate help. Most differences hinge on the underlying coagulation disorder but some, at the present stage of the epidemic, reflect feelings about the life styles of the other groups of people primarily involved.

In order to understand why the counselling of people with haemophilia is different from the counselling of others, it is necessary to understand the profound effect that the clotting disorder alone can have on individual and family health.

## The background of haemophilia

Haemophilia is an inherited disorder of blood coagulation. The genetic defect is present on one of the X chromosomes and it is this sex-linked recessive mode of inheritance that results in females (XX) being carriers, and males (XY) having haemophilia. There is thus an immediate analogy to HIV infection, which may be carried unknowingly in the cells of people who are otherwise healthy, and who look well.

Seventy per cent of haemophiliacs have a family history of the disorder but in 30 per cent it arises *de novo*, the most celebrated example of this being Queen Victoria who passed the defective gene to her daughters Alice and Beatrice, who were carriers like her, and to her son Leopold who had severe haemophilia. Like other carriers of genetic disease Victoria suffered the guilt of knowing that some of her descendants, notably those in the Russian and Spanish royal families, had been burdened by a defect passed on to them directly from herself. At least she was spared the remorse of many of today's carrier mothers who feel that their haemophilic sons also become infected with HIV as a direct result of their actions in giving them treatment for their bleeding episodes.

Clinically haemophilia presents as recurrent bleeds into joints and muscles. These closed bleeds, which account for over 95 per cent of all bleeding episodes, continue until the pressure exerted by the tissues surrounding the bleeding point equals the pressure of escaping blood. This means that joints become swollen, tense and exquisitely painful. Eventually the bleed stops and the blood within the joint is slowly reabsorbed, iron and other breakdown products passing into the synovial membrane which responds to the irritation by becoming hypertrophic. The function of the healthy synovium is to secrete an oily fluid into the major joints of the body, helping to provide friction-free movement. As with all secretory tissue this membrane is richly endowed with blood vessels and it is these that rupture and haemorrhage. Hypertrophic disruption of the membrane not only increases the likelihood of repeated bleeds, but also prevents secretion of synovial fluid, and friction-free movement is lost. Thus the long-term sequela of the underlying disorder of coagulation is a chronic, painful arthropathy.

The fact that the great majority of bleeds in haemophilia are internal is of fundamental importance when assessing the risk of spread of a blood-borne disease like HIV infection. Contrary to popular belief, haemophiliacs do *not* bleed uncontrollably from scratches, small cuts or pin-pricks; the body's protective mechanisms for these insults are intact. Nor do they bleed externally any more than other people, nose bleeds or blood in the urine being the most usual manifestations. The chances of contamination of the environment and therefore of other people from someone with haemophilia are therefore negligible.

Frequency of bleeding varies with age, being commoner in childhood and adolescence. On average the severely affected haemophiliac has 35 spontaneous bleeding episodes a year. Most of these are recognised within a few minutes of starting, the patient experiencing an 'aura' of unease in the joint. Treatment at this time aborts the bleed and allows an immediate return to normal activity.

Because early treatment prevents disability and because it must be given before the appearance of any physical signs, the foundation of modern haemophilia therapy is one of trust between doctor and patient, and the patient's family. In the early days of the epidemic, AIDS had a profound effect on that trust, and a great deal of time and repetitive counselling have been needed to restore rapport with the families.

There are two types of haemophilia, haemophilia A and haemophilia B. Haemophilia B is five times less common than A, and in Britain is also known as Christmas disease after the first patient to be found affected. In haemophilia A the biological activity of the clotting protein factor VIII is absent or reduced. In haemophilia B factor IX is affected. Treatment of both conditions is usually relatively straightforward, the defect being corrected by injection of the relevant factor into a vein.

**Treatment as the source of infection**

The source material for both factor VIII and factor IX is human blood. In the 1950s and 1960s haemophiliacs needing treatment had to be admitted to hospital to have their factor VIII or IX dripped into them in the form of whole fresh blood or plasma which had been frozen shortly after donation and thawed just before use. The materials had to be freshly prepared because the factors have a short life at body temperature, half the administered dose disappearing within 12 hours. The logistics of therapy were therefore difficult and patients missed much of their education and subsequently their employment prospects because they were in hospital so often. Their alternative was not to treat the majority of bleeds, but inevitably this led to severe crippling within a few years. As a result many of the older generation of haemophiliacs were already disadvantaged, both socially and physically, before the advent of AIDS.

In the 1960s it became possible to separate factor VIII from most other plasma components with ease. The resultant material, cryoprecipitate, was of small volume and could be given by syringe or fast-running drip, and bleeds could be treated without having to admit patients to hospital. Unfortunately cryoprecipitate has to be stored in a deep-frozen state in order to preserve its factor VIII content and once thawed several packs have to be pooled together to make up the correct dose. The answer to this problem lay in freeze drying, and the era of commercially viable concentrate production began.

Using plasma, or cryoprecipitate derived from it as source material, factor VIII and factor IX are fractionated out into highly concentrated, low volume doses. Freeze drying stabilises each dose in a single vial which can then be stored at room temperature and mixed with sterile water to reconstitute biologically active material.

In the 1970s the ease of storage, preparation and use of concentrate revolutionised haemophilia care. Patients (or their parents) were taught how to treat themselves at home and the bonds which had previously tied families to hospitals were severed. Haemophiliacs on home therapy with factor VIII or IX were similar to diabetics on self-administered insulin and, like diabetics, some were soon using their injections to *prevent* bleeding episodes, a form of management called prophylaxis. This, and the early treatment of bleeds before any significant damage had occurred, resulted in the normal physical and social growth of affected children. The incidence of severe arthritis declined and haemophiliacs began to compete as equals with their non-affected peers at school and work, and in many sports.

In order to achieve this remarkable advance in medical care and improved quality of life, the blood plasma of many donors was required. Factor VIII in particular is a labile protein, each step in fractionation lowering the yield of biologically active material in the end product. Therefore, unlike single-donor cryoprecipitate which, when pooled, might expose the adult patients to 10 or 15 donations, the concentrates required multiple donations, and a prerequisite of the development of the fractionation plants was the supply of large volumes of source material, up to 30,000 donations fuelling one run of concentrate production. Volunteer donor systems, like that serving the United Kingdom, could not compete with the commercial sector which could draw on the plasma of paid donors chiefly living in the United States, and in

1973 the importation of factor VIII concentrates into the UK was approved by government.

Exposure to multi-donor concentrates must increase the risk of disease transmission. It soon became clear that viruses could survive both fractionation and freeze drying, as the incidence of hepatitis B and hepatitis non A non B (NANB) in the haemophilic population rose. Vaccination against hepatitis B now protects recipients of material which, although contaminated, has escaped both donor surveillance and stringent laboratory testing of individual donations. Specific tests do not yet exist for the viruses of NANB and surrogate testing by liver function test on donor blood is only partially successful in the elimination of risk. But although the price of such treatment may be chronic liver disease, the balance is still tipped very much in the haemophiliac's favour. Prior to the modern era of therapy afforded by concentrates early disability and premature death were commonplace, and before HIV infection the great majority of those with severe haemophilia could expect to live a good quality life of normal longevity.

**Specific problems relating to HIV positive haemophiliacs**

To date the majority of those infected with HIV have been either sexually active adults or the children born to infected mothers. In contrast those infected as a result of contaminated blood or blood product transfusions may be of any age, in the UK the highest prevalence of infection being in adolescence (Table 7.1; UK Haemophilia Centre Directors, 1986). This has meant that counselling has had to be tailored to age and to the wishes of parents, as well as to the circumstances and understanding of older patients and their partners. Because infected haemophilic youngsters appear to face a bleak future it is not surprising that many parents have not wanted to burden them with an early diagnosis. However, the advent of anti-viral therapy, and the use of regular prophylactic intravenous gammaglobulin will result in having to arm children with knowledge of their infection earlier than most of us would perhaps like. But whether or not secrecy is preserved, those caring for young people must be alert to the strengths and weaknesses of the family as well as to the needs of the infected children. Above all else this means time: time spent just listening, time spent answering questions, time spent sorting out the vagaries of childhood illnesses and fads from the more sinister manifestations of AIDS-related disease, time spent in homes as well as hospitals and, increasingly, time involving family doctors and their staff.

**Table 7.1**  Percentages of HIV antibody positivity by age in a cohort of 1268 patients with severe haemophilia A

| AGE | INFECTED | AGE | INFECTED |
|---|---|---|---|
| under 5 years | 12% | 30−39 | 66% |
| 5−9 | 35% | 40−49 | 63% |
| 10−14 | 68% | 50−59 | 51% |
| 15−19 | 65% | 60−69 | 33% |
| 20−29 | 68% | 70 and over | 20% |

Overall 59 per cent of those with severe haemophilia were infected.
Adapted from: UK Haemophilia Centre Directors (1986).

Most Haemophilia Centres adopted an open-door policy for their families before the HIV epidemic. Haemophiliacs could phone or call in for immediate help with bleeds or other problems at any time. This service had to be hospital-based because this was where the therapeutic materials for haemophilia were stored and dispensed, prescription often requiring laboratory investigation and guidance. However, the treatment of acute episodes in hospital is only one facet of a haemophiliac's life, and as a result many Haemophilia Centres try to bring together all the facets by providing comprehensive care. With the active participation of doctors, dentists, nurses, physiotherapists, social workers and members of other professional groups and the lay Haemophilia Society, the aim of this approach is to *anticipate* and hopefully solve problems relating to subjects as diverse as joint replacement surgery, bullying at school, careers guidance and genetic counselling. This multidisciplinary approach has served the families well, and has been suggested as the template for the care of others with AIDS in the community (Jones, 1987). One of the great strengths of this approach is that the core team with direct responsibility for patient care remains the same and whatever the circumstances there is always a familiar face for the patient and his family to respond to. This is particularly important when admission to hospital becomes necessary, especially if the patient is already confused or in early dementia. The worst place for anybody with AIDS-related disease to be nursed is in isolation in a small white room in an unfamiliar hospital by staff he does not already know and without immediate access to a telephone so that he can talk to his family or friends at any time.

A shortcoming of the haemophilia model, partly because of the bias to hospital care and partly because of the rarity of the disorder, has been the lack of involvement of most general practitioners. With HIV infection this is beginning to change — a welcome advance, given the crucial and pivotal role the family doctor will have in the management of the epidemic as it spreads from the high risk groups into the general community.

It is unfortunate that the pattern of the AIDS epidemic in the West has had such a profound influence on our response. The close link between AIDS, male homosexuality and intravenous drug abuse has led naturally to the disease becoming the prerogative of the sexually transmitted disease and drug addiction units. The strict confidentiality that has to operate in these clinics, coupled with the prejudice felt, and reacted to, by these minority groups, has tended to remove AIDS from the remit of many doctors and to reduce the effectiveness of health education within the community. It has also resulted in the isolation of infected individuals, sometimes unable to confide in their families about their sexuality, or in those most equipped to help them. Infected people living in large cities may have recourse to one of the voluntary organisations or to local hospital staff used to coping with the problems of HIV infection; those in other areas often suffer in silence. For them AIDS is a sad, lonely and secret disease.

These attitudes colour the lives and thus the counselling of haemophiliacs and their families. Those living in small communities may not want their family doctor, previously trusted with their medical record, to be aware of their infection in case that record is seen and commented on by someone else working in the surgery. Young men may not disclose their haemophilia to girlfriends or to employers because of public awareness of the association between haemophilia and AIDS. Parents are wary in enlisting the help of school teachers to keep an eye on infected children who may be experiencing difficulties in learning or behaviour. Even uninfected, HIV antibody negative children suffer because it is difficult to reveal their status without implying that other children are positive.

## Anticipating some of the problems

Although counselling or social work intervention may be needed at any time the stress of HIV infection or AIDS increases at certain stages in the life of the haemophiliac. Anticipating these stages and gently guiding people before the associated problems arise helps them to cope more effectively.

## The schoolboy

In our experience it is very rare for younger boys to be told by their parents about their HIV infection. However, because both school teachers and peers know about their haemophilia, assumptions may be made and the child harmed by segregation or bullying. Much of this is readily preventable and parents should be counselled to consult their child's Haemophilia Centre doctor immediately a problem they cannot deal with themselves arises. Among the difficulties which may present in school as a result of HIV infection are delayed cognitive development and failure to thrive; an increasing number of children are failing to grow normally. As immune competence fails in these children live vaccines are contra-indicated, and prophylactic immuno-globulin, given either intravenously in order to prevent infections in general or as specific immune globulin, may be needed. Other difficulties which are more easily resolved by talking to and reassuring staff have been fear of casual contact, and concern about sports and trips abroad. Bullying has affected some children but most haemo-philic boys are remarkably robust and taunts of 'Aidsy' are met with the physical retaliation they deserve!

## Adolescence

Boys maturing to be at ease with their bodies, their sexuality and their relationships with other people in the context of their haemophilia now have the additional burden imposed by the threat of AIDS. Abrupt or insensitive counselling of young men who are beginning to 'feel different' from their peers because of their inherited disorder adds to their alienation. It can be avoided by the gradual establish-ment of trust afforded by seeing each boy informally and in privacy on several occasions without parents or siblings, and by careful physical examination without the paraphernalia of gloves or other protective clothing. This both demonstrates his normality and helps to reassure him that his doctor is not frightened by the infection.

Additional reassurance should come from talk about planning for a future career. HIV infection does not preclude adolescents from taking competitive exams and entering higher education or long-term em-ployment. At the present stage of our knowledge it is not possible to suggest individual prognoses and the introduction of anti-viral agents may well halt or at least slow down the progression of the disease. Above all, it is very important that hope is kept alive and that the youngster's life is allowed to proceed as normally as possible.

We have always counselled haemophilic adolescents about the inheritance of their disorder so that they and their future wives can make up their own minds about starting a family. This counselling has included advice about contraception and informal and free access to condoms. AIDS has meant that this help has had to be extended to encompass 'safe sex', a term of ominous significance which intimidates youngsters not yet aware of the joys of 'ordinary' sex. We do not yet know what effect the knowledge that they may infect girlfriends or wives and their babies is going to have on the long-term psychological and social health of haemophiliacs. Our limited experience is that youngsters seem to cope remarkably well with the news, at least in the short term. Some have decided to marry and have children despite long, detailed and repeated explanations of risk from staff often more worried about the future for their patients than the patients are themselves.

One rather worrying aspect of these decisions, which could be interpreted as a form of denial, is that the young couple may become isolated from parents opposed to the marriage. This is especially tragic in extended families with a long history of haemophilia and in which several relatives are infected with HIV, because the disruption caused adds to the uncertainty of the disease. It also creates additional work for the Haemophilia Centre team, who may have to assume responsibility for the follow-up and treatment of the wives and children of their original patient.

### The adult

Infected haemophiliacs who were already married at the start of the epidemic have had to work their way through a very frightening and often bewildering series of questions and doubts. Had they already infected their wives? Were the children safe? What were the chances of spread of infection in the future, and were these increased by continuing treatment for their haemophilia? How would knowledge of HIV infection affect employment? Could they still get insurance cover and plan for the future stability of the family and the family home?

These and many other questions relating to the health and financial security of the family are often posed by men feeling the remorse of 'having let the wife and children down' by exposing them both to infection and to an uncertain future. This guilt should be recognised early and talked over openly in counselling because it can lead to increasing isolation of the patient within his own family. Typically an initial reaction is to withdraw from having sexual intercourse, and to be fearful of handling young children. Repeated reassurance is needed, and is helped by seeing the whole family together in a relaxed and informal atmosphere, reserving more formal counselling sessions for husband and wife alone.

Despite the reassurance afforded by government statements on security of employment for infected people, knowledge of HIV infection presents a very real threat to some jobs. The problem arises most frequently in jobs involving contact with the general public, caterers, publicans, teachers and health care workers perceiving especial difficulty. Whilst the public remain unconvinced of the absence of casual spread of AIDS their preference may be to drink in the pub not owned or run by a severely affected haemophiliac. This, of course, provides another reason to conceal the underlying disorder and, yet again, isolates the individual from his community.

## Everyday health and activities

As a result of their chronic arthritic pain most severely affected haemophiliacs have relatively easy access to analgesic drugs. Some have become reliant on alcohol or hypnotics in order to ease this pain, particularly at night. Still others react to their stress by resorting to heavy smoking. In the context of HIV infection two factors are important here. Firstly, the addition of stress imposed by the knowledge of HIV positivity can result in further reliance on drugs and secondly, there is general agreement that most, if not all, of these substances taken in excess may be co-factors in helping to tip antibody positive people into the overt disease of ARC or AIDS.

In common with the counselling given to other groups about life style, haemophiliacs should be encouraged to lead healthy and active lives. Whilst advice about good diet, plenty of exercise, and sound sleep might appeal to the younger generations this is easier said than done for older people. In particular, families already suffering financial hardship because of loss of work simply cannot afford the recommended high protein diets unless they are lucky enough to obtain state assistance. Voluntary organisations like the Haemophilia Society are of immense importance in helping to cope with this aspect of HIV infection, as indeed they are in helping with many other aspects of individual and family support. Group, behavioural and relaxation therapy have a part to play but sometimes the depression commonly associated with HIV becomes so profound that only medication can help and it is important that anti-depressant therapy is considered early in the course of the disease.

**Fear of death**

Some of the most frequent questions asked by infected people relate to
the nature of death from AIDS. One of the effects of all the publicity,
and of the secrecy surrounding the disease, appears to be a perception
by some patients that HIV-related death is in some way horribly
different from death from other causes. Patients express their fears by
asking if they will 'look different' or 'go mad'. They are curious to
know what happens at and immediately after death. Will their relatives be allowed in the room and be able to touch and hold them?
Does there have to be an autopsy and a public inquest with all the
resultant publicity and harassment of widow and other relatives? Will
they have to be cremated?

The answers are, of course, that death from AIDS is as quiet and
dignified as any non-accidental death, that patients look no different,
that they will not be left alone to die and that they can be held and
comforted by their relatives, that they can be buried and that there is
no need for autopsy or inquest in the normal course of events. The
only difference from the majority of deaths is that the body is sealed in
a cadaver bag soon after the event (as with other infectious diseases
like hepatitis B) so that the family must take their leave of their
relative at the bedside, and will not be able to view him later.

The concern about 'going mad' is likely to increase as knowledge
about the high incidence of dementia in AIDS becomes more widespread. People need to be reassured that AIDS encephalopathy and
dementia usually result in a quiet decline in mental facilities rather
than in disruption or violence. However, it is the neurological and
psychiatric manifestations of AIDS that will present the major difficulties in future health and social care. Incontinence, occasional aber-
rant behaviour which requires sedation, and an increasing need for
constant supervision mean that many families will be unable to cope
with relatives dying at home.

Finally, patients need to be reassured that strenuous efforts at resuscitation will not be undertaken if death within a few weeks seems
inevitable.

**Bereavement counselling**

The care of the haemophilic family does not cease on the death of the
index patient. Firstly, the hereditary nature of haemophilia dictates
long-term follow-up of obligatory or putative carriers. Secondly, most

(but not all) families will be dependent on help from Haemophilia Centre staff for at least the first six months of bereavement.

The intricacies of the UK Social Security system mean that very detailed counselling and practical help should be available for widows and other dependants. Benefits previously available to the patient, and therefore enjoyed by his family, will be withdrawn. As these often include provision both of transport and of a telephone, remaining members of the family who cannot afford their replacement may be isolated at just the time they need to communicate with and seek the solace of others.

We have found informal group meetings of widows, and occasionally of widowers or bereaved fathers, especially helpful. This group, like one run for the mothers of infected children, meets regularly with a social worker to compare experiences and provide individual comfort. Although most meetings take place in the evening in the hospital, the occasional foray into the nearest wine bar or pizzeria is not unheard of. It is salutary to find that it is the sense of humour and friendship of those who have lost relatives because of contamination of their treatment that helps support the staff who prescribed it.

## The staff

Staff health is of paramount importance if patients and their families are to be helped. Members of staff in Haemophilia Centres will have known their patients for many years, and may have been present at the births and marriages of people now dying of AIDS. In this context, which is unique in the epidemic, teamwork is essential and administrators must be made aware of the need for adequate levels of staffing and accommodation, and adequate provision for holidays, sport and relaxation. As well as treating HIV-relative illness, staff remain responsible for the full gamut of haemophilia care. Home therapy programmes must be maintained, regular follow-up assessments, including musculoskeletal measurement, kept, and major reconstructive and dental surgery undertaken. In common with other teams we have explored the need for staff counselling by outside agencies, including psychiatric or psychological colleagues, but have rejected it in favour of the resources which were already present within the team prior to AIDS.

In the early days of the epidemic staff members were tested for antibody because we had no accurate knowledge about casual spread. The fact that everyone was, and has remained, seronegative within the context of an informal medical setting in which simple hygiene provides the only protection, has been very reassuring. Staff wash their hands with soap and water after examining or attending to an infected patient, wear gloves when taking or administering blood, and wipe contaminated surfaces down with sodium hypochlorite. Dentists are encouraged to wear eye and mouth protection as well as gloves, and patients are warned about this in advance. In the operating theatre or delivery suite those staff immediately concerned with the procedure wear disposable theatre clothing, plastic aprons and eye protection. Infected people requiring inpatient care are nursed in the open ward unless cubicle or barrier nursing is required because of their presenting illness; for instance it is inappropriate to nurse someone with herpes zoster in the same open ward as other immunocompromised patients.

The medical and nursing care of people with AIDS and their families is straightforward, safe and rewarding. The sooner HIV-related illness is approached and treated as a disease within the mainstream of medical practice the better it will be for everyone involved, especially our patients.

### References

UK Haemophilia Centre Directors (1986) 'Prevalence of antibody to HTLV III in haemophiliacs in the United Kingdom' *British Medical Journal*, **293** pp. 175−6.

Jones P. (1987) 'AIDS − planning for our future' *Social Work Today*, 9 Feb, pp. 10−12.

# Chapter 8

# Drug Abuse and HIV

GERALDINE MULLEADY

The process of pre- and post-test counselling for injecting drug users is much the same in its essentials as that for individuals in other risk groups (see Chapters 3 and 4). In this chapter I have, therefore, looked at specific issues which are different when dealing with injecting drug users, including some of the additional questions which need to be asked when counselling individuals in this group.

Counselling drug users cannot be separated from the framework of services which are available to them or from issues surrounding injecting practices, prescribing practices and the legal and practical issues relating to the availability of syringes. Therefore these issues are also covered in detail below.

Many counsellors may, with the appearance of HIV, be coming into contact with injecting drug users for the first time. I have tried to provide information on the background to injecting drug abuse and on the social and injecting behaviours of drug users which may be unfamiliar to them.

## Introduction

We are now seeing a sharp increase in the incidence of AIDS among injecting drug users (IDUs) in Europe (Ancelle-Park *et al.*, 1987; McEvoy, 1986). Intravenous drug abuse is quoted as a risk factor for 21 per cent of AIDS deaths in the United Kingdom (CDSC, 1988). Although there is some evidence of a slowing down of seroconversion rates in the gay population, this trend is not evident among IDUs and heterosexuals. Edinburgh continues to show the highest levels of HIV infection among IUDs in the UK (Robertson *et al.*, 1986; Brettle, 1987), although only limited numbers of IDUs in other areas have been tested, mostly from highly selected groups attending drug dependency or genitourinary medicine clinics (Jesson *et al.*, 1986; Webb *et al.*, 1986; Mulleady and Sherr, 1988). However, there is evidence of a slow but steady increase in this group. For example, at St Mary's Drug Dependency Unit (DDU) in 1986, 18 per cent of those tested were HIV antibody positive. In 1988 this had risen to 32 per cent. Since treatment agencies are only likely to be in contact with a minority of drug users (Hartnoll *et al.*, 1980), there is serious cause for concern.

As well as evidence of HIV transmission within the drug-using community, we are also seeing cases of HIV transmission from this group to their non-drug-using sexual partners. Many IDUs have sexual partners who are non-drug users (Stimson *et al.*, 1988). Most paediatric AIDS cases in this country and the United States have been born to women who either have intravenous drug use as their main transmission risk or are the sexual partners of at-risk males (Brettle, 1987; Novick and Rubenstein, 1987). Women of child-bearing age account for approximately one-third of drug users in Edinburgh (Brettle, 1987).

IDUs until recently have been under-researched in terms of their behaviour, cultural influences and treatment effectiveness. Both our own stereotypes and the jargon which surrounds drug abuse serve to increase its mystery for the general public.

Many drugs apart from heroin can be injected, e.g. amphetamines, cocaine. Syringe-sharing and sexual transmission are the two mechanisms of spread of HIV for this group. I will discuss the issue of sexual transmission later on.

The practice of 'flushing', 'washout' or 'booting' increases the chances of HIV transmission from syringe-sharing. This technique involves the drug user pumping blood in and out of the syringe in order to ensure injection of as much drug as possible. As a result of this practice, a small residue of blood will be left in the syringe (approximately 0.5 ml). If the syringe is then used by someone else, transmission of blood-borne infections may occur.

In some areas 'shooting galleries' exist (Des Jarlais and Friedman, 1987). These are places where the IDU will go to inject drugs. He may rent or borrow a syringe on the premises, which may have been used by many others. These places are more common where there are constraints on the availability of clean syringes, e.g. Edinburgh, New York. There does not appear to be evidence of a social culture of syringe-sharing among heroin users. Frequency of injection and the use of 'shooting galleries' are factors associated with HIV exposure among IDUs.

Injecting drug users have always suffered from physical problems as a result of their drug use, either from syringe-sharing and unsterile technique or from contaminated drugs: hepatitis, endocarditis, septicaemia and abscesses are common. Collapsed veins, as a result of injecting, can make it very difficult for health care staff to obtain blood samples. Continued injection of street drugs is associated with T4 cell loss (Des Jarlais and Friedman, 1987). This may be a useful deterrent for some HIV positive IDUs. In New York, they have found evidence of a dramatic increase in recorded deaths among IDUs from non-opportunistic infections such as endocarditis, tuberculosis and non-pneumocystis pneumonia. These deaths may also be related to HIV infection.

It is essential to have some awareness of the local drug scene since this will influence the preventive and treatment measures which will be appropriate. There will be regional variations, both in the preferred drug and the route of administration. For example, in Edinburgh the predominant route of administration of heroin is via injection (Kohn, 1986; Haw, 1985); in Liverpool, smoking or 'chasing' appears to be more common (Parry, 1987). The cultural context will also be important, influencing the preferred drug and route of administration. In Amsterdam, Surinamese people make up a large percentage of the heroin users. Their preferred route of administration is 'chinezing' (chasing). They have a high regard for their physical integrity and discourage injecting (Buning *et al.*, 1987); hence, approximately two-thirds of Amsterdam's heroin users 'chineze'. In London, whereas cannabis is a commonly used social drug among the Caribbean community, the use of heroin and especially injected heroin is frowned upon (Pearson *et al.*, 1985). Variations in the drug using subculture will depend on a complex set of circumstances which will include traditions, supply and cost constraints, local police policy and availability of syringes.

Our knowledge of the existence of the 'recreational' drug user is also vague: individuals who are not dependent on their drug of choice are unlikely to come to the attention of treatment agencies. They may also be unlikely to perceive risk reduction advice as applicable to their situation. It is possible that the recreational amphetamine or cocaine user will be more likely to inject in a social situation and therefore more likely to share syringes. Until such time as more drug treatment agencies are able to offer treatment programmes to those dependent on drugs, other than heroin, we are unlikely to learn about the extent of recreational drug use.

The IDU will usually proceed through a series of stages in his progression from using occasionally to being dependent and needing the drug regularly. Even at the dependent stage, he may be able to exercise a considerable degree of control over his habit (Strang *et al.*, 1987). Hence the need for individual assessment of each IDU. For some, being an IDU can provide a sense of purpose and identity. It can be a full-time absorbing and stressful occupation, one for which we have few viable alternatives to offer. The stress of coming off drugs can be minor in comparison to the changes that are necessary if a drug-free life style is to be maintained. A recent study has shown that the period immediately after discharge from a treatment centre is one of high risk for relapse and that aftercare services are needed to provide support for IDUs at this stage (Gossop, 1978). It is precisely this area which is under-developed in the drug treatment field.

Drug users will frequently be involved in criminal activities in order to finance their habit. This can involve dealing drugs, shoplifting, fraud, burglary or prostitution. Many IDUs will spend time in prison. Prisons will vary regarding their policy of coping with HIV positive people. Frequently, this involves segregation. Also variable are the prisons' facilities to cope with sick inmates. This will be an increasing problem with respect to the IDU with AIDS. In some cases, with the client's consent, HIV status has been divulged in Court and has resulted in leniency of sentence, but this is by no means universal. Probation services are often involved with the IDUs and can provide a useful link in their overall care.

Prior to the epidemic of HIV, treatment of drug problems was predominantly the domain of the Drug Dependency Clinic. Because of HIV, this situation is likely to change. Many GPs and hospital staff will become involved as a result of sick IDUs coming under their care. This will be a necessary development as without increased resources traditional drug treatment services will be unlikely to be able to cope with increased demand. However, other health care professionals may have had limited contact with drug users when they have come under their care for physical problems. Few will have dealt in detail with issues related to drug use.

Drug users are a heterogeneous group of people; the intervention that is appropriate for a given individual will depend on that person's level of risk. Risk taking will include both injecting drug use and sexual behaviour. Care of the user will include management of the drug problem and provision of appropriate physical care.

### Injecting drug use

*Interviewing the clients about drug use*

It may be appropriate to glean the following information:

- What drugs do they use?

- Do they inject?
- If so, how frequently?
- Do they know how syringe-sharing can transmit HIV?
- Do they consider themselves to be at risk?
- Have they ever borrowed someone else's syringe?
- Have they ever lent their syringe to someone else?
- Do they restrict sharing to their sexual partners?
- Do they know who their partner shares with?
- How often do they change syringes?
- What methods of sterilisation, if any, do they use?
- Can they obtain clean syringes?
- Where do they get clean syringes from?
- Do they think that they would be able to change to a safer route of administration, e.g. oral, inhalation?
- Into what part of the body do they inject?
- Do they use alternative injection sites?
- Are they aware of good injecting practice?
- Do they have any physical problems as a result of injecting?

### Reducing risks associated with sharing

The evidence so far available suggests that substantial numbers of IDUs have modified their injecting behaviour. In New York in 1984, 54 per cent of a sample of IDUs reported that they had reduced risk injection practices (Des Jarlais *et al.*, 1985). Selwyn *et al.*, (1985) similarly found a 60 per cent reduction in needle-sharing.

In San Francisco, 73 per cent of IDUs had made at least one change in their drug-related behaviour in order to avoid HIV exposure (Newmeyer *et al.*, 1988). In Amsterdam, Buning, Verster and Hartgers (1987) found that of 150 IDUs, needlesharing had reduced from 70 per cent in the early 80s to 20 per cent in 1987. At St Mary's DDU, we found that of 74 IDUs attending the clinic, 65 per cent reported that they had shared syringes previously but were not doing so now due to AIDS (Mulleady and Sherr, 1988).

In some areas, local pharmacists may be the chief supplier of clean syringes. You will need to know which pharmacists, if any, are willing to supply syringes and if so, whether they are happy for you to refer IDUs to them. Syringe Exchange Units have been established in some areas; it is useful to have their details available for the IDU. A major evaluation of Syringe Exchange Units in the UK has indicated that the majority of clients who attend these units are not receiving treatment for their drug problem (Stimson *et al.*, 1988). Even if they are, they may still be injecting non-prescribed drugs. A study in San Francisco found that 53 per cent of drug users contacted in the community would not enter treatment 'even if it was available tomorrow' (Watters *et al.*, 1986). It is necessary to accept that some IDUs will not want treatment for their drug problem. Syringe exchange may therefore be more acceptable to them.

Apart from injecting advice and equipment, the range of services Syringe Exchange Units offer varies considerably. These may include drug counselling and referral for treatment and detoxification, medical and family planning care, free condoms, information on welfare and housing, legal advice, HIV testing and health education.

Where there is no exchange scheme and access to clean syringes is limited, sterilisation of equipment may be the only alternative. Some confusion seems to exist about the appropriate advice to give drug users should they request information on sterilising injecting equipment. In the United States, many out-reach programmes distribute bleach to drug users with advice on the procedure to follow (Watters *et al.*, 1986). In order to be effective the bleach needs to penetrate the dried blood. For this reason, and because of the instability of bleach in solution and risks of injecting bleach, the Home Office recommend a two-stage process which involves flushing the syringe twice with a solution of washing-up liquid and cold water and then dismantling the syringe and immersing it in boiling water for at least 5 minutes.

In ascending order of efficacy the syringe can be:

(1)  Flushed repeatedly with cold water.
(2)  As above, but with a mixture of washing-up liquid and cold water.
(3)  Dismantled and the parts boiled for 5 minutes.

The procedure does seem to be rather involved, requires access to a lot of facilities, and is probably time-consuming, especially for someone who is desperate for a fix. However, until more evidence is available on the sterilising techniques commonly employed, it is difficult to ascertain how feasible this advice is. Obviously, increased availability of syringes will reduce the need for sterilising equipment. However, there may be situations where the IDU finds him or herself without access to a clean syringe and under these circumstances it is probably useful for him to know how to sterilise a syringe adequately, especially if this involves techniques which the IDU has used previously. More significant may be the possession of the necessary social skills to refuse to share, or to sterilise equipment, offered by a drug-using friend.

**Sexual behaviour**

*Interviewing the clients about sexual issues*

It may be useful to have information on the following:

- Do they have a regular sexual partner?
- Any irregularities in menstrual cycle, for women?
- How often do they have sexual intercourse?
- What are their preferred activities?
- Have they ever/regularly used a condom?
- Do they know how?
- Do they use contraception of any kind?
- Have they ever attended a family planning clinic or GP for family planning advice?
- Any unplanned pregnancies?
- Activities engaged in − safe/unsafe?
- Have they ever used prostitution as a source of funding for their habit?
- How recently?
- If yes, do they work for themselves?
  If not, do they have sex with their pimp, do they use a condom with him?
- Ever visited an STD clinic or been treated for an STD?

*Dealing with sexual issues*

Many drug workers report that they find it easier to discuss drug issues than sexual issues with IDUs (Stimson, 1988). IDUs frequently report a loss of interest in sex as a result of heroin use, they may not therefore see sexual risk reduction as applicable to them. However, many IDUs report that they are sexually active (Stimson *et al.*, 1988; Mulleady and Sherr, 1988). It is possible that this is unplanned and therefore more likely to take place without the use of contraception. It is also possible that as a result of risk reduction advice which emphasises the need to reduce syringe-sharing, many IDUs do not readily recognise the need to modify sexual behaviour.

Many of the HIV positive IDU women at St Mary's DDU do not use contraception (Mulleady and Sherr, 1988). Amenorrhoea is common and as a result they do not consider pregnancy to be a significant risk for them. We also see many couples where one partner is antibody positive and the other negative. Frequently, they are resistant to the idea of safer sex. The reasons they give for this vary but are mainly involved with their fear that they will somehow damage their relationship, which is more important to them than their health. This is especially true if the antibody positive individual is asymptomatic, since the problem is not a physically apparent one. In these cases there is a definite need for increased access to family planning services. If possible this service should be brought to the IDU. Both the City Hospital, Edinburgh (Brettle, 1987), and St Mary's provide an 'on site' family planning clinic. Many more sites should be involved in the free distribution of condoms.

The management of the pregnant IDU is a complex and sensitive issue. They may attend inconsistently for antenatal care. They may also turn up late in the pregnancy. The mother has to cope with the increased attention of outside agencies and the fear that these professionals will be trying to take the baby away from her. The baby may have to be withdrawn from opiates in hospital. Consequently, mother and baby are separated early on. The mother may feel a strong sense of guilt about this. She also has to try to care for her baby and cope with her dependence problem at the same time.

Added to this, we now have HIV, the fear and the unknowns that positive mothers are faced with, both for themselves and for the baby. Obstetric and paediatric care should be sensitive to the special needs and problems of working with these mothers and their children. Edinburgh have pioneered a model of community care for these families which has resulted in effective delivery of post-natal care. This is discussed in Chapter 10 on paediatric HIV infection. Adoption and foster care is required when parents become ill. It is helpful if these facilities are established before they need to be used.

## Management of the drug problem

Drug treatment services are in contact with only a small proportion of drug users (Hartnell *et al.*, 1980); if IDUs were encouraged to seek treatment, under the present circumstances facilities would be unable to cope. Many GPs are now treating IDUs (Glanz and Taylor, 1986), and it is vital that this trend should continue. Staff of inpatient wards may also be involved in the detoxification of IDUs. Where possible, close liaison with drug workers should take place. It is important that staff are aware of their own limitations and, equally, that they set limits for the IDU, provided that these have a logical basis.

IDUs sometimes seek to play agencies off against each other. Tactics that the IDU may use involve either praising your efforts, usually to the detriment of some other helping agency, or focusing on your shortcomings and inability to really understand the problem (Levine and Stephens, 1971). The HIV positive IDU may need to express anger at his situation, and you may be the only safe person he can talk to. The IDU can be demanding of attention. This may cause management difficulties on busy inpatient wards. They are also unreliable in their attendance: if your surgery or clinic operates on an appointment system this can be disruptive. IDUs will have a tendency to turn up in a crisis. This makes effective management more difficult but how we respond to that crisis will be crucial in establishing an effective working relationship with the client. It is helpful if both the drug worker and the IDU have a realistic attitude towards what they are likely to be able to achieve, although this may be limited. If there were any easy solutions to the problem of drug abuse treatment, no doubt someone would have discovered them by now.

One of the most important issues for the current IDU is the amount and type of drugs available to him on prescription. It will be necessary to establish the type of drug which the IDU perceives as the problem, the duration of use, and previous treatment experience, if any.

## Drug treatment services

There are a wide variety of drug treatment facilities which can be broadly divided into prescribing and non-prescribing agencies. Prescribing agencies will offer a substitute to heroin, most commonly oral methadone, more occasionally injectable methadone. A prescribing agency may be a drug-dependency unit or a GP. Non-prescribing agencies are often street-based and offer advice, support and sometimes referral for treatment. Residential care may offer time-limited detoxification from drugs and longer-term rehabilitation, abstinence from drugs being the ultimate goal. Street agencies and residential units are more frequently non-statutory organisations.

Currently, many DDUs have waiting lists. This is often seen as a method of weeding out the unmotivated as it is assumed that the individuals who drop out whilst on the waiting list were not motivated to come off drugs. Obviously, this is a crude technique to use. DDUs have primarily seen their role as helping those who want to come off drugs, nudging the IDU in the desired direction. HIV has challenged this. It now appears necessary to reduce damage, to try to keep drug users uninfected until such time as they may decide that they want to come off drugs. This involves a significant alteration, both in terms of the drug workers' view of their role and organisational changes necessary within treatment agencies. It may be appropriate for another tier of 'harm reduction' agencies to be developed in order to provide this service, but it is essential that these are not developed to the neglect of traditional treatment agencies.

Much debate has taken place about the role of drug treatment clinics in harm reduction. Predominantly this has been focused on prescribing policies, with methadone variously considered as either the universal evil or universal panacea. That this synthetic opiate has received so much attention possibly indicates our anxiety to do something that will succeed in 'making' IDUs reduce their HIV transmission risks. Clinics may offer short-time limited reduction programmes, flexible reduction programmes and maintenance.

It is worth considering methadone from an historical perspective from which are derived most of the current arguments for and against its usefulness. Studies attempted to determine whether methadone maintenance was an effective treatment in its own right with drug abuse conceived of as a 'metabolic disease' or would it only be useful as an adjunct to other forms of treatment? Methodological problems were common to most of these studies. Therefore the results are dubious (Gossop, 1978).

There is little evidence that dosage levels are crucial (Goldstein, 1971; Connell, 1975): one study found that low dosage maintenance (20–70 mg) did better than high dosage in terms of social adaptation measures and reduction in illicit drug use. Methadone treatment is popular with drug users. However, its ability to retain clients in treatment has also been questioned. Williams and Lee (1975) found that only 25 per cent of their sample remained in treatment. Indeed, Hartnell *et al.* (1980) compared oral methadone with intravenous heroin maintenance and found no difference between the two groups in terms of use of illicit opiates, employment and patterns of health. Crime was a significant source of income for both groups. Furthermore, the heroin group showed a better attendance rate (76 per cent of the heroin group compared with 29 per cent of the methadone group after 12 months).

Whatever the research results, most were obtained prior to the epidemic of HIV. It is therefore clearly inappropriate to apply their findings without regard to the present situation. Current research on the role of methadone maintenance treatment in reducing transmission-related behaviours has indicated that drug users on such programmes inject less frequently than those who are not (Des Jarlais and Friedman, 1987). It is essential that drug users have increased access to treatment, but the treatment programme as a whole needs to be considered, of which methadone is clearly only one component. It is also necessary to promote counselling, medical and family planning care, housing, rehabilitation, skills training, self-help and advocacy, effective health education and welfare. We require a range of treatments to which the IDU has easier access.

Increased access to treatment programmes could be achieved by expansion which would reduce the perennial problem of waiting lists. This could be further facilitated if time-consuming assessment procedures were streamlined. Such a model has been adopted at the Northern Road Drug Clinic in Portsmouth. The programme is designed in three stages. The drug user has quick access to stage one of the programme, where he collects his methadone from the clinic daily within a set time period. At the time of collection, if he wishes, the drug user has access to a casual open-ended discussion group which uses motivational interviewing techniques (Van Bilsen, 1986). At this stage there are no further programme constraints. Should the client decide he wants to reduce or come off methadone he can proceed to stage two where he can pick up methadone daily from a local chemist and attend the clinic for urine assessment and counselling. There is also a third option of more flexible access to methadone and reduced frequency of attendance at the clinic. The programme is community based, with staff making regular home visits. This change in practice was brought about as a result of the clinic's response to HIV, and has increased the rate of referrals. Although this programme may not be universally appropriate, certain components could be adopted by most clinics. It is a rare example of a treatment unit prepared to radically change its policies and procedures.

There is a need for increased co-ordination of our approach to drug treatment, incorporating sensitivity to local needs. Our present system is unable to respond effectively to the changing circumstances of the people we provide the service for.

## Self help and self advocacy

Friedman *et al.* (1987) found that IDUs were more likely to reduce risk-taking behaviour if they saw other IDUs trying to protect themselves. This amplifies the importance of peer group behaviour in influencing risk reduction. Self-help organisations have been slow to develop among IDUs and may require a greater input from drug workers, at least initially. A number of self-help groups already exist, such as Narcotics Anonymous. The Junkiebonden in the Netherlands has been in existence for some years and was formed originally as a pressure group to influence government policy on drug use issues. Similar groups have developed in the United States, specifically with regard to HIV risk reduction among IDUs, e.g. ADAPT (Association for Drug Abuse Prevention and Treatment) (Des Jarlais and Friedman, 1987).

These groups are likely to have more impact on IDU behaviour than any other since they will be able to communicate effectively within the sub-culture and have a good rapport. They are also essential since drug users may feel isolated from support groups who have no experience of the problems and life style of the drug user.

A number of small support/self-help groups for HIV positive IDUs and their partners have developed throughout the United Kingdom (Mulleady and Riccio, 1988). These provide an essential forum for information and support. Many are in the early stages of development, maintained by a few committed individuals. Drug workers need to encourage and support the development of these groups. As workers, we can learn useful information about the services that may be required for effective intervention. The following points are useful if considering setting up such a group:

- Siting is important and should as far as possible be on neutral territory.
- A group leader who acts as a facilitator of communications between group members can be of invaluable assistance. The facilitator needs to be well informed on all aspects of HIV and AIDS.
- The stage of drug use (i.e. abstinent, those on a methadone prescription, occasional users) does not appear to be a basis for separate groups.
- The stage of illness of group attenders appears to be more crucial and is more likely to be an appropriate reason for separate groups (i.e. asymptomatic, ARC, AIDS).
- Practical and accurate information, as well as emotional support, needs to be available.
- It may be appropriate to engage 'expert speakers' from time to time to discuss specific issues.
- Sexual behaviour is a frequently raised issue. The group should provide a safe and comfortable forum for its discussion.
- It is helpful if the group has some degree of structure and that its aims are established and agreed on at the outset. Aims can be renegotiated as and when appropriate.
- An HIV self-help group should always attempt to reduce anxiety levels, enhance individual coping skills and self-esteem, and encourage harm reduction.

**Outreach work**

This model of service is not new. It has received increased attention with the need to reach drug users in the community. It is possible that only the more organised IDUs ever make use of drug agencies, therefore outreach work may provide access to the more chaotic user. The success of this method of working relies heavily on the skills of the outreach worker. By its very nature, it can be stressful work to undertake, and adequate support should be available to the workers. It has been suggested that the main purpose of outreach work is to inform IDUs about existing drug services and to encourage them to use them. However, for IDUs who choose not to avail themselves of these drug services, the outreach worker will be the only helping agency that they come into contact with. This makes the content of the service delivered by the outreach worker all the more significant. The content will be influenced by a number of factors: the setting for the contact; people present; what the IDU wants/is willing to listen to; the detail of information he is willing to disclose; the IDU's behaviour in terms of HIV transmission risk; access to local services; conditions/culture of local drug use scene.

In effect the outreach worker may function as a 'mobile drug agency' and as well as information and advice, may choose to operate a limited syringe exchange service and distribute condoms.

The major effect of outreach projects that have been evaluated so far has been to encourage IDUs to enter treatment (Jackson and Neshin, 1986). This entitled the drug user to a three-week free detoxification. Of 607 coupons given out, 76 per cent were redeemed at the treatment centre; 41 per cent of these IDUs had never been in treatment before. In San Francisco bleach was distributed by outreach workers: Watters *et al.* (1986) found that whilst only 3 per cent of IDUs used bleach for sterilising their equipment at the commencement of the programme, six months later 76 per cent reported that they did. A number of these programmes have specifically utilised ex-users for outreach work (Friedman *et al.*, 1988). Drug users and ex-users are individuals who may have high status in drug using circles; they could use their knowledge in order to reach the largest possible audience.

Liaison with other agencies is an essential component of outreach work. In Westminster, we have a large educational input to the local police in order to advertise our services. Effective lines of communication must exist with other outreach projects in order that duplication work and disputes can be kept to a minimum.

Since the major effect of outreach work observed so far has been to encourage IDUs to enter treatment, increased accessibility to treatment is an essential component of this service.

### Therapeutic communities

Drug-free therapeutic communities can provide many of the services already discussed as well as giving syringes to those clients they know are leaving to continue injecting drug use. They have the advantage that they will have clients who are in residence and therefore may be able to develop more sophisticated training packages for those residents who choose to stay. They will also have the chance to work with drug users who are not under the influence of drugs and will therefore have the opportunity to explore the more emotive and stressful issues for the client.

Many residential units have programmes which are based on confrontation and of their nature are stress-inducing. In order to accommodate HIV positive IDUs and PWAs, it may be necessary to 'tone down' the confrontative component of the rehabilitation programme. It is the author's experience that mood swings can undermine attempts to remain drug free, and the attitude, 'What's the point in the struggle, I'm going to die anyway' tends to emerge at times of depression. The appearance of symptoms of HIV is also particularly distressing for the IDU who has managed to become abstinent and to embark on a new life. Mood swings tend to undermine self-esteem which for many drug users is low anyway. A difficult decision for the therapeutic community is how far they are willing or able to provide physical care for the IDU with AIDS when he becomes debilitated by the illness.

### Physical care

Many drug users attending Syringe Exchanges and Treatment Agencies have physical problems which require treatment. Drug users do not always receive adequate medical care, for a variety of reasons. They have a tendency to turn up when it suits them, often in a crisis which requires immediate attention. They are not necessarily welcomed by many health care staff who may have fixed ideas about what drug users are like. We need a commitment to the provision of better medical care for drug users. Accessibility is facilitated if medical services can be provided 'on site'. Drop-in surgeries for physical problems or family planning advice where no appointment is necessary may go some way to alleviating the problem of poor attendance. Another alternative is to have a bleep system to call for medical assistance when the need arises.

The drug user may not return for subsequent appointments. Therefore maximum use of this 'one-off' contact must be achieved. These services need to be 'sold' — made attractive to drug users. Most drug users will not have a GP and may have difficulty finding a GP willing to take them on.

In prescribing agencies, it is probably easier for health care staff if a clear distinction is made between physical treatment and drug treatment. It is necessary to understand that care for physical problems may not be the drug user's priority. Catering for their habit will probably be their priority, and unless the two issues are separated it may be difficult to provide adequate physical care.

Facing up to a medical examination can be very traumatic for the HIV positive person; many of our clients default on their medical appointments and later admit that this is because they do not want to know the significance of their physical symptoms. Having said this, once they manage to attend for the examination, they often feel relieved that they know what they are up against.

It is also clear that offering an HIV positive person drug therapy such as AZT or Interferon has a profound psychological impact. This is especially true if the client has recently commenced a methadone programme, may have increased appetite and be feeling better generally: a sense of the unreality of HIV often ensues. When offered AZT, it is no longer possible for the client to deny the significance of his physical condition.

Whatever the problems of delivering an effective medical service, it is clear that the choice of the drug user will prevail, however illogical or self-destructive his decisions may appear to us. Good liaison and clear lines of communication between drug workers and health care workers are essential in order to manage these difficulties should they arise, and ensure accurate information and effective management of the drug problem.

## Antibody testing

It has been suggested that HIV antibody testing can have a significant influence on transmission-related behaviour in IDUs. Only limited evidence is so far available (Casadonte *et al.*, 1986; Cox *et al.*, 1986; Marlink *et al.*, 1987). In the short term a dramatic reduction in needle transmission behaviour was found, following feedback of antibody test results. It is important to note that these studies took place in the context of a treatment unit, where testing was voluntary and pre- and post-test counselling and support was available. These results should be approached with caution since even with adequate support mechanisms, feedback of positive test results can lead to a significant increase in the levels of both depression and anxiety (Casadonte *et al.*, 1986) and increases in illicit drug use. Testing in the absence of support services is more likely to be harmful than lead to reductions in risk behaviour. It has been the author's impression that even in the context of a treatment unit people who are antibody positive experience serious problems in modifying their injecting and sexual behaviour, whereas those who test negative see this as a 'clean bill of health' or that HIV risk adds a reckless edge to their drug use. HIV antibody testing can be an important part of a drug treatment service. It is not a solution to the problem of transmission-related behaviour in drug users.

The HIV positive IDU will have the burden of his drug use to cope with as well as all the issues associated with being HIV positive. He may respond to this by positively attempting to gain some control over his habit, or he may continue to use drugs in an attempt to blot out his feelings about HIV — or, more frequently, he alternates between these two reactions. A number of IDUs have expressed concern that the stress involved in coming off drugs may cause them to progress to full-blown AIDS.

### Community care

According to Miller (1987), PWAs who experience the greatest difficulty in adjusting to their situation have one or more of the following factors in common:

- Poor accommodation.
- Few or poor family ties.
- Low peer acceptance.
- Guilt over past behaviour.

Many of these factors apply to the IDUs seen at St Mary's DDU — housing and financial difficulties being the most common problems. It is essential that we offer practical help. Since many of the drug users seen have housing problems and lack of network of carers in the community, they may spend longer in hospital, putting pressure on already overburdened hospital wards.

In working with drug users infected with HIV, what has clearly emerged at this clinic is that the majority of the work involves assisting with practical issues such as housing, welfare, diet and legal problems. These are time-consuming and frustrating from the point of view of both the worker and the client. One of the most difficult problems is the issue of welfare benefits and the liaison difficulties with DHSS departments.

Many bereaved families of IDUs have great difficulty in coming to terms with the circumstances of their son's/daughter's death. We have found that they often want to believe their son/daughter was off drugs, even if circumstances indicate that this was patently not the case. Care must be taken to determine the family's awareness of HIV, and their degree of involvement in the drug problem. If it is appropriate, the family should be offered support. We have found that even a 'one-off' meeting can do much to improve the relationship between the IDU and his/her family.

## Prevention of initiation

An individual is often introduced to heroin by his peers (Friedman *et al.*, 1988). If it is taken by the intravenous route then it is likely that the syringe will be shared. We do not have a national, co-ordinated, school-based drug education programme; if the subject is addressed it is often left to teachers who have not been given any specific training. Measures we take to reduce harm in drug services only address the problem when it has developed. Therefore, much more effort is required to educate children and adolescents about what they can do safely in a realistic way. Emphasis must be placed on skills training. We have good evidence that prevention programmes based on fear arousal have not been very successful in the past, particularly if fear is associated with a low probability event or if there is a long time period between the risk drug use and the adverse consequences (Friedman *et al.*, 1988). If we are able to target specific groups we must ensure that the targeting has maximum impact (Sherr, 1987).

One interesting development in the field of harm reduction is the Sniffer Project in New York. This aims to reduce the likelihood of injecting for drug users who take heroin. It involves group training in the skills necessary to cope with potentially 'risky situations'.

An attempt needs to be made to contact IDUs earlier in their career. Training is necessary for staff as well as clients and a multi-media approach can be used, with one-to-one sessions, groups, outside lecturers, workshops, videos, leaflets, journals, and open days.

## Conclusion

For the intravenous drug user, HIV is yet another problem to add to many others. It is difficult but necessary to accept that some drug users will choose to continue to use illegal drugs and we have a duty to be realistic about this and ensure that they do this with minimum risks to themselves and their community. However, we must be able to offer treatment for drug abuse to those individuals who request it. Good communication with other workers is also essential, particularly where a drug user may be involved with numerous people from a variety of agencies, all basically trying to achieve the same thing. The models discussed will need to be applied in an aggressive and co-ordinated way in order to have maximum impact. So far this has not been the case: our approach to the problem of HIV and drug use in the United Kingdom has been piecemeal and slow. We have only to look at the situation in New York to know that time is not on our side.

## References

Ancelle-Park, R., Brunet, J.B. and Downs, A.M. (1987) 'AIDS and drug addicts in Europe' *Lancet*, **ii**, 626–627.

Brettle, R.P. (1987) 'Drug abuse and human immunodeficiency virus in Scotland' *Journal of the Royal Society of Medicine*, **80**, pp.276–278.

Buning, E.C., Verster, A.D. and Hartgers, C. (1987) *Amsterdam's Policy on AIDS and Drugs* Presented at National Institute on Drug Abuse Meeting, Washington, D.C., May 1987.

Casadonte, P., Des Jarlais, D.C., Smith, T.S., Novatt, A. and Hemdal, P. (1986) *Psychological and Behavioural Impact on Learning HTLV III/LAV Antibody Test Results* Presented at the International Conference on AIDS, Paris, June 1986.

Centre for Disease Surveillance and Control (1988) *Acquired Immune Deficiency Syndrome: United Kingdom: 1982 – January 1988*. 5 February.

Connell, P.H. (1975) Skandia International Symposia, Stockholm, pp.133.

Cox, C.P., Selwyn, P.A., Schoenbaum, E.E., O'Dowd, M.A. and Drucker, E. (1986) *Psychological and Behavioural Consequences of HTLV III/LAV Antibody Testing and Notification Among Intravenous Drug Abusers in a Methadone Programme in New York City*. Presented at the International Conference on AIDS, Paris, June 1986.

Des Jarlais, D.C. and Friedman, S.R. (1987) 'HIV infection among intravenous drug users: epidemiology and risk reduction' *AIDS*, **1**, pp.67–76.

Des Jarlais, D.C., Friedman, S.R. and Hopkins, W (1985) 'Risk reduction for the Acquired Immune Deficiency Syndrome among intravenous drug users' *Annals of Internal Medicine*, **103**, pp.755–759.

Friedman, S.R., Des Jarlais, D.C. and Goldsmith, D.S. (1988) 'An overview of current AIDS prevention efforts aimed at intravenous drug users' *Journal of Drug Issues*. In Press.

Friedman, S.R., Des Jarlais, D.C., Southeran, J.C., *et al*. (1987) 'Self organisation among intravenous drug abusers' *International Journal of Addiction*, **22**, pp.201–220.

Glanz, A. and Taylor, C. (1986) 'Findings of a national survey of the role of General Practictioners in the treatment of opiate misuse: extent of contact with opiate misusers' *British Medical Journal*, **293**, pp.427–430.

Goldstein, A. (1971) *Journal of Psychedelic Drugs*, **4**, p.177.

Gossop, M., (1978) 'A review of the evidence for Methadone maintenance as a treatment for narcotic addiction' *Lancet*, April, pp.812–15.

Gossop, M., Green, L., Phillips, G., Bradley, B. (1987) 'What happens to opiate addicts immediately after treatment: A prospective follow-up study' *British Medical Journal*, **294**, pp.1377–80.

Hartnell, R.L., Mitcheson, M.B., Battersby, A., Brown, G., Ellis, M., Fleming, P. and Hedley, N. (1980) 'Evaluation of heroin maintenance in controlled trial' *Archives General Psychiatry*, **37**, pp.877–884.

Haw, S. (1985) *Drug Problems in Greater Glasgow*. Standing Conference on Drug Abuse, London.

Home Office Statistical Bulletin (1986) *Statistics of Drug Addicts Notified to the Home Office* HMSO, 19 December.

Jackson, J., and Neshin, S. (1986) New Jersey Community Health Education Project *Impact of Using Ex-addict Educators to Disseminate Information on AIDS to Intravenous Drug Users* Presented at the International Conference on AIDS, Paris, June 1986.

Jesson, W.I., Thorp, R.W., Mortimer, P.P. and Oates, J.K. (1986) 'Prevalence of anti-HTLV III in UK risk groups, 1984/85' *Lancet*, 18 January, p.155.

Kohn, M. (1986) 'The virus in Edinburgh' *New Society*, 2 May, pp.11–13.

Levine, S. and Stephens, R. (1971) 'Games addicts play' *Psychiatric Quarterly*, **45**, 4, pp.582–592.

Marlink, R.G., Foss, B., Swift, R., Davis, W., Essex, M., Groopman, J. *et al*. (1987) *High Rate of HTLV III/HIV Exposure in IVDAs from a Small Sized City and the Rate of Failure of Specialised Methadone Maintenance to Prevent Further Drug Use* Presented at the Third International Conference on AIDS, Washington, D.C., June 1987.

McEvoy, M. (1986) *Surveillance: The Role of the Communicable Disease Surveillance Centre* Proceedings of Intercept AIDS Conference, Newcastle Upon Tyne.

Miller, D. (1987) *Living with AIDS and HIV* London: Macmillan Press.

Mulleady, G. and Riccio, M. (1988) 'HIV infection and drug users: Setting up support groups' Submitted for Publication, *British Journal of Addiction*.

Mulleady, G. and Sherr, L. (1988) 'Lifestyle factors for drug users in relation to risks for HIV and AIDS' Submitted for Publication, *British Journal of Clinical Psychology*.

Newmeyer, J.A., Feldman, H.W., Biernacki, P. and Walters, J.K. (1988) 'Preventing AIDS contagion among intravenous drug users' *Medical Anthropology*, In Press.

Novick, B.E., Rubenstein, A. (1987) 'AIDS – the paediatric perspective' *AIDS*, 1, pp.3–7.

Parry, A. (1987) 'Needle swop in Mersey' *Druglink 2*, 1, p.7.

Pearson, G., Gilman, M. and Mc Iver, S. (1985) *Young People and Heroin* Health Education Council.

Power, M. (1987) *The Influence of AIDS Upon Patterns of Intravenous Use, Syringe and Needle Sharing, Amongst Illicit Drug Users in Britain* NIDA Conference, May 18, Washington D.C.

Robertson, I.R., Bucknall, A.B.V., Wersby, P.D., Roberts, J.J., Inglis, J.M., Peutherer, J.F. and Brettle, R.P. (1986) 'Epidemic of AIDS related virus (HTLV-III/LAV). Infection among intravenous drug abusers' *British Medical Journal*, 292, pp.527–529.

Selwyn, P.A., Cox, C.P., Feiner, C., Lipschutz, C. and Cohen, R. (1985) 'Knowledge about AIDS and high risk behaviour among intravenous drug abusers in New York City'. Presented at the Annual Meeting of the American Public Health Association, Washington, DC, November 1985.

Sherr, L. (1987) 'An evaluation of the UK Government health education campaign on AIDS' *Psychology and Health*, 1, pp.61–72.

Stimson, G.V., Aldritt, L., Dolan, K. and Donoghoe, M. (1988) *Injecting Equipment Exchange Schemes: A Preliminary Report on Research* Monitoring Research Group, Sociology Department, University of London, Goldsmiths College.

Strang, J., Ghodse, M. and Johns, A. (1987) 'Responding flexibly but not gullibly to addiction' *British Medical Journal*, 295, p.1364.

Strang, J., Heathcote, S. and Watson, P. (1987) 'Habit moderation in injecting drug addicts' *Health Trend*, 19, pp.16–18.

United Kingdom Home Office (1986) '*Tackling Drug Misuse – A Summary of the Government Strategy*' United Kingdom Home Office, 2nd edition, p.5.

Van Bilsen, H.P.J.G. (1986) 'Heroin addiction, morals re-visited' *Journal of Substance Abuse Treatment*, 3, pp.279–284.

Watters, J.K., Lura, D.M. and Lura, K.W. (1986) *AIDS Prevention and Education Services to Intravenous Drug Users Through the Mid City Consortium to Combat AIDS: Administrative Report on the First Six Months.*

Webb, G., Wells, B., Morgan, J.R. and McManus, T.J. (1986) 'Epidemic of AIDS-related virus infection among intravenous drug abusers' *British Medical Journal*, 292, p. 1202.

Williams, W.V. and Lee, J. (1975) 'Methadone Maintenance: A Comparison of methadone treatment subjects and methadone treatment drop-outs' *International Journal of Addiction*, 10, pp.599–608.

# Chapter 9

# Counselling and Pregnancy

JOHN GREEN

## Background

The information available about the risks of pregnancy to mother and baby presented by HIV infection is currently unsatisfactory in several respects. It is likely that this will improve in the next few years as a number of prospective studies report. The factual aspects of counselling in HIV infection can only be as good as the information available at the time that it is carried out. Therefore, for any counsellor in this field, it is vital to keep abreast of current research papers.

The information contained in this chapter is based on what is known at the time of preparation, and the advice is based on that information. If and when new information becomes available it will be necessary to consider the suggestions offered in the light of that information. The area of pregnancy throws into stark relief one of the key issues in counselling. We can only provide the information to patients which we have ourselves, however inadequate and incomplete that may be. For the woman who is pregnant and who is contemplating a termination it is just not possible to say, 'We don't know, come back in two years and we might be able to tell you'. It is only possible to say, 'Here is the evidence, here's what it tells us and here's what we don't know'.

Currently the evidence available suggests the following:

### Risks to mother

Early reports (Lapointe *et al*. 1985; Scott *et al*. 1985; Sprecher *et al*. 1986) suggested that the HIV positive mother might herself be at greater risk of going on to develop AIDS. Later studies have not confirmed this risk (Berrebi *et al.* 1988; Braddick *et al.* 1988; Ciraru-Vigueron *et al.* 1988; McCallum *et al.* 1988; Schaeffes *et al.* 1988). The difference in findings between studies is probably accounted for in part by the different initial state of health of the mothers in different studies. One difficulty with some currently available studies is the lack of an adequately matched group of non-pregnant infected women to provide a comparison group. Studies which do not contain such a comparison group are difficult to interpret.

The data available is consistent with the hypothesis that the health of the woman at the time of pregnancy may be a factor. A woman who is in poor health to start off with and who is already showing symptoms of HIV infection, whether overt symptoms or the signs of poor immune functioning, may be more likely to progress to ill-health. There is no evidence available currently that pregnancy tends to cause progression to frank disease in asymptomatic women who are otherwise well.

If it is correct that some women may be at risk through pregnancy and others not, the data is still not available to decide precisely what clinical immunological or virological criteria should be used to decide which women fall into which group.

### Risks to the child

Early studies suggested that a mother infected with HIV virus had over a 50 per cent chance of passing that virus on to her baby either in the womb or at birth (Friedland and Klein 1987; Scott *et al.* 1985). Recent studies (Peckham 1988) suggest that the risks are lower, perhaps of the order of 20–30 per cent. The early studies used mothers who had already had babies with AIDS.

The best current guess is that the risk of transmission of HIV from mother to fetus is related to the immunological and virological status of the mother. Virus levels in the blood vary at different times in infected individuals. There is reason to suspect that virus in the blood is highest during two periods. The first is just after infection, before an antibody response develops to the virus. The second occurs when the individual starts to become sick as antibody levels against the core of the virus start to reduce and, possibly, other reductions in immunological efficiency occur.

Based on these considerations it is suggested that the mother may be most likely to pass on the virus to the fetus either when she has just recently been infected with HIV, or when she herself is either becoming symptomatic and showing signs of immunological decline or actually has AIDS. This does not imply that a mother who is clinically and immunologically free from abnormalities *cannot* pass on the virus to the fetus, but the risks may be rather lower.

It is clear that the gross health status of the mother cannot be the only factor in the transmission of HIV. Even for mothers who have already had one infected child the risk of subsequent children being infected is probably not more than 50–60 per cent.

Even if a child is born infected with the virus the chances of that child going on to develop AIDS are difficult to assess (see Chapter 10). Given a virus which persists for life it will not be possible to assess the life-time risks of AIDS or of HIV-related encephalopathy for many years.

### Effects of termination

It is not known what effect a termination will have on the prospects of a symptomatic woman who becomes pregnant. If pregnancy does, indeed, cause a progression to AIDS in susceptible women it is not clear whether later pregnancy is more of a factor than early pregnancy in causing progression. Hence the value of termination in protecting the mother's health is unproven.

The above background shows some of the difficulties involved in counselling women who are pregnant and who have HIV infection. The only intervention which can be offered to a pregnant woman under these circumstances is termination. Her decision is likely to be influenced to some extent by the information provided to her as well as by a whole host of other considerations. Two years ago the only evidence available suggested that the pregnant woman was at risk of herself progressing to AIDS and had a 50–50 chance of the baby having the HIV virus. It was known that this evidence *might* not apply to all HIV infected pregnant women, however there was little hard evidence that it didn't. Currently the evidence suggests that for some women the risk of progression to AIDS being provoked by pregnancy may be lower or even in some cases non-existent; however it is difficult to say with any certainty who is and who is not at risk. The risk of transmission, at least for the asymptomatic woman who has not previously had a baby with AIDS, also appears lower, though still significant.

There are other issues involved. A woman who is pregnant, asymptomatic and in good general health who has a termination is unlikely to be in a better situation to have a baby in the future. Her physical health and immunological status are only likely to get worse or, at best, stay the same. Therefore the probability of difficulties is likely to be greater rather than less in the future. Age may be a factor here. A woman of eighteen who is HIV infected, pregnant and determined that she wants a child at some point, may take a different decision from a woman of 38 in the same position. The first might hope that within her years of fertility an effective treatment may be available for AIDS, the second might find this less likely.

Similar considerations apply to the HIV seropositive woman who is not yet pregnant but who wishes to have a baby. There are all sorts of reasons why a woman who is HIV positive would be unwise to become pregnant in the first place, but supposing she is still determined to become pregnant, is it better to have that pregnancy now, while she is in good health and the risks to her or the baby may be lower, or to wait in the hope of some sort of treatment becoming available?

The mother's health is also a consideration for another reason. The mother may herself become ill at some point after the birth of the child. Under these circumstances who will look after the child, what will happen to it? It may even be difficult to find someone to look after the child for short periods while, say, the mother is in hospital. Some of the difficulties involved in the care of the seropositive child and family are covered in Chapter 10.

## Identifying mothers at risk

Early studies of pregnancy and HIV used mothers who were identified either because they had AIDS themselves or because their child developed AIDS. However, today most health workers will want to try to identify the pregnant woman who is infected as early as possible. There are several reasons for this:

- So that the woman can be counselled concerning possible termination.
- So that both the woman and the baby can be monitored in terms of general health.
- So that planning can begin for the care of the child after birth.
- In the future, if a successful treatment can be found, in order that the child can be offered that treatment as soon as it is available.

There are basically two possible approaches to identifying women who are infected:

**Mass screening** Every woman can be offered the HIV antibody test on a routine basis, as is done for syphilis in the UK.

The advantages of this approach are:

- There is less risk of a woman being missed who is at risk without knowing that she is at risk, for instance a woman in an area of low heterosexual prevalence who has been the partner of an infected bisexual man without knowing it.
- Such an approach may offer a better indication of prevalence of the virus amongst pregnant women without known risk factors generally. However, there are other ways of finding this information out. For instance all women identified as at low risk could be asked to provide anonymous non-identifiable samples for antibody testing as well as being offered the test if they wish to have it. This approach also provides a non-threatening way into discussing issues surrounding the test.

The disadvantages of this approach are:

- This book stresses repeatedly the importance of appropriate pre-test counselling and the arguments appear no less compelling when applied to pregnant women. In an area of low general prevalence the resources required to counsel every pregnant woman about the HIV test, and the laboratory costs for the testing, are likely to be enormous and may identify no women who could not have been identified by other means.
- In the population at large there is considerable anxiety about HIV and AIDS. Some women at little or no risk may become highly anxious about the HIV test and suffer unnecessary distress.
- Not every woman offered the test may accept it, at least if pre-test counselling is being carried out properly. It is possible that some women who are most at risk may refuse the test.

**Risk-based identification** The test can be actively offered to women on the basis of risk behaviours identified either in them or in their partners.

The advantages of this approach are:

- It is an efficient use of laboratory and counselling resources.
- Women anxious about their health with no risk will not be unnecessarily worried.

The disadvantages of this approach are:

- It may miss women who do not know that they are at risk. Ideally the partner would also be interviewed, but this is often not possible for a variety of reasons.

- It requires staff to ask all women detailed questions about their risk factors, although assessment of risk factors needs to be a part of pre-test counselling even where mass screening is undertaken.

Which of these approaches is adopted will be likely to depend on the prevalence of the virus in the general heterosexual population. In areas where heterosexual transmission is common, offering the test to all pregnant women as a matter of routine, with appropriate counselling, is likely to be the most useful strategy. Where prevalence is low except in individuals with known risk factors then it is likely to be most sensible to actively offer the test only to women who are identified as being at risk on the basis of their behaviour or that of their partners.

There is, of course, a difference here between actively offering the test to a woman identified as being at risk (i.e. asking her to consider the possibility of having it) and its being available to anyone who wants it on demand. It is clearly important that anyone who thinks she is at risk in the population, however unlikely that may be in terms of her behaviour, should be able to have a test if she wants it.

Where risk-based identification is the method adopted it may be sensible to carry out periodic non-identifiable anonymous testing with consent on samples of women identified as being at low risk to ensure that cases are not being missed.

## Pre-test counselling

Regardless of whether a screening approach or a risk-based identification approach is being used the key element is the assessment of risk. Assessment of risk will be based on an understanding of the situation with respect to spread in that area or in comparable geographical areas at that time. Clearly who is at risk will differ in, for instance, Nairobi and in Stockholm at the time of writing because of the different pattern of spread in the two places.

In a European city with low levels of heterosexual spread the key risk factors would currently be:

- A woman with a history of injecting drug abuse involving sharing syringes with other users.
- A sexual partner or sexual partners within the last few years who is bisexual.

- A sexual partner who engages in, or has engaged in, intravenous drug abuse with syringe-sharing within the last few years.
- A woman with a history of recent blood transfusions in a high prevalence area prior to the introduction of donation screening. Someone who has had blood transfusions in Europe or North America would not normally fall into this category unless they had other reasons to suppose they had received an infected donation. A woman whose partner fell into this group might also be at risk.
- A woman whose partner is an infected haemophilic man.
- A woman who has had sex in an area with high levels of hetero-sexual spread or whose current or recent past partners originate from such areas.

In the above list 'last few years' is something which has to be deter-mined locally because it depends on the estimated time of appearance of significant levels of HIV infection in an area in those practising particular risk behaviours. In the Paddington area of London, for instance, there is no evidence of infection in intravenous drug abusers who ceased sharing syringes before late 1982. Even in 1984 the infection rate was probably less than 2 per cent. So a cut-off point of 1981 for classifying someone as at risk on the basis of sharing syringes locally in Paddington would be expected to be effective.

Ideally, of course, it is helpful to interview the father-to-be as well as the pregnant woman, since it is possible that the woman may not be aware of all the partner's risk behaviours. However, this is not always possible for practical reasons. Where the woman appears uncertain about the answers to some questions it is likely to be useful to make considerable attempts to interview the man concerned. However, even in the absence of an interview with the father-to-be the chances of missing a case currently in, say, London are likely to be extremely low. Most women, for instance, are aware of whether their partner has been an intravenous drug abuser, at least recently.

The sort of questions above should be asked of every pregnant woman in Western Europe in today's climate. However in an area of significant heterosexual spread the considerations are different, the assessment of risk in such areas is covered in Chapter 18.

Pre-test counselling of women identified as being at high risk will follow the pattern set out in Chapter 3. It is, however, important to point out to a woman that no specific medical intervention can be offered to an infected woman except termination. It is also important to discuss the advantages of identification of the infected mother outlined earlier in this chapter. A woman who does not, under any circumstances, want a termination may well decide that she does not want to be tested and that is, of course, her right. Similarly, in countries where termination is either illegal or culturally unacceptable a woman may elect not to be tested.

In areas where screening is offered to all women as a matter of routine the woman is likely to find less in the way of difficulties with insurance and employment since she can say it is a routine part of the antenatal procedures. However should she turn out to be positive she will, of course, have the same problems with these things as anyone else found to be infected.

In areas where screening is offered to all women as routine there is also likely to be another issue involved. It is important to give a woman an estimation of what her personal risk is likely to be based on the questions asked. This is likely to reduce undue anxiety about the likely outcome. Pre-test counselling is also likely to take a shorter time with the lower risk woman since a lot of the issues will not apply directly to her and there is likely to be less discussion about them between counsellor and patient. However, it is important not to skimp on pre-test counselling. Any hospital which introduces routine screening with its attendant counselling load is assuming almost by definition that it is going to pick up seropositive pregnant women whom it could not otherwise easily identify through risk-based identification. This can only mean that it is expected that some apparently low-risk women will turn out to be infected and this in turn means that every pregnant woman needs careful pre-test counselling.

### Counselling for possible termination

The woman who turns out to be seropositive should be offered the possibility of counselling for termination in countries where this is legally acceptable. Where termination is available there should be expertise in counselling about termination for other issues and it is not intended to review here what is a whole area of counselling in itself. Instead the main differences and additions will be covered.

Firstly, in counselling for termination it is important to let the woman decide what she wants to do. This means giving her the information to allow her to make the choice which is right for her. As was noted earlier, the information available at the moment is in many cases unsatisfactory as a basis for the woman to make a decision. It may be, in the near future, that the information will improve. In particular, if it becomes possible to assess which women are most likely to infect their foetuses and which put their own health at risk then it will be possible to offer better advice. At the moment the connection between immunological functioning and/or symptoms and risk to baby and mother's health seems the most likely hypothesis and this can be put to the woman as just that — a hypothesis, but not as absolute truth. This implies that the woman should be given some assessment of her physical health and immunological status if this is available. At the least she needs to know whether there is any sign that she is symptomatic.

When termination is being considered it is important to consider not just the risks of transmission and any possible risks to the mother but also the practicalities. Can the mother cope physically and mentally with a potentially sick child? Is there anyone available to help with the care? Is there anyone available to cope with the child if the mother herself becomes ill or dies? In putting these issues to the woman it is important to maintain some balance in presentation. In many cases the answers to these questions may be 'yes'. The hospital itself, if it has planned ahead for the care of seropositive babies and mothers, will sometimes be able to help and the help which is on offer from the hospital needs to be outlined in a sensible way to the pregnant woman.

It is also important to note that there may be other reasons why a woman may elect to have a termination. In discussing it with a woman it is all too easy to concentrate on the dramatic issue of HIV and forget all the other reasons. Asking the wrong question can easily lead to the wrong answer.

In many cases of termination, while the issue is extremely distressing to the woman concerned, there is at least one ray of hope: many will be able to have another baby later. For the HIV seropositive woman terminating because of HIV this may not, as noted above, be the case, at least in the older woman and possibly in the younger one also.

It is, as has been mentioned elsewhere in this book, difficult to provide a balanced view of complex and frightening issues to a patient. Counselling seropositive women about HIV and termination combines two of the most emotive and difficult issues there are into one nightmare issue for pregnant woman and counsellor. And yet it is important that they both should find their way through the problems and, ultimately, that the woman should take the decision *she* wants about her future.


### The woman who does terminate

The actual termination of pregnancy of an HIV seropositive woman needs considerable tact from medical and nursing staff. They are likely to take a range of precautions associated with infection control. It is important to explain these to the woman before the termination takes place and to discuss them with her. To have a termination is bad enough for many women; to feel in addition that one is a dreadful risk to everyone around is an additional burden that should be avoided.

The woman who elects to terminate needs at least three different strands of counselling, not necessarily from different workers.

### Post-termination counselling

Firstly, the woman is likely to need considerable support and counselling about the termination. Particularly where she has contracted the virus sexually or through drug abuse, she may blame herself. Guilt occurs even in those who have contracted the virus through blood transfusions or other means which they could not conceivably have avoided. The counsellor should try particularly vigorously to help the woman deal with guilt. A woman who caught the virus sexually or through drug abuse has not set out to catch the virus. Sex doesn't cause HIV infection, it is caused by a virus which *happens* to be sexually transmitted. After all, most children probably catch measles by playing with other children; if they didn't play with other children they wouldn't catch it, but no-one would dream of blaming a child for catching measles.

There is also likely to be mourning which needs to be gone through, not just for the child but also for the children the woman may never have. This needs to be handled with sympathy and tact and the woman needs to be given the time and opportunity to grieve.

Although both guilt and mourning reactions are very, very common there is sometimes a feeling that they are 'normal' reactions, with the implication that any woman who doesn't have them must be abnormal and is storing up difficulties for the future. There is no scientific evidence for this hypothesis at all. Forcing women to fit the model of how the counsellor thinks they should feel can be terribly destructive. It is important to take the lead from the woman and to exercise common sense, as always in counselling.

A careful eye has to be kept on the woman to ensure that she does not become depressed or anxious after the termination. If she does then appropriate psychological or psychiatric intervention may be called for. A woman who becomes severely depressed should not be denied medication simply because such a reaction is thought to be normal.

The above issues are likely to be familiar to those who have been involved in counselling around termination in other contexts.

## Counselling about HIV

The issues here are covered in Chapter 4, on post-test counselling.

## Counselling about contraception

Clearly, a woman who is HIV seropositive and has just had a termination is going to need good advice on contraception.

## The woman who doesn't terminate

Many women who find that they are infected with HIV and pregnant will not terminate. They will want to go ahead with the baby. In some cases, of course, the woman will seek advice only when it is too late to have a termination anyway.

For the woman who elects not to terminate the important issues in counselling are likely to be those related to planning for the future. She is going to have a baby and she needs to be in the best psychological and physical state to look after that baby.

For the seropositive woman the period of the pregnancy is an anxious one. She does not know whether her baby will be infected when it is born, and indeed it will probably not be possible in most centres to tell her whether it is infected for at least the first year of life. She does not know whether it will become sick after the birth. This uncertainty is added to worries about her own health. Where the baby's father is also infected she may be worried about his health too.

It is important to provide the woman with as much feedback as possible about her own health and reassurance about the general state of the foetus where this is possible. It is particularly important to give the woman feedback about the results of any routine tests carried out during pregnancy – it is always easy to carry out a test on a pregnant woman and then forget to tell her when the results come back normal.

In terms of forward planning there is much to be discussed with the mother: the planning of regular health monitoring for baby and mother, the planning of arrangements in case the mother becomes sick and the baby has to be looked after, even the planning of ways to ensure that the mother has someone who can look after the baby for short periods to give her a break. The sort of services needed are covered in more detail in Chapter 10, which can provide the basis for forward planning.

Good planning is also essential for the birth itself. It is probable that, in most settings, some degree of extra infection control precautions will be taken with a woman known to be seropositive or thought to be at high risk and the purpose of these precautions and what they will be like should be explained to the mother so that she knows what to expect. There is no reason why special precautions should be inconsistent with childbirth being a positive experience for the mother, but it does take planning and forethought.

## The woman planning pregnancy

Sometimes women seek advice before they become pregnant. For the woman known to be infected or at high risk this can be an opportunity to get help and advice in deciding what to do. More often the issue of pregnancy will come up in other contexts where women at risk or infected are being counselled. This is, clearly, a crucial discussion between counsellor and woman.

It is not uncommon for a woman to feel that she has been at risk in the past but that that risk has now been eliminated. For instance in the following case:

> Jane was 28 years old. During her early twenties she had spent some time in Amsterdam and gone through a period of experimentation with drugs including some experience of injecting drugs. Never actually dependent on drugs, she had eventually drifted away from their use and had now got married and wanted to start a family. She had always used someone else's syringe when injecting drugs and, in the light of the publicity about AIDS, sought advice as to what she should do.

This sort of case involving ex-users is not uncommon. The first issue is to consider with her whether she should have the test. In her case there would be very considerable advantages since she has eliminated her risk factor (although it is important to ensure that she has no other risk factors — her husband doesn't use drugs currently, for instance). These advantages would be part of pre-test counselling. However it is also important to ensure that the whole of pre-test counselling is covered. With luck she may turn out to be negative and can get pregnant without worrying, on the other hand the luck may be the other way, her limited drug injecting has all been high risk, she might just be infected and it is important not to downplay this. She needs to be prepared for both a positive and a negative result if she decides to be tested.

Suppose that Jane was still taking drugs and sharing syringes and wanted to get pregnant: what would the situation be then? Clearly quite apart from questions about HIV, there are questions about the wisdom of someone injecting drugs becoming pregnant at all. However, looking only for the moment at the issues around HIV, there are obviously a number of problems.

Firstly, there is no point in testing her, finding her to be negative and her then continuing to share a syringe. Ideally she will give up drugs, but that *is* the ideal — she may get pregnant and still go back to drugs. Clearly from all points of view if she does decide to get pregnant the counsellor is going to have to counsel her that (i) she should cease drug use, but that (ii) if she does use drugs she should not inject, or, if she cannot follow this advice, (iii) that she should not share. Handling this mixed message is difficult, but it is one which must be handled. It must be handled because it is realistic. Drug users, whatever their good intentions, come under pressure both from their habit and from their friends to keep on taking drugs.

Clearly under these circumstances the woman could be tested now but if the result was negative it would be wise for her to leave at least six months of sharing-free time before having another test and *then* deciding on whether to get pregnant.

The third sort of case is the woman who knows that her sexual partner is infected:

Zara was 35 years of age. Her haemophiliac husband had known that he was infected for three years. He was well. She had, herself, already had a test and this was negative. When they had sex she used dual contraception, she had elected to stay on the pill and also to use a condom. She now wanted to have a child.

This sort of situation is also not uncommon. The difficulty is, obviously, that in the process of getting pregnant Zara may manage to get infected at the same time. There is also the question of whether her husband might get ill in the future, but they had thought that one through. One safe alternative is for Zara to have artificial insemination by donor (AID). While this looks like a good option few women actually want to take it. They usually want to have the baby of the man in their life, not a donor's baby, however anonymous and forgettable the 'other man's' part in the procedure might be. At this stage it is worth going through the issues about nurture versus nature — a child is psychologically more the offspring of the parents who bring it up than it ever is a product of the chromosomes that built it. A child born via AID will still be *their* child. Even so, many women find this line of argument an emotionally unsatisfying one.

In this sort of case there is often a key issue. For many women whose husband is sick or may become sick the bearing of a child fills a special place. If the husband dies the child will be a living reminder of their relationship, something of the relationship will live on, a small thread of immortality for the husband and what they had together. AID just can't meet this need.

Discussion of the risks involved in getting pregnant in such cases often involves some degree of 'bargaining':

'Suppose I only have sex with him when I am ovulating?'
'Can't I be artificially inseminated with my husband's semen?'
'Can't you filter the semen somehow? Or test it to make sure it's safe?'

The answer is that it is not possible to remove the risk of infection and it is clear that there is a risk of infection even from a single exposure to infected semen, however that semen is introduced. At the moment there is no way of ensuring that semen is safe (other than making sure the producer of the semen is not himself infected) or of removing the virus from semen. The best advice for Zara was that she could not become pregnant by her husband without at least some degree of risk of infection.

She might just possibly reduce that risk slightly by restricting un-protected intercourse to her fertile period, though what difference this would make, if any, is hard to assess. There is no evidence that being artificially inseminated with her husband's semen would confer an advantage, it might mean fewer occasions of exposure but on the other hand there have been a number of cases of infection of women through infected semen donations (admittedly involving the same donor).

At the end of the day, however good the counselling, some women who are infected or at risk will decide to become pregnant. Probably a larger number still, especially intravenous drug abusing women, will not make a decision at all. What they will elect to do is to 'take a chance', they will not use contraception or, if they are currently using contraception, will begin to become more erratic in its use, placing a difficult decision in the lap of the gods. Sooner or later the gods usually decide in favour of pregnancy.

Deciding to become pregnant even though one is infected may seem an incredible decision. However, it is a very human one. Many women desperately want to have a child. While the counsellor should probably try hard to dissuade a woman who is infected from becoming pregnant, both for her own sake and for that of the child, ultimately it is the woman who will decide. If she decides in favour of becoming pregnant then the counsellor needs to accept that situation and get on with helping the woman to make the best of the situation.

As noted above, for the woman who decides that, in spite of being infected, she wishes to become pregnant, there is then a decision about timing. Should she have a pregnancy now, while she is well, or should she wait for medical science to come to her rescue at some indeterminate point in the future? It is an issue which can only be talked through in the light of the limited evidence presented earlier.

## Overview

The issues surrounding pregnancy are amongst the most difficult in HIV counselling. The situation is made even more difficult currently by our lack of knowledge about certain key issues concerning risks to mother and child. As knowledge improves, our ability to help our patients to make informed decisions about their lives is likely to increase. However, it is hard to see, in the absence of effective treatments for HIV infection, that this area is ever going to be an easy one in which to work.

## References

Berrebi, A., Puel, J., Tricoire, J., Grandjean, H., Herne, P. and Pontonnier, G. (1988)'The Influence of pregnancy on the evolution of HIV infection.' Data presented at the IVth International conference on AIDS, Stockholm, June 1988.

Braddick, M., Datta, P., Embree, J., Ndinga-Achola, J., Kreiss, J. and Plummer, F.A. (1988) 'Progression of HIV following pregnancy.' Data presented at the IVth International Conference on AIDS, Stockholm, June 1988.

Ciraru-Vigneron, N., Lung, R.N., Bercau, A., Sauvanet, E., Bitton, C., Brunner, C., Buizard, B., Lisautier, J.L. and Ravina, J.H. (1988), 'Prospective study for HIV Infection amoung high risk women?' Data presented at the IVth International Conference on AIDS, Stockholm, June 1988.

Friedland, G.M. and Klein, R.S. (1987) Transmission of the Human Immuno-deficiency Virus. *New Eng J Med*, **317**, pp.1125–35.

Lapointe, N., Michand, J., Pekovic, D., Chausseau, J. and Dupuy, J.M. (1985) 'Transplacental transmission of HTLV III virus.' *New Eng J Med*, **312**, pp.1325–6.

McCallum L.R., France A.J., Jones M.E., Steel, C.M., Burns, S.M. and Brettle, R.P. (1988) 'The effects of pregnancy on the progression of HIV Infection.' Data presented at the IVth International Conference on AIDS, Stockholm, June 1988.

Peckham, C. (1988) 'Consequences of HIV Infection in pregnancy.' Results from the European Collaborative Study. Data presented at the IVth International Conference of AIDS, Stockholm, June 1988.

Schaeffes, A., Grosch-Woernes, I., Friedmann, W., Kunze, R., Mielke, M. and Jiueuez, E. (1988) 'The effects of pregnancy on the natural course of HIV

Infection'. Data presented at the IVth International Conference on AIDS, Stockholm, June 1988.

Scott, G.B., Fischl, M.A., Klimas, N., Fletcher, M.A. Dickinson, G.M., Levine, R.S. and Parks, W.P. (1985) 'Mothers of infants with the Acquired Immunodeficiency Syndrome.' *J Am Med Ass*, **253**, pp.363—366.

Sprecher, S., Soumenkoff, G., Puissant, F. and Degueldre, M. (1986) 'Vertical transmission of HIV in a 15 week fetus'. *Lancet*, **ii**, pp.288—289.

# Chapter 10

# Paediatric HIV Infection

JACQUELINE MOK

## Introduction

Since AIDS was recognised in children in 1982, the number of cases known to the Center for Disease Control (CDC) in Atlanta has increased. At the end of 1986, 394 children with AIDS were reported to the CDC. This number only represents the severe end of the clinical spectrum, so that an unknown number of infected children exist. Children who are asymptomatic although infected will present problems in management.

In the United Kingdom (February 1987), only 12 cases of AIDS have been described in children under 14 years of age. With the increase in heterosexual spread of the disease, women have become infected. In Edinburgh, 50—60 per cent of the injecting drug user population are seropositive for HIV. Since one-third of IDUs are women of child-bearing age, babies have been born to IDUs. Concern about the management of these infants has led to a special clinic being established in January 1986; this chapter reports on the experiences gained in the care of babies born to seropositive mothers.

## Paediatric high-risk groups

Seventy-five per cent of paediatric AIDS cases have acquired the infection from their mothers. Maternal risk activity includes intravenous drug abuse and sexual promiscuity, while other risk factors are being sexual partners of men in high-risk groups and having sex in countries with a high prevalence of heterosexual HIV infection. Some children have been infected through blood and blood products.

The possible routes for virus transmission in children infected from their mothers are:

- Transplacental passage.
- Through the birth canal during delivery.
- Postnatally via breast milk or close mother–child contact.

Clear evidence has been presented to favour the first route, i.e. that perinatal HIV infection is a congenital virus infection. However, the exact risk of perinatal transmission from an infected mother to her infant is not known, with studies reporting transmission rates from 0 per cent (0/3) to 65 per cent (13/20). Transmission rates were highest when the woman had previously delivered a symptomatic child.

### Antenatal screening

The current practice in most antenatal clinics is that screening for HIV antibody takes place only on clinical grounds, with the woman's informed consent and following counselling.

Obstetricians will test the woman who is believed to belong to a high-risk group, or if she is the sexual partner of a man in a high-risk group. Failure of the woman to disclose her risk activities, or lack of suspicion on the doctor's part, may result in some women having unidentified HIV infection.

Proponents for routine antenatal screening argue that pregnancy accelerates HIV disease in the mother, and quote the high risk of transmission of HIV to the foetus. It is thought that identification of an infected woman would allow termination of pregnancy to take place. However, most women are infected through intravenous drug abuse and it is debatable whether this group will present early enough in pregnancy for termination to be considered. The more common experience is for these women to arrive in labour!

Where there is believed to be a high incidence of heterosexual spread of HIV (e.g. in Edinburgh), then it might be acceptable to screen routinely during antenatal care. It is hoped that knowledge of the prevalence of HIV amongst a defined population such as in an antenatal clinic will help towards the planning of resources. If such a policy is adopted, then it is imperative that resources for pre-test as well as post-test counselling are readily available. There is no place for 'slipping blood off' for HIV antibody testing without the patient's consent or knowledge that this has been done.

## The HIV seropositive woman

Early reports from the United States suggested that pregnancy accelerates the progression of AIDS in women. However, the study populations included women with more severe HIV infection, or women who were identified following the birth of a child with AIDS or ARC. The results should not be extrapolated to all HIV seropositive women, although in the absence of other evidence, the current advice is against pregnancy, or that termination of pregnancy should be considered. Follow-up studies of seropositive women following both termination and childbirth are in progress, and it is hoped that questions on the effect of pregnancy will be answered.

While clear evidence indicates intrauterine infection as the most likely route, the exact risk of virus transmission from infected mother to foetus is not yet known. Intrauterine transmission has been shown to occur as early as the 15th week of pregnancy, but little is known of the factors which may contribute to virus transfer. One case is known where only one of non-identical twins was infected, suggesting that selective virus transfer occurred. Where women had already delivered a child with AIDS, the risk in subsequent pregnancies was reported as 65 per cent. Again, this high risk of virus transmission probably does not apply to all seropositive women, but no other data have been produced. The risks of pregnancy causing deterioration of disease, and of intrauterine infection of the infant, can only be ascertained after careful prospective studies which are only just under way. Until more is known, it is prudent to advise a seropositive woman not to become pregnant, or to offer termination of pregnancy should she be seen early enough for this to be considered.

Some seropositive women have chosen to have a child despite adequate counselling. In these circumstances, the obstetrician and midwife should be prepared for the delivery of the infant. Although some centres still deliver these women by elective Caesarean section, no evidence exists to suggest that this route avoids infection. As perinatal HIV is acquired congenitally, there is no justification in elective Caesarean section. During delivery, protective clothing should be worn because of the copious amounts of amniotic fluid and blood present. These should include water-resistant gowns, gloves, and masks. Goggles or safety spectacles should be worn if there is a risk of eye splash. All equipment required for the delivery should be available in the room.

The paediatrician should be informed of the impending delivery. Resuscitation of the infant, if required, should take place in the same room, with specially identified equipment which can then be sterilised.

Mouth suction should be performed with a large syringe attached to the mucous extractor. The infant should be nursed in the same room as mother and again, because of the presence of blood and body fluids, nursing staff should wear gloves and waterproof gowns when handling the infant. If the infant requires special neonatal care, this should be given with isolation facilities and dedicated equipment. While clearer data are awaited, the current advice is that seropositive women should not breast-feed their infants because of the isolation of HIV from the non-cellular fraction of breast milk and one case of possible transmission from mother to infant via breast milk. However, a general policy advising against breast-feeding could have adverse consequences for infants in developing countries.

### Definition of HIV infection in children

Detection of HIV antibody in an adult or older child is a sensitive and specific indicator of HIV infection, since in the majority of such patients, virus culture is positive. The presence of passively transferred maternal antibody in young infants tends to limit the usefulness of a positive antibody test in this age group. Although the Edinburgh experience is that infants lose maternal antibody from 9 to 12 months of age, other centres have reported persistence of antibody up to 15 months. For this reason, infants below this age with a risk of perinatal infection present difficulties with definition. It has been argued that the only definitive evidence for infection in a young infant is the identification of HIV in blood or other tissues. However, the sensitivity of the culture system may be low so that a negative virus culture does not necessarily exclude infection. More specific antibody tests, or antigen testing, are now being used in adults, and may prove helpful in young children. At present, careful documentation of clinical signs and immunological abnormalities on a longitudinal basis remain important tools in defining paediatric HIV infection.

### Routine surveillance

As symptoms and signs of HIV infection do not usually occur in early infancy, and until more is known about the exact risk of virus transmission from mother to child, all infants who have had perinatal exposure to the virus should be considered at risk of HIV infection. These infants should be monitored closely for clinical and immunological abnormalities.

At the same time, the mothers and infants should be allowed to attend normal child welfare clinics for weighing and general advice on infant care issues. No special precautions are necessary in the handling of these infants if all health care staff are conscientious in good hygiene practices, so that all spillages of blood and body fluids from every baby are treated as if potentially infectious.

## General advice on daily activities

### Personal hygiene

This means thorough handwashing after handling body secretions. Those who are not the baby's natural mother may wish to use household gloves when changing nappies, especially when the skin on the hands is broken.

Heavily soiled sheets, clothing and Terry nappies should be washed separately at a high temperature. While disposable nappies are convenient, they are not absolutely essential as the virus is destroyed in a hot wash. Soiled disposable nappies should be burnt or double-wrapped in polythene bags. No special disinfectants are necessary for either the bath or toilet.

Although HIV is not transmitted through sharing toothbrushes or combs, it is good practice never to share these implements. Toys which a baby chews should, if possible, be kept just for the baby and should be washed regularly with hot water and washing-up liquid.

### Feeding

The baby's bottles should be sterilised in the normal way, with cups, plates and cutlery washed as usual with hot water and washing-up liquid. If the infant vomits, soils or wets, the spillage should be washed off the skin or clothes with soap and water. For these reasons, carers may prefer to wear a waterproof apron when feeding or changing the baby.

### Other activities

The infected infant or child should be allowed to lead a normal life, and be treated no differently from others. Sport and outdoor activities should be permitted, including swimming, provided there are no medical contra-indications. There is no danger of anyone acquiring HIV infection from swimming pools, although the child with AIDS may have to be protected from acquiring other infections by swimming.

Children who are healthy carriers of HIV should be permitted to attend youth clubs, discos and other organisations.

### School

No case of HIV infection has been transmitted in the school setting. Children who are HIV carriers or AIDS sufferers should attend normal schools if their health permits. Staff in educational establishments should be sensitive to the child's and family's need for privacy and confidentiality. The number of people who need to know should be limited to those who will be dealing directly with the child, so that precautions can be taken to safeguard the child.

Some families have, understandably, chosen to withhold the child's HIV status from school staff because of the risk of that information being passed on unscrupulously. Such situations have led to the infected child or other children being withdrawn from school.

### Trauma

Some schools have adopted a general policy where a pair of household gloves are available in the first-aid box, so that all children are treated the same when blood or body secretions are handled. Teachers have to be reassured that gloves are only required when dealing with large amounts of spillage — so that no child is left bleeding while gloves are sought! Splashes of blood or secretions should be washed immediately with copious amounts of water and soap. The wound should then be covered with a waterproof dressing until healed.

## The child who is potentially immunocompromised

### Immunisation

The risks of vaccinating children with HIV infection are not yet defined, but potential risks may exist if such children are not vaccinated. Measles infection amongst immune-depressed children is usually severe and fatal.

Concern has been raised about the immunisation of infected infants, owing to the immunological abnormalities which have been reported in symptomatic children. In theory, the antigenic stimulation produced by vaccination as well as the replication of live, attenuated vaccine viruses may produce serious adverse reactions. There have also been reports of abnormal responses to tetanus and pneumovac immunisation

in children with HIV infection. On the other hand, children have received routine immunisations prior to AIDS being diagnosed, without
any adverse reactions. The current recommendations are that infected,
symptomatic children should not receive live virus or bacterial vaccines
(oral polio, measles, mumps, rubella, BCG). These children should be
immunised with diphtheria, pertussis and tetanus (DPT) and inactivated
polio vaccine. Following significant exposure to measles or varicella,
hyperimmune gammaglobulin should be administered. Children who
remain asymptomatic should be given DPT and inactivated polio vaccine
(because the mother may be immunocompromised), followed by measles
vaccine at 15–18 months if they remain immunologically intact.

In the case of infants with perinatal exposure, the mother's hepatitis
B status should be checked and the infant given hepatitis B immuno-
globulin and vaccine if necessary.

### Acute infections

HIV seropositive children, although clinically well, could have immunological dysfunction. This means that any acute illness could run a
protracted course. Carers should be warned that medical attention
should be sought sooner rather than later. The child should also be
kept away from known cases of measles or chicken pox.

### Day and foster care

Every child should be considered on an individual basis, with careful
weighing up of risks and benefits before he is placed in day or foster
care. In perinatally exposed children, the mother is usually infected so
that her own health may not permit her to look after her child. Also, as
many of the mothers' risk activities include intravenous drug abuse,
there are other psychosocial problems which mean that the child has
to be placed in care. Thus the benefits are obvious; the risks of the
child acquiring potentially fatal infections are greater than him trans-
mitting HIV to other children.

Foster parents are carefully chosen, and should be well informed of
the very low risks involved in looking after an infected child. They
should also understand the implications of immune-suppression, i.e.
regarding immunisations and otherwise trivial illnesses. A high
standard of hygiene is encouraged. One particular foster mother carries
with her a 'handy bag', where she keeps a pair of household gloves,
several disposable cloths, polythene bags, dressings and plasters so

that she has everything to hand in case of emergencies. Staff in children's centres should think about having such an 'emergency pack', especially if children are taken on an outing.

Foster parents and day carers should be warned that it is not always possible to identify a child's HIV status, and that good hygiene practices should be performed at all times for all children who come under their care. Other parents who use the same facilities should be educated in a general way about the possibility of an unidentified HIV carrier being placed. That way, members of the public are made aware of the problem without the need to identify any one child or family.

## Adoption

### All infants

The question now asked by medical advisers of adoption agencies is whether all infants being placed for adoption should be routinely tested for HIV antibody, along with tests for syphilis. As already discussed, the HIV antibody test is unhelpful in the definition of infection in young infants because of the presence of maternal antibody. A positive antibody test in an infant only implies maternal HIV infection, with an unknown risk to the infant. Many centres report the persistence of maternal antibody up to the age of 15 months, and this could mean unnecessary delay in placing an infant. A negative antibody test in the absence of any maternal risk factors is more meaningful in young infants, although infants have been reported to be seronegative but virus positive. These facts would make HIV antibody testing of very little use for the purposes of adoption, and I would not recommend routine HIV antibody testing on all infants placed for adoption.

### High risk infants

Often, infants are placed for adoption because of psychosocial reasons. In many cases, the mother's habits and life style are considered to have put the infant at high risk of HIV infection. Where possible, the mother's HIV status should be determined, as current tests are more reliable in an adult. If the mother cannot be traced, then the infant may have to be tested and the results interpreted in the light of the above discussion. Tests of immune function may be more useful. All this will cause unavoidable delay in placement, especially if the prospective adopters wish to be assured that the child is not infected.

*Infants of known HIV infected mothers*

The present state of knowledge does not permit the risk of perinatal transmission of HIV to be quoted with absolute certainty. While careful prospective studies are under way, there are now infants born to mothers with HIV infection who have been freed for adoption.

Prospective adoptive parents have to be informed of the uncertain future for the child, as regards HIV infection. As mentioned earlier, the presence of maternal HIV antibody makes this test unhelpful in infants under 15 months of age. Identification of the virus would be definitive evidence of infection, but currently available culture systems are not sensitive enough, so that a negative virus culture does not necessarily rule out infection. Specific antibody tests and antigen tests have not yet been evaluated in children and infants. Also, little is known about the pattern of HIV antibody production in young infants who may have been infected *in utero*, nor have reservoirs of infection been clearly identified.

Should the infant be placed in an adoptive family, the parents ought to be counselled on issues of general care as well as specific issues. At worst, they will have to cope with a child with chronic ill health including neurological deterioration. This will affect other children in the family who will also need support. Finally, the death of the infected child will necessitate bereavement support.

On the other hand, the infected child could be an asymptomatic, healthy carrier. When he is old enough to understand, he will have to be told the implications of his HIV status, and helped to cope with adolescence, social pressures and relationships. If the present prejudices against HIV infected individuals prevail, then there is the risk of the whole family being ostracised from the local community.

## HIV education in schools

The captive audience in schools provides an ideal opportunity for informing youngsters of the facts about HIV infection, and the precautions one can take to prevent being infected. The subject of AIDS should be taught to schoolchildren in context with health education and social education as well as sex education. All staff at primary and secondary schools should be sufficiently well informed about HIV infection to be able to answer children's questions appropriately, however and whenever they arise. At the same time, staff will have to re-evaluate their own attitudes and prejudices against promiscuity, homo-sexuality and drug abuse. It is hoped that an enlightened teaching staff will mean a more tolerant society as schoolchildren grow up, with less stigma surrounding HIV infected children.

## Suggested reading

ACIP (1986) 'Immunization of children infected with human T-lympho-trophic virus type III/lymphadenopathy associated virus' *MMWR*, **35** pp.595−606.

Epstein, L.G., Sharer, L.R., *et al.* (1986) 'Neurologic manifestations of human immunodeficiency virus infection in children' *Pediatrics* **78** pp.678−87.

Rogers, M.F. (1985) 'AIDS in children: a review of the clinical, epidemiologic and public health aspects' *Pediatric Infectious Disease*, **4** pp.230−6.

Rubinstein, A. (1986) 'Schooling for children with acquired immune deficiency syndrome' *Journal of Pediatrics* **109** pp.242−4.

Shannon, K.M. and Ammann, A.J. (1985) 'Acquired immune deficiency syndrome in childhood' *Journal of Paediatrics* **106** pp.332−42.

# Chapter 11

# The Worried Well

JOHN GREEN

The term 'worried well' is one that has undergone a shift in meaning. Originally it simply meant someone who was worried about AIDS but was untested and had no symptoms. Today it is used to refer to someone who is excessively worried about AIDS or HIV infection, despite being known to be uninfected or being objectively at little or no risk.

To most clinics offering the test the worried well individual is a familiar sight. Often highly anxious, they seem to have little to worry about in reality:

> Mary was a 58-year-old woman who had been celibate for six years since her husband died. Following a mild bout of illness, probably influenza, she became worried that she had contracted HIV infection. She worked in a busy shop and felt sure that she had been in contact with someone who was infected and that they had passed on the virus to her by giving her money with 'body fluids' on it, possibly someone had licked their fingers before giving her a bank-note. She worried about HIV for much of every day, it was seldom far from her thoughts and she interpreted every minor illness as the result of AIDS. At the time of coming for testing she had already put her affairs in order and was coming for final confirmation of what she already 'knew' to be a fact, that she was infected and would soon die.

Sometimes individuals who are worried well do have some very small theoretical risk of being infected:

> Jim had travelled widely on business. He had, on two occasions over the past three years, had sex with a prostitute in New York in a hotel; on both occasions there had been some oral sex first but intercourse had been with a condom. Over the past year, with all the information about AIDS in the media, he had become convinced not only that he had become infected with HIV but that he had infected his wife and also his children with HIV. At the time of presenting he was in a thoroughly wretched state of anxiety and depression.

Careful examination of the cases of those who are worried well shows that they fall into several overlapping categories.

### Misunderstanders

These are individuals who have simply misunderstood the way in which the virus can be transmitted. In most countries health education campaigns run by governments and voluntary groups find themselves up against misinformation in some sections of the media and against the rumours which exist in just about any community about dramatic events which are affecting that community. Generally such individuals can overcome their fears with clear, precise information and are much reassured by a discussion of the issues.

### Hypochondriacs

In every age and in every place there are people who worry about their health to the extent that they believe that they have whatever disease happens to be fashionable or attracting attention at that time. It is interesting to match up what is being written about in the newspapers or covered on television against what people feel they have at any given time. In the past few years there have been bursts of people with food allergies of various sorts, with post-viral syndrome, with legionnaires disease, even with problems associated with strip-lighting following publicity on these problems. This is not to say that these problems are not real ones, nor that some people do not suffer terribly from them. But undoubtedly many people present at hospitals utterly convinced that they have these problems when, in fact, they do not.

It is likely that many people in the population feel generally unwell for much of the time. They seek for an explanation of this, initially from their doctor, later, when he or she cannot help, through their own reading and research. They are often extremely well-informed about the illness which they feel they have. Sometimes if they are convinced that they do not have one illness they will switch to another:

Alan, a gay man, became convinced that he was infected with HIV despite repeated blood tests which were negative. After many sessions of counselling he was finally convinced that he was not infected. After the end of the treatment he contacted the hospital to say that he was sure that he had contracted legionnaire's disease.

### The guilty

A surprising number of people in the population suffer from chronic unresolved guilt. In particular, guilt about past sexual behaviour is very common. Few of these people seek any sort of counselling or advice about their feelings but the appearance of AIDS has provided a focus for many of them, something concrete to match up to their guilt:

> In 1981 Peter had had a brief affair with a woman at work at a time when his marriage was going through a bad patch. He felt her to be promiscuous at the time and had vaguely disapproved of her. He had terminated their relationship. He had always felt very guilty about this affair and had striven to be a model husband when it ended. The woman had subsequently moved to another firm. Recently quite by chance he heard that she had become seriously ill. He immediately thought of AIDS and gradually became more and more convinced that he had caught HIV from her and had passed this on to his wife and, probably, to his children. The family dog had been unwell and he half-wondered whether he might not have passed the virus to the dog through some cut on his hands, even though he knew this to be ridiculous.

There is little doubt that the guilty form a very large proportion of the worried well.

## AIDS as an addition to psychiatric conditions

A small proportion of the worried well turn out to be individuals suffering from psychiatric conditions with concerns about AIDS as a more or less incidental feature. Worries about AIDS occasionally appear as features of schizophrenic delusions or as part of a paranoid delusional system. Rarely they appear as a monosymptomatic delusion.

More commonly they appear as features of either depressive illnesses or as part of obsessional states, particularly those obsessions concerned with cleaning. The issues of both depression and obsessions are covered in more detail in Chapter 12.

It is, however, worth separating out those worried well in whom AIDS has become incorporated into a pre-existing psychiatric condition from those frequent cases in which other types of worried well patients have, as a result of their concerns, become depressed, or anxious or obsessional.

In a busy clinic dealing with individuals who are very ill with HIV-related conditions it is easy to ignore the worried well and to treat them as a nuisance. In fact a disturbingly high proportion of them turn out to be quite depressed or highly distressed. Worries about AIDS can often produce levels of depression and anxiety far higher than those seen in individuals with AIDS itself. Suicidal ideation is not uncommon and suicide attempts, some successful, are far from uncommon.

One of the difficulties with the worried well is that as a result of their fears they tend to become anxious. Anxiety and depression themselves can produce symptoms which appear to the patient to be those associated with AIDS. Fatigue, sweating, anorexia and weight loss, diarrhoea, a feeling of malaise, nausea, breathlessness as a result of hyperventilation, all these are not uncommon in the anxious depressed patient. These natural sensations are a confirmation of the patient's worst fears.

### Dealing with the worried well

Pre-test counselling is likely to be much the same with the worried well as with those who are objectively at higher risk. It is likely to be briefer in those who have no risk. The level of risk should be established early on in pre-test counselling, of course. The time taken for pre-test counselling is likely to be less simply because some of the issues discussed will not be particularly relevant to the person with no risk. They will not, for instance, require a detailed discussion of some risk behaviours because they simply do not engage in them.

On the other hand it is important not to skimp on pre-test counselling for several reasons. Firstly, good pre-test counselling is an educative process which will prepare the patient to understand why he is not at risk. Secondly, someone who is at low risk at the moment may, of course, start to engage in higher risk behaviour in the future and pre-test counselling provides an opportunity to educate. Thirdly, it will prepare him to understand the blood test results when they come back. Fourthly, because pre-test counselling in itself serves to reassure patients that they are not at risk it reduces the anxiety level of the patient while they wait for the test results. Finally, it is worth bearing in mind that being worried about HIV does not in itself serve as a protection against getting it. Some people who appear highly anxious do, in fact, have some degree of risk. A few of them will turn out to be infected.

At pre-test counselling a few people who had misunderstood will elect not to be tested. However, by the time they come for testing most worried well have become so anxious that they elect to go on and be tested.

At post-test counselling the counsellor is almost certain to be holding a negative test result for the worried well patient. It is important at this stage to discuss the patient's worries with him in detail and to try to reassure him that the test result is accurate. This can only be done by relating the negative result to the fact that he has been at no risk or at minimal risk. With many worried well patients the test result in itself does not serve to reassure more than temporarily. In most countries with testing facilities there are numbers of worried well individuals who travel from test site to test site seeking repeated blood tests simply because they do not believe the results they have been given.

It is important to discuss with anyone whose result is negative any risk behaviours they may actually have and to seek to ensure that these are reduced. It is also important to ensure that those who are unnecessarily worried now understand the true facts about the virus.

At post-test counselling it is also important to try to assess how likely it is that the patient is actually reassured. If he is not reassured it is important to assess whether he has actually understood the information he has been given.

For patients who still appear anxious about HIV even after counselling, and even after they have understood the facts about AIDS, it is particularly important to try to discover the reason why they remain worried. The patient should be assessed for anxiety, depression and obsessions and carefully questioned about past contact with psychiatric services in a way that does not imply that the counsellor feels that the patient is mentally ill.

At this stage there are two choices available to the counsellor. Either he can undertake to try to help the patient himself, or he can refer the patient on for specialist help. The decision is likely to be made on the basis of the level of anxiety and depression, on the basis of the counsellor's confidence that he can deal with the problem, and on the amount of time the counsellor has. Clearly, a patient who is very depressed or actively suicidal is in need of specialist help as a matter of urgency.

It is important to any counsellor to have good mental health facilities as a back-up. Referring on worried-well patients in need of psychiatric support appropriately is an important skill for the counsellor. It is important to be frank with the patient and to stress that he appears anxious and depressed (if he does) and that sometimes these feelings can make it difficult to accept the results of a blood test, but that if they can be dealt with the patient will feel better and, hopefully, stop worrying about HIV.

Patients who have come thinking they have AIDS are sometimes rather unhappy about the suggestion that they should be referred for psychiatric help. It needs tact on the part of the counsellor and, if they do decide to be referred, it needs knowledge of HIV and tact on the part of the mental health worker who takes the referral. Sometimes the counsellor may feel it best to see a patient a few times himself until he feels that the patient has built up sufficient trust to agree to being referred. It also helps greatly if the referral can be made to a mental health professional whom the counsellor can vouch for and discuss with the patient by name.

If the counsellor decides to try to help the patient himself he will be aiming to use the same sort of skills which are used in dealing with anxiety, depression and obsessional behaviours and thoughts in the HIV positive patient. The types of approaches which can be used are dealt with in detail in Chapter 4.

In addition to dealing with any anxiety or depression, discussing the patient's worries with him can be of considerable value. In particular, those who are guilty about some past sexual episode may want to talk over the issue with the counsellor to try to find some resolution in their own minds. This can be a very valuable process but it is always important to keep an eye on the patient and to make sure that he is, in fact, becoming less worried or guilty. If he is just using the service as a prop but not making any progress the counsellor is still going to need to pick up the issue and to think in terms of referral.

Individuals who are worried well can often be frustratingly difficult to deal with. However it is surprising just how successful simple interventions can be with those who are not suffering from major depressive symptoms or other major psychiatric conditions:

Anthony was a 36-year-old man who had no previous psychiatric history. Following the break-up of his marriage three years before he had gone through a very bad period. He had stopped going out socially, his only social contact being at work. He lived alone and spent most of his leisure hours reading or watching the television. He had had one brief affair with a woman he met in a pub. It had been an unpleasant experience because they had split up under strained circumstances with her accusing him of being an 'inadequate person'. He had not liked her and had only had sex with her for the company. Later he had noticed her in the pub with several different men, and formed the view that she was 'promiscuous'. Shortly after breaking up with her he began to worry about AIDS and this anxiety built up until he was thinking about the issue most of the time.

On assessment Anthony was sleeping a normal amount, eating well and, though he felt life was 'pointless', he denied suicidal intentions. He did not enjoy much in his life but he did have a few things which brought him pleasure. He felt himself, accurately, to be mildly depressed. He was also anxious. When he thought about AIDS he sometimes felt rather dizzy and, while he did not have panic attacks during the day, he was troubled by vivid and unpleasant dreams and sometimes woke in the night sweating heavily.

He was somewhat reassured by the information he was given about AIDS. However, he still continued to worry that he might have it, despite realising rationally that this was not so. He benefited from discussion of his life with the counsellor. The counsellor also taught him relaxation skills which he found very helpful in reducing his physical anxiety symptoms. At the same time he was encouraged to increase the level of pleasurable activity in his life. The counsellor and the patient drew up a list of activities which he enjoyed and could carry out, including visiting places he enjoyed going to. At the same time he began to build up his social life, inviting people at work round for dinner, taking every opportunity to go out with them and looking up old friends he had lost contact with.

His level of anxiety began to reduce and he became more cheerful and less depressed. He also began to feel that he was coping much better with his life. After six sessions he reported that he only thought about AIDS occasionally and was enjoying life much more. It was agreed that he would continue to work on his own but come back in three months for follow-up. In the intervening period he could come back if he felt that things were not going well. At follow-up he reported that he was continuing to feel better, that he thought about AIDS infrequently and that when he did think of AIDS it no longer worried him as much as it used to. He had begun to go out with a woman with whom he got on very well. He had high expectations of the relationship and these seemed to be justified from his account.

Sometimes it is difficult in the middle of the HIV/AIDS epidemic not to feel rather resentful about the time and energy the worried well can absorb. However they, like those who have HIV-related diseases, do have a real problem and like those with the disease itself they have a right to the efforts of the counsellor to try to reduce distress and to promote well-being.

# Chapter 12

# Dealing with Anxiety and Depression

JOHN GREEN

## DEALING WITH ANXIETY

Some degree of anxiety is virtually universal in individuals who have a positive antibody test result. Even for someone who has adjusted to being infected there are likely to be occasions when he becomes anxious, perhaps when a friend dies of AIDS or when he reads something disturbing about AIDS in the newspaper or when he feels that he is not well. However, anxiety can be long-lasting and intense and it can make people's lives unpleasant. Since anxiety can usually be reduced with the right intervention it is important to assess for it and to intervene if anxiety is long-lasting or if there are frequent bouts of anxiety.

Anxiety has four different components, a somatic (physical) component, a cognitive component (changes in thought patterns), an affective component (changes in feelings) and a behavioural component. Particularly in someone who is only mildly anxious, one or more of these components may be missing. Moreover the actual pattern of anxiety differs quite a bit from person to person. People who are very anxious usually, but not always, have elements of all four components.

Table 12.1 shows the symptoms of anxiety. It is important with all seropositives to check whether they have these symptoms and how frequent and intense they are.

Looking at the physical symptoms of anxiety it is clear that many of them are, individually, seen in physical illnesses. For instance, individuals with pneumocystis also show shortness of breath. Those with meningitis have headaches. Those with opportunistic infections of the gut have diarrhoea. This overlap between the symptoms of physical disease and anxiety can cause people to worry that they are physically

**Table 12.1**   Symptoms of anxiety

**Somatic Symptoms**

| | |
|---|---|
| Muscular | Tension headache<br>Pains in muscles and joints<br>Shaking<br>Feelings of tension in the muscles |
| Cardiovascular symptoms | Increased heart rate<br>Sensation of heart pounding<br>Peripheral vasoconstriction causing cold hands and feet and whiteness in extremities<br>Flushing |
| Breathing | A feeling of tightness in the chest<br>Difficulty in breathing<br>Excessive yawning<br>Overbreathing (hyperventilation) |
| Sweating | Sweating on palms and soles of feet<br>Excessive sweating in axillae<br>Generalised sweating |
| Dizziness | |
| Blurred vision | |
| Loss of libido | Loss of desire<br>Impotence<br>Lack of arousal<br>Lack of vaginal lubrication<br>Failure to reach orgasm |
| Sleep disturbance | Delay in getting off to sleep<br>Very light fitful sleep<br>Frequent waking<br>Disturbing, vivid dreams |
| Gastro-intestinal | Nausea<br>Lack of appetite<br>Diarrhoea<br>Frequent bowel movements |
| Frequency of micturition | |

**Affective Symptoms**

| | |
|---|---|
| | Feelings of anxiety<br>Feelings of panic<br>Feelings of being 'out of control' |

**Cognitive Symptoms**

| | |
|---|---|
| | Difficulty in concentrating<br>Preoccupation with problems<br>Narrowing of attention<br>Excessive worrying over minor issues<br>Feeling that things are out of control |

**Table 12.1** (*contd*)

| Behavioural Symptoms |
| --- |
| Avoidance of particular situations<br>Rapid speech<br>Jerky or sudden movements<br>Increased levels of overall activity |

ill when in fact they are showing normal symptoms of anxiety. It is also the basis of some of the difficulties with dealing with the worried well.

In assessing for anxiety one is, as with all other assessments, looking for a *pattern* of symptoms. Where there is any doubt about whether physical symptoms are the result of anxiety or of disease they should always be thoroughly investigated to reassure the patient as well as to ensure that nothing is missed. However, frequently physical symptoms are obviously the result of anxiety because of the pattern shown which does not resemble physical illness and because the patient is able to identify the link between physical symptoms and cognitive, affective and behavioural symptoms.

In fact anxiety comes in two different types: as a sort of steady or fluctuating high background level of anxiety, or in the form of intense bursts of very high anxiety — panic attacks. Many people have a mixture of the two types. Sometimes people have one panic attack and then never have another. In some there may be very frequent panic attacks, sometimes only lasting a few minutes at a time but repeated over and over again.

There are several steps to take in dealing with anxiety.

**Explaining to the patient what is happening to him**

The symptoms of anxiety, the physical ones in particular, are very dramatic. Many patients think that they are physically ill when they have them, sometimes people in panic attacks even think that they are going to die or go mad. They need to be given a clear explanation of the meaning of the symptoms.

A careful examination of Table 12.1 will show that many of the symptoms of anxiety are those of general excitement. Indeed physiologically the changes seen in anxiety are much the same as those seen in someone violently in love or very angry. They are the result of a generalised physiological reaction which has been called the 'fight or flight' response because it prepares the body for action. The exception is symptoms like tension headaches, which are the result of prolonged increased muscle tension, and sleep disturbances which are the result of the carry-over of anxiety from the day.

It is helpful to explain this to the patient, as with Paul:

PAUL: 'So, why do I get these physical sensations?'
COUNSELLOR: 'They are intended to prepare your body for rapid action, for fighting or for running away.'
PAUL: 'But I don't have anything to fight or run away from.'
COUNSELLOR: 'That's right, but your body doesn't know that, it has the same primitive response to all sorts of stresses. Somewhere, part of your mind knows you are under threat, but it doesn't know quite what threat, so it prepares you for any eventuality.'
PAUL: 'But why do I get these particular symptoms?'

The answer is actually very straightforward. Each of the symptoms of anxiety serves a purpose. In general they are aimed at making rapid vigorous muscular effort easier or more efficient.

There is a rise in heart rate and in cardiac output (pounding heart) to increase blood flow. When someone engages in violent physical activity he needs increased blood flow to the muscles. In the fight or flight response this occurs in advance of the physical effort so that the person is prepared for when muscular activity starts. At the same time blood is shifted away from non-essential areas so that it can be concentrated on the muscles; the blood vessels of the hands, feet and skin contract so the person goes pale and his extremities cold. Blood is diverted away from the stomach and this contributes to the feeling of 'butterflies in the stomach'.

There is increased sweating on hands and feet because wet skin is tougher than dry skin and slightly damp skin grips better. More general sweating is aimed at preparing in advance for the sweating needed to dissipate heat generated by muscular effort.

Emptying the bowels and bladder has obvious advantages. Loss of appetite is partly the result of changes in blood-flow away from the stomach, and partly has survival value. If our ancestors were being chased by lions it paid not to stop to eat a banana. It also paid not to stop to have sex, hence the effects on libido. Basically all appetites and needs are reduced and concentration is shifted onto the main aim, survival, the changes in concentration being particularly obvious in some anxious subjects.

There is an increase in muscle tension designed to prepare for vigorous rapid muscular action. If this is sustained over long periods it can lead to tension headaches and muscular pains.

The breathing changes are interesting in themselves because they can often be quite crucial to the experience of anxiety. Most people when they are anxious overbreathe; some people overbreathe quite substantially. Overbreathing is aimed at increasing the oxygen content of the blood, it simply means breathing too much for the immediate needs of the body. Obviously it prepares for the increased oxygen requirements of active muscles.

However, if overbreathing is sustained for long periods it causes excessive loss of carbon dioxide. This, while a waste product, is crucial to blood chemistry. This can lead to an interesting situation:

- When carbon dioxide loss becomes excessive the brain acts to shut down the breathing and bring blood chemistry back into balance. It does so in part by increasing muscle tension in the chest. The patient thus feels a 'tightness' in the chest.
- In part because of the disrupted blood chemistry the patient feels that he is not getting enough oxygen and tries to breathe more rapidly.
- The patient struggles to breathe while the brain struggles to cut down on breathing.

It is an interesting struggle, which occasionally results in the patient fainting, upon which breathing returns to normal and he is fine. However, this is unusual. Generally overbreathing occurs on a much less dramatic scale, with the patient complaining of episodes of breathlessness and tightness in the chest. Episodes of dizziness and faintness can often be traced to overbreathing.

It is important to go through the reasons for the symptoms of anxiety with a patient. It can make a tremendous difference to the success of intervention in anxiety.

It is also important to make it clear to the patient that anxiety can spread. Someone who is already anxious about one thing will be likely to react with greater anxiety to something else which would, in the normal course of things, elicit only a small amount of anxiety. This is particularly the case when there is a strong physiological component to the anxiety.

## Teaching relaxation techniques

Relaxation techniques can be extremely helpful in dealing with anxiety. All patients who are anxious should be taught relaxation methods. The basis of this is covered in Appendix A.

## Talking over why someone is anxious

Often anxiety is the result of real worries in someone's life. This chapter is all about finding out what problems people have and trying to help them to deal with them. Helping people to deal with their problems is likely in itself to reduce their anxieties. Just talking over worries — ventilation — in itself is often extremely effective in reducing anxiety. As people talk they are able to put their problems into perspective.

However, sometimes anxiety appears as a result of something that nothing can be done about, for instance as a result of the very fact of being seropositive. Or it can actually get in the way of solving problems so that it needs to be reduced before the patient can take any action. Or it can take on a life of its own. Anxiety can feed on itself; just being anxious can make people more anxious, particularly if they are interpreting anxiety symptoms as the result of physical disease.

## Looking for things which make anxiety worse or better

It often helps to try to find out under what circumstances anxiety is reduced or increased:

COUNSELLOR: 'Are there times when you are less anxious?'
PATIENT: 'Yes, when I'm with other people, talking to them, I forget myself and my symptoms disappear'.
COUNSELLOR: 'What about things which make you more anxious?'
PATIENT: 'Well, I get anxious when I am on my own in the house during the day, if I go out and do something I tend to feel better. It's when my mind is unoccupied that I feel most anxious'.

This sort of situation is very common. Often anxiety is greatest when someone has nothing to do and therefore has time to worry. The patient can be helped to become more active. However different people get anxious under different circumstances and it is important to look for what these are.

In some cases giving up doing things actually makes anxiety worse. This tends to be the case when they have panic attacks in particular situations, for instance when they are in company, or going into busy social situations. In these circumstances avoiding those situations may lead to the patient finding it increasingly difficult to go into them, and so may actually increase overall anxiety. Increasing the amount of time a person spends in these situations will, over time, reduce anxiety. They should be encouraged to make active efforts to put themselves into such situations as frequently as possible. They should not leave an anxiety-provoking situation until their anxiety level drops, as it always will. They should remind themselves what the symptoms they are experiencing really are, i.e. symptoms of anxiety, that although it is unpleasant it will do them no harm and they should, if possible, use relaxation techniques to reduce their anxiety.

In finding out what the factors causing changes in anxiety are it is often helpful to get people to keep a diary. Most people find it easy to make a rating of their anxiety level on a simple scale:

1 – No anxiety
2 – Slight anxiety
3 – Moderate anxiety
4 – Strong anxiety
5 – Overwhelming anxiety

They can use the scale to make a diary. The diary should record what they were doing, how anxious they felt, what they did about the anxiety and what difference this made. A diary entry of this sort is shown below. They should also record the date and time of each recording (not shown below). It is easy to make up sheets of paper divided into the headings shown and give them to the patient.

| What doing | Rating | What did then | Effect |
|---|---|---|---|
| Reading newspaper article about AIDS | 4 | Got up, went out for walk | Anxiety dropped to 2 within ten minutes |

It is important in giving someone a diary:

• To explain the rationale, otherwise many patients just won't do it since it is rather time-consuming.

COUNSELLOR: 'This diary will help us in two ways. First of all, we'll be able to see the sort of things which make you more anxious and the sort of things which help to reduce your anxiety. It's often not all that obvious what these are. But if we get a record over several days we can often pick out a pattern, even one you may not have noticed yourself. Secondly we are going to try to work together to reduce your anxiety. We want to make sure that what we are doing really is having an effect. By keeping a diary we'll be able to see what impact we're making and, if we are not making an impact one way, we'll be able to change to attack the problem in another way. Does that make sense to you?'
PATIENT: 'Yes, I understand that'.

- To take an example of a time when the patient has been particularly anxious and to fill in the diary with him to make sure that he grasps what needs to be done from a worked example. He can then take the example with him as a guide to what he should be doing. An example is often worth a thousand words of explanation in filling in a diary.

Diaries are useful not just in anxiety but in trying to help in a range of other sorts of problem. For instance, a similar diary can be used to monitor length of sleep and factors affecting the quality of sleep in someone with sleep problems. Or it can be used in recording how many rows a couple have, what they row about, how intense these are and what ends the row and how they feel afterwards. They not only help to elicit what affects particular psychological reactions, they are also vital in measuring whether possible solutions to particular problems are working or not.

## Drugs

There are a number of drugs available which can reduce anxiety. These all have problems. Some can induce drowsiness which may make driving or operating machinery hazardous or increase feelings of fatigue. However, there are three particular problems with them which severely restrict their usefulness. The first is that they are not a cure for whatever is causing the anxiety and so when they are stopped the anxiety tends to return. Secondly, many anxiolytics cause dependency in a large proportion of patients who take them. Thirdly, after a time they become less effective in relieving anxiety in many of those who use them.

These characteristics mean that the use of anxiolytics for more than a few weeks at most is undesirable. They can be helpful for very short-term control of high levels of anxiety until other interventions can be made to work. However they are not in any way a cure in themselves.

### Referral

Because anxiety is often a highly treatable condition it is important to refer on to specialist mental health workers patients who either appear particularly anxious or who fail to respond to simple interventions such as those outlined above.

## DEPRESSION

There is no-one who does not from time to time get depressed. Certainly anyone faced with having HIV or AIDS is likely to have hours or days when they are depressed. Periods of depression may come and go, interspersed with periods when they don't feel depressed at all.

However, depression can be more than a passing mood. It becomes a matter of concern either when it lasts for more than a few days at a time or when bouts of depression are very frequent or when it is very intense. This chapter addresses itself to this sort of depression rather than passing moods of mild depression. This sort of depression undermines people's ability to deal with the problems of everyday life, it makes life a misery for them and, ultimately, it can lead people to commit suicide, although even amongst people who are very severely depressed only a small proportion are actively suicidal.

When dealing with people with AIDS, seropositives, the worried well or partners and carers, it is important that the counsellor should assess for depression and should keep a careful eye on proceedings to make sure that the individual concerned does not become depressed.

It is a mistake to assume that prolonged or intense depression is 'natural'. Amongst people with AIDS we are seeing only a minority show depression at a level which requires specific intervention during the course of their illness. There is some evidence to suggest that professionals sometimes fail to intervene in cases of depression in those with life-threatening disease simply because they regard the individual's depression as natural. People with AIDS are simply ordinary people, usually with no history of psychiatric problems, faced with the strains that having AIDS can bring. It would be a major surprise if they showed very high levels of severe depression.

**Assessing depression**

As with anxiety, the symptoms of depression can be split into four main headings: somatic symptoms, affective symptoms, cognitive symptoms and behavioural symptoms.

In assessing for depression it is important to look for a pattern. A single isolated symptom does not usually mean that someone is depressed. In general the greater the number of the symptoms listed below shown by an individual, the more depressed he is. However the *intensity* of the symptoms has also to be taken into account; someone with slight anorexia, a slightly depressed mood and slight gastro-intestinal symptoms is hardly likely to be severely depressed.

It is also worth bearing in mind that many people who are depressed are also highly anxious and so it is common to find a mix of the symptoms of anxiety and depression. It is, thus, important to look for the symptoms of both.

**The symptoms of depression**

*Affective symptoms*

*Depressed mood*
The single most common feature in depression is people complaining that they feel depressed. People can often give you a good estimate of just how depressed they are by comparing their current mood with their mood at other times when they have been depressed in the past.

However there is something of a snag in only using people's subjective estimates of whether they are depressed or not. Because people's thinking about themselves and the world changes when they become depressed they may not see themselves as being depressed at all, or they may underestimate the extent of their depression. Instead they may see things about them as being hopeless and pointless and see this as being realistic, or they may see themselves as being worthless.

It is important to ask about mood, not just currently, but over the past few weeks.

*Changes in how enjoyable things are*
A moment's thought about what it is like to be depressed (and most people have been at least a little depressed at one time or another) will show that one of the key elements in depressed mood is that things no longer seem pleasurable. Everyday things which normally give pleasure no longer give pleasure, instead they become a chore. People who are

depressed may become extremely bored. Ultimately lack of enjoyment in things can lead to people simply stopping doing anything.

One of the most important questions to ask someone about depression is, 'What have you enjoyed doing over the last two weeks?'. This does not simply mean big things, but also small pleasures, watching television, drinking coffee, talking to friends, doing the garden. Someone who can think of nothing or very little that he has enjoyed doing is very likely to be depressed.

*Loss of libido*
Lack of interest in sex is common in depression. Sex itself may become unpleasurable. There may also be a lack of arousal, a man may find it difficult to get an erection or ejaculate, a woman may not lubricate properly or may fail to reach orgasm. It is a *change* in these things which makes a difference. Some people have long-lasting sexual problems which are quite unrelated to depression.

It is important to ask whether there have been any changes in the patient's interest in, or enjoyment of, sex recently.

*Irritability and increased emotional lability*
People who become depressed are often much more irritable; things which would not normally bother them may make them very angry. They change not just in terms of how easily they are angered but also, often, in terms of how easily they are upset or moved to tears.

It is important to ask whether the patient has become more irritable recently or whether he has found himself more easily upset than usual.

## Cognitive changes

When people are depressed their view of themselves and of their world changes in several ways.

*Loss of self-esteem*
People who are depressed often feel worthless and unlovable. They look at themselves in a very negative way, seeing only their failures and shortcomings. Depression should always be suspected in a patient who seems to be taking an unrealistically harsh view of himself.

These changes are sometimes combined with a change in perception of their own body. They feel not just personally but also physically unattractive. They may start as a result to neglect their appearance. Or they may start to exaggerate some real blemish. They may, for instance, feel that a small KS lesion on the face is not only glaringly obvious to everyone, but also that what it is is obvious to everyone.

It is important to ask patients how they feel about themselves, whether this has changed recently and whether they feel less attractive than they used to.

## Guilt

People who are depressed sometimes start to feel guilty about things which they have done in the past which objectively were quite minor or which were not their fault at all.

Sometimes this can be quite severe. One patient had absent-mindedly driven away from a petrol station without paying several years before. When he became depressed (but not when he wasn't) he was racked with guilt about this and made repeated attempts to give himself up to the police. They sought to reassure him, one policeman admitting that he had done the same himself, prior to driving the patient home. He even 'confessed' to the garage owner, who made him coffee and told him to forget it. None of this made him feel any less guilty.

However, guilt is often more subtle. Patients blame themselves for infecting others, or blame themselves for engaging in particular high-risk sexual activities and getting infected, although many could not have known that they were at risk or putting others at risk. They may, indeed, in some cases have behaved unwisely but their feelings of guilt are out of all proportion to what they have done.

Gay men sometimes blame themselves for being gay when they become depressed and reject all aspects of being gay, including other gay men.

It is important to ask patients whether they feel guilty about anything.

## Feelings of failure

The person who is depressed often feels a failure. Looking back over a successful and happy life he may tend to see only the bad things, the things which have gone wrong for him and the things he failed to do. One patient, when asked about his career as a salesman, talked about an order he had lost and implied that he was likely to lose his job as a result. Further questioning showed that he was the most successful salesman the company had and that not only was the order in question small but the loss had not been his fault at all.

It is very difficult to come up with a single question or few questions to elicit a person's view of his past. However the information usually comes out in discussion and in history-taking. The counsellor can compare the objective details of someone's life against the patient's assessment of that life. This often reveals the gap in the patient's perceptions.

*Loss of hope*
For people who are depressed the future looks bleak. There is nothing to look forward to. They anticipate that anything they do will end in failure because of their lack of ability to carry out the task. Depressed people often say things like, 'I'll try it, but I know that I won't be able to do it'. In fact there is very little loss of ability to carry out tasks in people who are depressed, they just *think* that they will fail. This feeling of *helplessness*, that nothing they can do will make any difference, failure is inevitable, is common in depression.

It is important to ask patients what they are looking forward to in their lives. Unrealistic expectations of failure are usually very obvious when talking through with patients what their plans for the future are.

*Feelings of changes in thinking*
People who are depressed very frequently report changes in how they are thinking. They report that they have difficulty in concentrating, cannot attend to one thing for more than brief periods and that when they are thinking about things their minds are painfully slow. They also very frequently report difficulties with their memory. Often they feel that something is wrong with their brain. The mental symptoms of depression are often misinterpreted by people with AIDS as early signs of encephalopathy, and cause intense anxiety. In fact, objective measurement of mental functioning usually shows no real change in cognitive efficiency.

It is important to ask patients whether they feel they are thinking less clearly than they used to. It is also important to reassure the patient about the nature of any changes they report.

*Obsessional thought patterns*
Obsessional thoughts and obsessional behaviours are sometimes seen in depression. Brooding on past behaviour or on negative and unpleasant thoughts is quite common. This is covered in more detail below.

**Somatic symptoms**

*Sleep disturbances*
Disturbances in sleep are common in those with depression. Particularly common in severe depression is waking up early and not being able to get back to sleep, often at 4 or 5 o'clock in the morning. Difficulties in getting to sleep are also seen, particularly in those who are also anxious,

which many depressed people are. The sleep problems are often combined with a feeling of great fatigue and tiredness during the day.
There may also be nightmares.

Occasionally people who are depressed show a great increase in the
amount that they sleep and spend a lot of their time in bed.

In assessing sleep disturbances it is important to look for *changes* in
sleep pattern. Some people are, and have always been, poor sleepers.
Patients should be asked whether they have noticed any changes in
their sleep pattern recently.

### Anorexia

Anorexia is common in depression, although the opposite state, eating
excessively, is also seen in some people, particularly those who have
always used food as a comfort. The anorexia in depression is characterised by a loss of appetite, loss of interest in food and a loss of
appreciation of food generally – it may not taste as it used to. Eating
is often an effort.

Again, it is the *change* in eating and attitude to food which matters;
some people have never had much interest in food. They may also be
anorexic because they have pain on eating because of some physical
condition, and this possibility should be excluded.

Patients should be asked whether there has been any change in
their appetite or enjoyment of food recently.

### Gastro-intestinal symptoms

Changes in bowel motility can occur. Constipation is fairly common,
sometimes linked to changes in eating. However, in the individual
who is very anxious diarrhoea is sometimes seen.

Patients should be asked whether they have noticed that they have
been constipated or they have had diarrhoea recently.

### Multiple physical complaints

People who are depressed sometimes report multiple physical complaints, headaches, joint pains, palpitations, stomach problems and so
on. These are often, when examined closely, symptoms of anxiety.
People who are depressed often interpret such symptoms as signs of
physical disease.

Patients should be asked about any physical symptoms they may
have. Naturally physical complaints are seen also in physical conditions
so any possible organic illness should be eliminated.

## Behavioural symptoms

### Lack of energy

People who are depressed feel that they lack energy, that everything is too much effort and too much trouble. They may be unable to 'get going' in the mornings or even to get out of bed. They may 'put off things until tomorrow'.

Patients should be asked whether they have noticed that they are any less energetic recently.

### Reduction in overall levels of activity

People who are depressed tend to do less than they used to. They go out less, they find they do less at work, they find that they do less at home, often simply sitting in a chair or in bed.

Patients should be asked whether they are doing less than they used to.

In extreme cases *retardation* is seen. The depressed person shows a slowing in movement and/or speech which is obvious to the observer. In very rare cases this may become so extreme that the patient simply sits mute in a chair or lies in bed doing nothing at all unless prompted.

## Suicidal thoughts and actions

Many people who become depressed contemplate suicide at one time or another. There is a spectrum of thoughts about suicide, from the person who feels that 'it's not worth going on' but has never actually thought of killing himself, through the person who has daydreamed about it, through the person who has made plans but has no intention of carrying them out, to the person who expresses an intention of killing himself or makes an attempt. It is a dangerous myth that people who intend to kill themselves don't tell anyone else but just go ahead and do it: the majority of successful suicides have told someone else that they were thinking of suicide in the days leading up to the attempt.

It is also a myth that suicides can be divided into 'real' attempts and 'cries for attention'. People who actually attempt suicide tend to take a calculated chance, with different people balancing that calculation in different ways. Some people take very little risk that they will die — they may take pills in front of others, for instance. Others take a greater risk: they take tablets knowing that it is likely (but not certain) that their partner will return before they die and find them. Others stack the chances firmly in favour of death. A man who shoots himself with a shotgun is certain he is going to die.

People who have made suicide attempts in the past are more likely to do so in the future. Past attempts may have been weighted heavily towards being found and saved. Future attempts may be weighted more towards dying.

It is important always to ask the depressed patient about suicide. Counsellors are often very reluctant and embarrassed to ask about this issue; they should not be, it can be a matter of life and death.

COUNSELLOR: 'When people get depressed they often think about killing themselves. Have you thought about that?'
PATIENT: 'Yes I have, I've even thought that if I was to do it, I'd take tablets'
COUNSELLOR: 'Have you thought like that recently?'
PATIENT: 'I thought about it quite a lot over the weekend'.
COUNSELLOR: 'How likely do you think it is that you will actually do it?'
PATIENT: 'I won't kill myself, but sometimes it comforts me to think about it as a way out if I get very sick.'

If someone is actively planning suicide and intends to carry out his plan he will, very often, tell you so if you are sympathetic. Often it is a great relief to him to tell you. An active suicidal intent is a psychiatric emergency and arrangements should always be made to bring in advice from specialist mental health workers.

Where someone is contemplating suicide but has no active intent a careful eye should be kept on him to monitor changes in his mood. If he becomes more depressed there is a danger that he may become more active in planning to kill himself.

## Interpreting symptoms

The list of symptoms above suggests the sort of questions that need to be asked. It is, of course, the *pattern* of symptoms which is being looked for. It is also helpful to ask patients about:

- When did the symptoms start and how long have they lasted?
- Are they constant or does the level of depression fluctuate?
- How intense are the symptoms?
- Have they been depressed at any time in the past?
- Have they ever had treatment for depression, if so what was it and how successful was it?
- Are they currently receiving treatment for depression?

## Using standardised measures of depression

There are a number of questionnaires which can be filled in by the patient and a number of observer-rating forms to assess depression. These can be very helpful in assessing depression because they usually make it possible to assess how depressed a patient is in comparison with others. They give a numeric value for the level of depression. They do not, however, remove the necessity to ask patients about depressive symptoms.

Introducing standardised methods as a routine part of assessing patients can be very helpful. There are many different scales, each with their advantages and disadvantages. In order to select the right scales to use it is helpful to discuss what should be used with mental health professionals who will be aware of what is available, will probably have or be able to obtain suitable instruments, and can usually advise on their use and interpretation.

## Taking action

The first decision is whether the counsellor should attempt to deal with the depression himself or whether he should pass on the patient for specialist advice to specialist mental health services. Anyone who is severely depressed or actively suicidal should always be the subject of urgent referral to specialist services.

There is a range of antidepressant medication available which can often be very effective in relieving depression. This does not necessarily in itself provide a complete answer but it can 'lift' very depressed patients sufficiently to make it possible to help them deal with their problems. In some cases psychiatric admission may be required.

For individuals who are mildly depressed and who are not actively suicidal there are steps which the counsellor can take to help. It is worth reviewing these.

### Putting things in perspective

As with anxiety it helps just to tell patients that they are depressed and to explain to them that the symptoms they are experiencing are those of depression. It is also important to tell them that, however they feel at the moment, they will feel better in the future. The symptoms above provide a framework to talk about the sort of experiences which go with being depressed.

It is also a fact that, at least in cases where people are reacting to some life event, with depression, they will eventually almost certainly feel better *even if no intervention is undertaken*. That is, depression does eventually tend to lift either of its own accord or because events in the person's life change so that the factors causing or supporting the continuance of depression disappear or become less important. This is the reason why the brief depressions we all get tend usually to pass off after hours or days and not to become fixed features.

It is important to reassure patients that they won't always feel like this, it is a passing phenomenon and in the future they will feel better.

## Sorting out problems

The chapters of this book look at various ways of helping people to solve their problems. Where depression is the result of specific problems dealing with those problems can in itself often relieve depression.

## Increasing activity

Our mood is maintained at least in part by the pleasures of life. Pleasant things tend to keep us on an even keel in terms of mood.

People who get depressed tend to get less pleasure from what they do. As a result they stop doing things. The result is that they have even less pleasure in their lives and get more depressed. It is a vicious circle and can lead to people going further into depression.

It is very helpful to get people to increase their overall level of activity. At first the things they do may not be pleasurable but they should be told that they will have to do more first and then they will start to find things more pleasurable later. There are several steps:

- Go through with the patient things that he enjoyed in the past (not necessarily currently).
- Make a list of these.
- Make up a simple diary sheet for the week with a slot for each hour, or use a new commercial diary.
- Go through with the patient and fill in something which he can do each hour. This need not be a particularly complicated or elaborate item; some examples might be:
  *Ringing up an old friend and asking how he is*
  *Eating some specially liked food for lunch*
  *Going to an exhibition*
  *Going out and buying a book*
  *Going to the cinema*

*Going for a walk in a favourite park*
Whatever is agreed needs to be realistic.

- Get the patient to tick off the items on the diary as they are done and also to make ratings on a simple five-point scale from unenjoyable (1) to very enjoyable (5) according to how much he enjoyed doing each thing. It is also helpful to get him to rate how well he feels he carried out each task (regardless of how well he enjoyed it) on a scale from 1 (not carried out well at all) to 5 (very well). These ratings help both the patient and the counsellor to keep an eye on progress.

- After the first week the patient should be encouraged to fill in his own diary either at the beginning of the week or each evening for the following day.

It is surprising what a difference such an apparently simple intervention can make. People's mood very often improves dramatically over a few weeks.

The most difficult part of the process tends to be getting people started. Because they are depressed they tend not to want to start out on the process. It is important to encourage them as much as possible. Once they get going it usually goes well enough to gather its own momentum because patients start to feel better.

### Identifying inaccurate thoughts

The cognitive symptoms list above shows that people who are depressed tend to have an inaccurate view of themselves. For instance they may feel that they are unattractive, when they are not, or that they have behaved badly, when they have not.

When this sort of thought is identified in a patient it is useful to challenge the thought, to explain that it is inaccurate and to look for ways of dealing with the inaccurate thought. The challenging of inaccurate thoughts is one of the elements of cognitive approaches to depression which are the subject of books in themselves. However there are elements from these approaches which can be easily used:

### Testing out

Quite often patients hold views which are not in accordance with reality but which they can test out to see if they are true. For instance, one patient expressed the view, 'Now I have AIDS I don't even bother seeing my friends any more, they wouldn't want to see me anyway'. He agreed that this was testable and that, while he was sure he was right, there was no harm in trying out his view to see if it was true. He was encouraged to select several friends he had been close to in the past and to invite them round for a meal (which a friend would help him cook). He rang around and, to his surprise, many people asked him why he hadn't been in touch before and said they would be pleased to come.

When getting patients to test things out it is, of course, important to ensure that they succeed. It was agreed in the case above that the patient would plan well in advance so that people were less likely to be already committed. The fact that not everyone he rang would be able to come for a meal on a given day was also discussed. Getting a friend to help him cook also ensured that the thing wouldn't fail because he was unable to make the meal.

### Writing down thoughts and talking them through
It can be very helpful to simply get someone to make a list of the negative thoughts they have about themselves and then for the counsellor and the patient coolly to go through and look at each of these in turn to examine how realistic they are.

> A successful businessman became depressed. He had had a career with many successes and few failures. However, he concentrated on the failures and ignored the successes. The counsellor and the businessman compiled a list of failures and the way that he had dealt with these, and also of successes. The successes markedly outweighed the failures but also it was clear that he had usually managed either to learn from failures or to turn them to his advantage.

### Rewarding and encouraging
For the depressed patient the world is a rather unrewarding place. However, few patients who are moderately depressed find it totally unrewarding, just more so than before. The counsellor needs to provide clear encouragement to the patient to solve his problems and to increase his activity levels or whatever else it is agreed the patient will do.

It is important that the counsellor should look out for things which the patient has achieved positively and then provide clear praise for the achievement. A partial failure is also a partial success and it is important to get the patient to look at the success element. Praise from the counsellor is also rewarding in itself. To hear someone say, 'You've done very well' is a boost to almost anyone's confidence and mood and, while it appears a simple point, it is surprising how many counsellors concentrate on what has gone wrong and fail to give praise for success.

*If the patient doesn't get less depressed*

It is unreasonable to expect that someone is going to move from being depressed to being happy or in a normal mood in a few days or even a few weeks. However, some progress should be seen over the first few weeks of intervention. If there is no progress, then is the time to refer someone on. If they start to get markedly worse then they should also be referred on.

## Obsessions

Obsessions come in two overlapping types, obsessional behaviours and obsessional thoughts.

### Obsessional behaviours

Nothing appears more odd initially than obsessional behaviours:

> Edward began to worry that he had left a plug in the electrics in his house when he went to bed at night and that this might cause a fire. He spent up to three hours per night checking and rechecking his electrics.

> Mary had sex with a man she said was 'very dirty' at a party. She began to worry that he had infected her with some disease and spent several hours a day checking her vagina with the aid of a mirror, trying to work out whether it looked normal or whether she had any sort of rash.

> After David became seropositive he began to examine his skin in minute detail, looking for signs of Kaposi's sarcoma. He started at the soles of his feet and worked upwards, always in the same order of checking. If he was interrupted or lost his place he would have to start again from the beginning. Sometimes he would finish and then feel he had 'not done it properly' and start again. This took up large parts of his morning.

In fact these sorts of behaviour have their counterparts in everyday life: the child stepping over cracks in the pavement or counting up to particular numbers, or the person going on holiday driving to the end of the street and then coming back to check that he has turned off the gas.

A key feature of obsessional behaviours is that people who engage in them *know* that they are unreasonable but still feel compelled to carry them out. The most common types of obsessional behaviour are:

- *Checking.* Checking gas or electrics or locks or checking for disease of one sort or another.

- *Cleaning.* Repeatedly and excessively cleaning, either objects or surfaces or one's own body, for instance the hand-washer who washes his hands for hours at a time, like Lady Macbeth.

No-one knows what causes obsessions. However, it is known that some cases of obsession are linked to depression and if the depression is treated the obsessions will disappear.

Despite the cause being unknown there are ways of dealing with obsessions. Obsessions tend to feed on themselves. The more they are done the more people feel the urge to do them. The answer is to encourage the patient not to do them. This seems fairly obvious but it sometimes works rather well, it is even given a name in textbooks — *response prevention.*

The key elements are:

- To discuss with the patient in a non-accusatory way the essential pointlessness and unreasonableness of the obsessional behaviours.
- To explain to the patient that the obsessions are self-sustaining and to provide a rationale for resisting them.
- To tell him that only by avoiding doing the rituals can he get rid of them and that this will inevitably involve him in some discomfort but that it will be worth while in the end.
- To encourage the patient to notice those events which tend to set off an obsessional chain of behaviour and, as far as possible, to avoid such events or situations. Keeping a diary in the way set out in the section on anxiety can help to pinpoint things to avoid.
- To encourage the patient to use distraction to avoid the obsessional behaviours. For instance, if a patient has an urge to wash the kitchen floor, he might be encouraged to go out for a walk. This takes him out of the situation and makes the behaviour less likely to occur.
- If the patient cannot avoid the situation where he will want to engage in obsessional behaviours he should resist them for as long as possible. The urge to carry out the ritual involved will, eventually, weaken (though it may return later). In order to deal with the urge engaging in some alternative activity is essential, carrying out relaxation exercises is often helpful.
- Obsessional rituals take a considerable amount of time. It is important to find alternative activities to fill the time that is freed by not carrying out the rituals, otherwise they will creep back into the free space.

Again, if these simple interventions fail it is important to seek specialist help for the patient.

In the case of David above, his checking of his body for Kaposi's sarcoma was reduced by a very simple programme:

- He only rarely checked at any time except in the mornings when he went to the bathroom to wash. He was encouraged to get up, get dressed and to go straight out without washing. This was a good deal less of a problem to him than getting stuck in the bathroom for hours.
- He had rigged up an elaborate system of mirrors so that he could see inaccessible bits of his anatomy. He was encouraged to remove *all* the mirrors in his flat.
- When he felt the urge to check he was encouraged to put off actually checking as long as possible by using relaxation techniques or by doing something else active and incompatible with checking such as cleaning the floor (which was not one of his obsessions), or going out or ringing a friend.
- Where the urge to check was overwhelming he was taught to put it off by engaging in self-talk along the lines of 'I'll wait five minutes before I check'. If he succeeded for five minutes he was encouraged to try to postpone it another five minutes.
- He booked occasional appointments with the doctor who gave him a full examination, 'so that he wouldn't have to check himself'.

This simple programme, over a period of a few weeks, more or less eliminated his checking.

### Obsessional thoughts

Obsessional thoughts are sometimes called 'ruminations'. They differ from everyday worries, with which they overlap, because of their rather stereotyped nature. They often involve a sort of 'mental checking':

Richard developed ruminations that he might have run someone over in his car on the way back from work, even though he knew this was ridiculous. He would sit in the evenings and go though his journey in minute detail over and over again trying to work out if he had injured anyone. These thoughts distressed him greatly.

Barbara, an antibody positive woman, developed a fear that she might in some way have infected someone else in her everyday life. She reviewed her day minutely to make sure that she had not cut herself or had a nosebleed and exposed someone to risk. She even thought over the possibility that she might have had sex with someone without remembering it. She knew these ideas were ridiculous but she felt obliged to go through the ritual of thinking about them.

Again, obsessional thoughts can be the result of depression, indeed they are very common in that form. Sometimes in people with AIDS obsessional thoughts are seen in the form of stereotyped worries about AIDS or obsessional attempts to remember anyone they might have infected in the past.

The first thing to try in dealing with obsessional thoughts is distraction. Patients should be encouraged to monitor their thoughts and, when they begin to start ruminating, they should interrupt their train of thought and occupy their minds with something else active— talking to someone, singing, adding up their bank balance, anything which distracts them.

Trains of obsessional thoughts are often easy to interrupt, although they tend to come back again. Some psychiatrists and psychologists have advocated that the patient should actually shout out loud 'Stop!', or they should pinch themselves or do something else dramatic to divert their attention as soon as they detect obsessional thoughts starting (called *thought-stopping*). Then they should distract themselves with alternative activities.

The following are suggested steps in dealing with obsessional thoughts:

- The patient and the counsellor should discuss the obsessional thoughts and try to sort out any underlying realistic worries the patient may have.
- If the patient is depressed he should be treated for this.
- If he is not depressed or the depression improves but his obsessional thoughts do not remit, distraction should be tried with or without thought-stopping.
- If he is anxious and anxiety increases his tendency to have obsessional thoughts, relaxation training should be tried.
- The patient should be encouraged to keep his mind occupied as much as possible since obsessional thoughts tend to be most common when people's minds are unoccupied.

Obsessional thoughts are notoriously difficult to treat. Quite often they disappear on their own but they can persist for months or years and make life a misery for the patient. New treatment approaches are being developed to try to solve the problem of obsessional thoughts, and if the patient fails to respond to simple interventions they should be referred on for specialist advice.

# Chapter 13

# Problem Solving

JOHN GREEN

## The problem-solving approach

People in the real world, unlike those reported in many textbooks, tend to have more than one problem and these problems tend to be mixed together. The result is that the counsellor is faced by a tangled web of problems which have to be sorted out before they can be tackled. For the patient the tangle of problems makes life particularly difficult. Because everything is mixed together he feels that there is no way in which he will ever find a sensible solution to his difficulties.

The problem-solving approach to helping people is simply a set of ways of breaking down a series of problems so that they become easier to deal with. Breaking down the problems into discrete blocks is a very valuable process for the patient because it allows him to get his difficulties into perspective and they no longer seem so insoluble.

The whole process of problem solving is carried out jointly with the patient. It is not a process in which the counsellor decides what are the problems and what are the solutions; it is a process in which the two work together. There are several good reasons for this:

- It is important to check that what is being written down is, in fact, correct. This is an opportunity to re-check that the counsellor has, in fact, grasped the problems.
- As problem solving goes along it will, in itself, generate questions which need to be asked and considered. A history is seldom perfect, some things will have been missed and other things will need clarifying.
- It is useful to go through the approach with the patient because it is a generally helpful way of looking at problems which the patient can use for himself in the future.

- It engages the patient in the task of *solving his own problems*, something which is absolutely vital. An individual is far more likely to implement solutions he himself has come up with.
- The process itself helps to sort out the problems in the patient's own mind.

There are several steps to taking a problem-solving approach.

### Taking a good history

The first step is to gather as much information as possible about the patient's difficulties. The sort of information-gathering covered in Chapters 3, 4 and 5 should provide a good basis on which to start.

In taking a history it is always helpful to take notes, if the patient doesn't mind. Naturally he will wish to be reassured that such notes are confidential.

At this stage a fairly good overall picture of what is happening should be available.

### Making a list of problems

The next step is simply to make a list of the problems the patient has. This list needs to be constructed with the patient, of course.

At this stage it doesn't matter if the same problem goes down twice in different forms. Nor is it necessary to try to sort out the links between different problems or to look for solutions. That comes later.

Making a good list of problems is more difficult than it appears at first sight. In fact, it is probably the single most difficult thing to do. Consider these statements about patients which are typical of the sort of thing that appears in notes or in discussions about patients:

'He is worried about AIDS'. [Worried about what aspect of AIDS? Is he afraid that he has it? Is he afraid that he will get it?]
'She is unable to cope because of her social problems'. [What sort of social problems? Unable to cope with what?]
'He is rather socially inadequate.' [What does socially inadequate mean?]
'She has sexual problems.' [Does she not want to have it? Or does she get pain in intercourse? What exactly is the problem?]
'He doesn't have any friends.' [Does he want friends? Does he lack opportunity to make friends? Does he find it difficult to make friends although he has plenty of contacts?]

'He has sleep difficulties.' [Sleeps too little? Too much? Can't get off to sleep? Wakes early? Wakes up often?]

All the above statements may be factually correct. However they are *unhelpful* because they don't give a clear enough description of what the problem actually is. Clear descriptions make it much easier to come up with solutions. Better problem descriptions might be:

'He is worried that he will get AIDS because he engages in casual unprotected anal intercourse'.
'She is unable to keep herself warm because she does not have the money to heat her flat and this makes her miserable.'
'He finds that in company he can't say what he wants because he is anxious that he has nothing interesting to say.'
'She has pain at the entrance to the vagina on penetration.'
'He does not meet people who he could make friends with.'
'He is unable to get off to sleep at nights because he worries about HIV, but he sleeps well once asleep.'

These problem descriptions, while far from perfect, do at least suggest further questions to ask and the lines along which possible solutions might be sought.

The following example of a case shows what might be done. The list of problems is rather shorter than it might be in reality since it is an illustration only:

David, aged 35, has ARC. He is anxious about his future and finds that he constantly worries about the possibility that he is going to get AIDS. It occupies his thoughts for most of the time. He checks himself every day in the mirror, looking for signs of Kaposi's sarcoma.

Previously self-employed, he gave up his job, which involved a lot of travelling, because he did not feel well enough to carry on. Since then he has spent most of his time at home reading the paper and watching the television. He finds himself frequently bored. He used to have an active social life around the clubs but now finds he tires easily and doesn't want to go.

He lives with Ted, who he has been living with for five years. They get on well but, recently, he has been unable to have any form of sexual activity with Ted because as soon as they start safer sex he starts to think about AIDS and becomes more and more anxious. He now finds he is unable even to cuddle Ted because he fears it might lead to sex. He suffers from spells of dizziness and sweating. These can occur at any time, but are more frequent when he is thinking about AIDS.

The problem list developed with the patient in this case was:

(1)  He constantly worries about AIDS, particularly when he has nothing else to occupy his mind.
(2)  He spends half an hour first thing every morning checking his body for Kaposi's sarcoma and this makes him very anxious.
(3)  He stays at home most of the time and finds that he is very bored and unhappy because there is little interesting to do.
(4)  He enjoys seeing people but, since he stopped going to clubs, he does not see many people.
(5)  As soon as Ted touches him when they are in bed he thinks they are going to have sex and he begins to think of AIDS and cannot get aroused.
(6)  He cannot cuddle Ted or be cuddled because he fears this might lead to sex.
(7)  He gets spells of dizziness and sweating; these are more frequent when he is thinking about AIDS.

These have been entered on the problem chart (Fig. 13.1) in an abbreviated form for reasons of space. On the full chart they would be entered in full. In the explanations below they have also been abbreviated, however the counsellor would normally use the full descriptions of problems.

### Looking for links and hypotheses

The next thing is for the counsellor and the patient jointly to try to form hypotheses about the ways in which different problems are linked together and about possible causes of particular problems.

In the case of problem 1, *his constant worries about AIDS*, it may be that:

- Because he has so much time on his hands which he is not able to use pleasurably and where his mind is unoccupied, he has time to worry excessively.
- The problem is linked to high overall anxiety levels, both as a result of these and also, probably, contributing to the maintenance of anxiety.
- Checking for KS may be contributing to maintaining thoughts of AIDS uppermost in his mind.
- The thoughts may be obsessional in nature. This needs further investigation (see Chapter 12).

| Problem | Links/Hypotheses | Possible solutions | Evaluation |
|---|---|---|---|
| (1) Worries constantly about AIDS | Linked to (3) and (4) because mind frequently not occupied. Linked to overall high level of anxiety. Linked to (2)? Obsessional thoughts? | Occupy time more effectively. Treat for anxiety. Try treatments for obsessional thoughts. | See text for explanation |
| (2) Checks for KS | May be an obsessional behaviour either contributing to or resulting from (1). | Treat for anxiety. Treat as obsessional behaviour. | |
| (3) Stays at home and gets bored | Contributes to (1) and (2)? | Go out more. Draw up list of enjoyed things which can be done at home and carry out. | |
| (4) Doesn't see many people since stopped going to clubs | Failed to develop alternative social outlets. | Start going to clubs again. Invite people round more. | |
| (5) Can't get aroused because of thoughts of AIDS | Linked to (1)? Result of high anxiety. | Embark on programme of sex therapy. Treat for anxiety and see if arousal returns. | |
| (6) Cannot cuddle Ted or be cuddled | Linked to (5). May not feel in control of sexual aspects of relationship? | As for 5. Develop rule with couple that cuddles outside bed don't lead to sex. Help him to be more assertive in relationship. | |
| (7) Spells of dizziness and sweating | Result of high anxiety. Physical problem exacerbated by anxiety? | Treat for anxiety. Get medical done. | |

*Fig. 13.1*   Problem chart

Or, in the case of problem 6, *he doesn't feel able to cuddle Ted or be cuddled*, it may be that:

- This is linked to problem 5, *difficulties in getting aroused in sex*.
- He may not feel in control in their sexual relationship, so that he does not feel that he can call a halt if things are going too far for his liking.

These links need to be developed by the counsellor with the patient so that any which do not fit the facts can be eliminated.

### Generating possible solutions

The next step is for the counsellor and the patient to go through looking for possible solutions to each problem. At this stage it is often helpful to generate a large number of possible solutions and not to worry too much about how practical each is. Later, unsuccessful solutions may form the basis for more successful solutions. Because of this, some workers advocate coming up with any solutions, however ridiculous, even solutions of the 'perhaps I could get a spaceship and go to Mars' type. However, I have not felt that going this far is very helpful and it tends simply to produce more totally unworkable solutions rather than ideas which can be turned to practical use.

On the problem chart it is possible to see some of the possible solutions generated for this case. In the case of problem 3, *staying at home and getting bored and unhappy*, possible solutions might be:

- Going out more.
- Drawing up a list of enjoyed activities which can be done at home and then planning a diary of these things. These might include past enjoyed activities but also some new ones. The patient might, for instance, want to take up painting.

In the case of problem 5, *not getting aroused in sex*, possible solutions might be:

- Embarking on a psychosexual therapy programme or finding a sex therapist to carry it out if the counsellor is not expert in the area.
- Treating general overall anxiety about AIDS and seeing whether the problem disappears.

## Evaluating solutions

The next step is for the counsellor and the patient to look at each possible solution in turn and to try to evaluate it. In making an evaluation there are several important things to think about. Using the solutions generated for problem 3 (above):

- What assets has the patient got to carry out a solution? For instance, if he has a lot of things which he likes doing which can be done at home then it should be relatively easy for him to make his time at home more pleasurable.
- What difficulties are there with the solution? Going out more may not be possible for a man who is in ill-health, cannot drive, is not near public transport and cannot afford a taxi. With difficulties the counsellor and the patient should look for practical solutions. Perhaps a friend could take him out in his car?
- Are there intermediate steps which need to be taken before a solution can be implemented? For instance, going out more may require an intermediate step of drawing up a list of places to go, or it may involve looking up old friends and telephoning them to arrange to meet.
- How practical is the solution? This should be the final decision when the above questions have been answered.

In Fig. 13.1 this section has not been filled in for reasons of space. However, against each possible solution it is helpful to jot down under each of the four headings above a line or two about what was decided.

With luck several different solutions may be possible for some problems. The decision then is which solution to try first, or whether to try a combination of different solutions.

## Drawing up an action list

The final step is to draw up an action list from the problem-solving chart with the patient. This needs to specify:

- What actions are needed to resolve the various problems.
- The order in which various things will be tried. Some things may be done first because they lead on naturally to the implementation of other solutions. At other times the most promising solution, or the quickest to implement, may be tried first and if that is not successful another solution tried.
- What steps are needed to solve a particular problem.

From the problem chart it might for instance be decided that the steps to take are as follows.

### Stage one

*Tackle the high level of overall anxiety and monitor the effects of this on the amount of checking for KS, frequency of spells of dizziness and sweating and on ability to get aroused in sex.*
Steps would be:

- Developing a relaxation strategy and a relaxation tape with the patient.
- Going through the procedures for reducing anxiety (Chapter 12).
- Keeping a diary to monitor levels of anxiety.
- Keeping diaries of frequency and duration of checking for KS, spells of dizziness and sweating and of level of sexual arousal during times he and Ted attempt sex.

*Develop a range of pleasurable activities which can improve the quality of time spent at home.*
Steps might be:

- Drawing up a list of activities which can be done at home which have been enjoyed in the past or which the patient would like to do.
- Drawing up a schedule for a week of such activities.
- Monitoring enjoyment and satisfaction of each of these.

*Arrange medical to ensure that there is no organic basis for sweating and dizziness spells.*

### Stage two

The next stage will depend in part on the results of stage one. The counsellor should always be prepared to try different approaches to solving a problem.

*Try to extend the number of people seen at home.*
Steps might be:

- Get out old address books and ring up old friends.
- Invite some friends round for a drink one evening.
- Arrange a dinner party and invite people round.

*Go out more socially.*
Steps might be:

- Draw up a list of places to go which are within the physical capacities of the patient, for instance going to a cinema or the theatre might be enjoyed and might be less wearing than going to clubs.
- Planning over the next two weeks when these things will be done.
- Making necessary arrangements to make these things happen— booking tickets, arranging transport and so on.

The reader might like to look through the other possible solutions in the problem sheet and to try to draw up similar plans for the next stage or stages.


## Overview

The problem-solving approach suggested above is, of course, only one way of tackling problem solving. However, whichever way the counsellor approaches problem solving, it is very helpful to work systematically through potential problems and to try to develop systematic solutions. Writing down problems and possible solutions is often very helpful for both the counsellor and the client. Problems which appear at first sight an unresolvable mass can resolve themselves into a series of manageable parts which can be dealt with effectively.

# Chapter 14

# Dying, Bereavement and Loss

JOHN GREEN

AND

LORRAINE SHERR

## Loss and bereavement

The literature on loss and bereavement relates largely to death itself, but this is not the only potential loss faced by those with AIDS; sometimes it is not the most important. However, lessons learnt from research into death and dying can be applied to the wider context of loss.

## Theory of loss

There is no prescriptive theory of loss — that is, no theory which says how people should feel about loss or how they should deal with it. There are only descriptive theories, theories which seek to categorise and describe things that people have seen when they have looked at people experiencing loss.

The best known theory (but by no means the only one) is that of Kubler-Ross (1970) who has set out a series of stages that have been observed in people facing loss. Such approaches can be very helpful in thinking about the issues surrounding death and bereavement.

However, particularly in the field of death and dying, workers have sometimes sought to use such descriptive theories as prescriptive theories. They have come to feel that unless people experience certain feelings or deal with those feelings in certain ways they will suffer psychological or even physical harm. Trying to force what happens to real people into rigid prescriptive theoretical models is at best unhelpful, at worst it prevents counsellors from seeing what is really happening and makes them see only what they *expect* to see.

Although descriptive models such as that of Kubler-Ross are helpful in thinking through the issues, our own clinical experience suggests they must be used with caution, since:

- One cannot assume that all individuals experience or ought to experience a similar set of reactions. Many individuals may experience some of the reactions — some may experience them all.
- Some may go through the stages in a different order, or entirely miss out a stage. There is no 'normal' grieving process and individuals show a wide variation in expression.
- Patients do not necessarily travel from the first stage to the last, they may move backwards and forwards between 'stages' at different times.
- It is not clear that some 'stages' are in fact 'stages' as opposed to reactions.
- Terms which are used specifically by particular writers are sometimes used in a broader, looser sense by workers in the field.

Theory is thus limited but can still allow for a framework which may be helpful in anticipating, guiding, helping and understanding and, within these constraints, may be a useful tool for counsellors.

Kubler-Ross felt that many patients showed an initial shock reaction to news of a loss. The shock made it difficult to take in information and difficult to think or plan rationally.

This reaction of shock was often, though not always, followed by a stage of denial. The concept of 'denial' is one which is often used by writers on loss other than Kubler-Ross. In general use it has sometimes become a vague catch-all term which is used to describe a whole range of different reactions. Stripped to its barest bones it is often used to mean the patient or relative not viewing the situation as negatively as others think they should. This is, of course, in contrast to the more precise usage of Kubler-Ross.

At its most extreme it may appear that the patient simply refuses to believe the diagnosis. We have not seen this extreme form of denial as a lasting response in our own patients, although it possibly appears as a very fleeting immediate response to being told they have AIDS: 'It can't be, I feel so well.' On the other hand there are sufficient cases in the literature to show that it does exist as an emotional response. However, at least some cases of 'denial of diagnosis' have rather simpler explanations:

A patient referred from a distant hospital was sent because he was believed to be 'suffering' from 'denial' in that he kept asking whether he had, in fact, got AIDS. On being questioned he said he was sure that he did, in fact, have AIDS but that no-one had said so in so many words. On contacting several doctors in the three hospitals he had previously been in touch with, each doctor ridiculed the view that he had not been told, each one saying that he had been 'told repeatedly'. Yet none of these doctors had told him himself! When the diagnosis was confirmed with the patient he said he was relieved to know and no longer showed any signs of 'denial'.

Less extreme forms of this sort of problem are probably not that uncommon. Cartwright *et al.* (1973) showed the discrepancies between the desire for information expressed by terminally ill patients and the provision offered by doctors. Such difficulties often referred to diagnosis and telling patients about the nature and prognosis of their condition.

While it cannot account for all cases of denial of diagnosis there are probably occasions where apparent denial is simply the result of poor explanation. It is easy for a well-educated professional to believe that he has adequately explained his condition to a patient when he has, in fact, completely failed to get the message across in an understandable form.

Probably a more common form of denial in people with AIDS is denial of the seriousness of a condition. In the early 80s, when few patients with a history of pneumocystis could be expected to live longer than twelve months, many patients, despite asking about this and being told the answer, took the view that they were 'going to beat this thing'. This is probably an example of the fact that denial can be a healthy reaction. Patients like this took the view that they *might* die, and made plans in case they did, but lived as though they were going to beat AIDS. There were no obvious adverse psychological sequelae to this stance, indeed such patients often appeared happier and more energetic in dealing with their condition. It is hard to believe that what was objectively an irrational view could be anything but beneficial *for them.*

It is interesting to note that it sometimes seems to be the professionals who find 'denial' more distressing than the patient. Perhaps it disturbs their framework of belief about the world.

Kubler-Ross suggested that, after shock and denial, many patients exhibit an anger reaction. Outbursts of anger will be familiar to anyone who has worked with the dying, and they can take many forms. People may be angry at themselves, others or medical staff. Indeed Parkes (1978) reported that 25 per cent of relatives of terminally ill patients exhibited anger towards staff. If irrational anger is shown towards them, staff must take care not to interpret it personally and patients should not face recriminations for angry outbursts from their relatives. Staff may pre-empt many such occurrences by open and honest two-way communications at all times.

However, anger is not always irrational. There may often be cause for anger. It is easy to attribute anger to the internal emotional state of the patient or relative when, in fact, they have good reason to be angry.

The next stage for many patients, in Kubler-Ross's formulation, is that of bargaining. The patient tries to strike a bargain, often with God but occasionally with their doctor, for more time along the lines of, 'Please, if I am good, give me more time'. This, in our experience, tends to be a rather fleeting reaction when it occurs and only occasionally does it take on major significance.

Kubler-Ross suggested that patients then tend to pass from the stage of anger into one of depression. Depression is a common feature in those experiencing loss. Times of brief transitory depression are almost inevitable in someone faced with death or other major losses. However when such depression is profound and prolonged it should not be dismissed simply as a normal 'part of mourning'. In many cases those suffering prolonged severe depression as a result of loss can benefit from counselling and support. Ultimately where there is severe and persistent depression which is not relieved by counselling it may be necessary to consider antidepressant medication (see Chapter 12).

For Kubler-Ross the final stage in the dying was acceptance, a coming to terms with the inevitability of death and an acceptance of it. However it is not clear that acceptance is a unitary thing. Some patients accept comfortably while they are still relatively well that they will die, and use this as the basis for living their lives from that point onwards.

For other patients acceptance of death is reached fully only when they have become very sick. Indeed for many patients who are in pain or tired of repeated infections death is no longer something to be feared — it is something almost to be welcomed. Even here, however, it is a mistake to assume that things are straightforward:

> Martin had had repeated infections over a period of three months. Always rather difficult and unpredictable to deal with, he also had considerable charm. He developed a respiratory infection and appeared to be certain to die. He himself was sure that he would die. He appeared to reach a comfortable acceptance of his impending death. He asked several people he had had difficult relationships with to come and see him and had a series of reconciliations with them. Shortly afterwards the treatment unexpectedly started to make an impact and within a few days he was well again. He then became exactly as 'difficult' as he had been before, including falling out with one of the people he had been reconciled with. He continued to be determined to fight his disease.

It could be argued that this is not 'true' acceptance because he moved away from it, but this would logically suggest that acceptance can only be judged when someone is dead and can't change his mind — which would make it a rather pointless concept.

People are immensely complex in their reactions to death, as in their reactions to life. They find many different ways to cope. Some individuals may rapidly find a way to cope and others may experience prolonged adverse reactions. There may be oscillations, gradual changes and abrupt changes. How people are coping may vary according to how well other aspects of their lives are going or according to other external factors. Anniversaries and special occasions can provide reminders which may bring on fresh mourning or cause changes in mood.

There is some evidence to suggest that multiple loss is more difficult to bear than single loss. If someone is faced with a sequence of losses he may find that his capacity to cope is further impaired and he needs extra support.

Ultimately descriptions such as that by Kubler-Ross of the reactions of those faced with death or other losses can be very valuable in providing the counsellor with signposts in unfamiliar territory. However, to date, all models are merely partial descriptions of very complex events with many unsatisfactory features. It is important for counsellors to use such models to help them to see more clearly what is happening to a person, not as blinkers to blind them to things happening to the person which are not in the model.

## Spectrum of loss

People with HIV can experience a wide range of losses other than simply those associated with the imminence of death. The following is a partial list of some of the losses which people faced with AIDS or HIV infection may suffer.

### 1. Loss of certainty

We all have a (spurious) certainty about what will happen to us next week or next month. Although people are mortal and life is uncertain, they tend to live as though life is certain and they are immortal, at least while they are young. Even filling in a diary for next month is an expression of faith. Someone with a potentially fatal illness is brought face-to-face with the fact that this sort of view is, to some extent, a self-deception.

## 2. Future hopes

Most people have a range of hopes for the future — promotion, that small house in the country, having a family, going to places. These hopes can be lost.

## 3. Relationships

People can be rejected by their family or partners or friends either because they have HIV or AIDS or because their sexuality or use of drugs is revealed for the first time. Under the strain of diagnosis relationships may break down. However there may be more subtle changes in the meaning of relationships as the other people involved change their behaviour and attitudes to the person who may be dying. A relationship based on equality may be unbalanced when the other person has to look after the PWA. The avenues to forge new relationships which might replace old relationships may also appear closed.

## 4. Health

People tend to take their health for granted, at least those who are younger do. The automatic assumption of good health is lost in someone faced by HIV or AIDS.

However, loss of health also means for some people a restriction on the range of activities which they can undertake. When a patient becomes easily tired or short of breath he may be unable to do the things he used to.

## 5. Control

People generally have an assumption (sometimes exaggerated) that they are in control of their lives. For the PWA or the individual with HIV there can be a considerable loss of control. In extreme cases they feel that they are the helpless victims of an attack by the virus.

However, there are also other control losses. They may lose control over their use of time because they find themselves forced to attend the hospital or clinic at particular times. If the issue of control is not understood by the hospital, patients may find themselves losing control over even their own bodies as others take decisions about their care. It is for this reason that decisions about care should always be *joint* between the clinician and the patient.

## 6. Sexual losses

The range of sexual expression is restricted for someone infected with the virus. He may miss the intimacy that penetrative sex represents for some people. If he is unable to function sexually because of organically caused impotence or inability to ejaculate, as occasionally happens, he may find that his sex life is virtually ended.

## 7. Life style

Changes in life style are common, particularly in PWAs. Losses in this area may include:

- Loss of standard of living through loss of earnings in those who become unemployed, or those whose earning ability is restricted.
- Loss of housing.
- Loss of ability to obtain mortgages and insurance.
- Loss of freedom to travel and settle in some countries.

## 8. Loss of body image

Particularly where this involves weight loss or extensive KS people may feel that they are no longer physically attractive, not just sexually, but also in everyday interaction with others. Often this feeling is unrealistic. Sometimes, however, it is realistic. There are steps which can be taken to help people to make the most of their appearance. Sometimes treatment is called for on cosmetic grounds where on strict clinical grounds it is unnecessary, for instance in the treatment of facial KS. The use of cosmetics to mask KS and other skin conditions, and even the purchase of new, well-fitting clothes to disguise weight loss, can sometimes help.

## 9. Loss of lovers

Those with AIDS or HIV sometimes experience the loss of lovers from AIDS too.

## 10. Loss of status

What someone does for a living is not just a source of income, it is also often a part of social status. A bank manager who suddenly becomes unemployed loses not just the income but also part of his place in society.

### 11. Loss of dignity and privacy

Particularly where extensive tests and clinical interventions are carried out there can be a perceived loss of dignity. Patients may find themselves festooned with pipes and tubes and with clinicians poking in every orifice with medical instruments. They may even be unable to go to the lavatory on their own and instead must call for a bed-pan.

Dignity and personal privacy are very important. Our dignity and privacy are a major part of our feelings about ourselves, and a major personal right. We have seen patients refuse treatment for particular conditions because, in spite of the best efforts of those working with them to minimise this loss, they can no longer tolerate the invasion of their privacy and the loss of dignity involved in treatment. If privacy and dignity are not respected by everyone dealing with the patient such refusals are likely to be even more common.

### 12. Loss of hopes for children

For the HIV seropositive man or woman there may be a loss of the hope of having a family.

### 13. Loss of security

Where there is prejudice against people with AIDS there is often a loss of the feeling of personal security. There is the fear that others will find out and that persecution will result.

## Counselling those facing death

The single most important thing to remember about people who are dying is that they are *living people*. They are just as alive as the person talking to them. There is a danger always of treating the patient as a 'dying person' rather than as just a person.

For the person who is faced with death most of his problems are the problems of living, not those of dying. However, there are some specific issues which are covered below.

### Discussing death

In discussing death with PWAs there are two different approaches, which will be appropriate in two different situations:

- There is the possibility for anyone who has AIDS that he may die in the near future. For most PWAs at most times it is simply not possible to answer the question, 'Will I die?' with any certainty. New treatments are being developed which may turn a probable 'yes' into a 'no' in the future. The patient may be a long-term survivor. However, both the counsellor and the patient know that most people with AIDS do die from the disease sooner or later. In discussing death with the patient it is important to acknowledge this and to answer any questions honestly and straightforwardly on the balance of probabilities.

PATIENT: 'Will I die from AIDS?'
COUNSELLOR: 'I don't know, no-one knows. It is quite likely that in the future you may die from AIDS. On the other hand you may not, because...'

An assessment of probabilities will take into account not just currently available treatments or those the counsellor knows may come into use in the future and the possibility of being a long-term survivor, but also the current clinical state of the patient. Clearly a man with a history of repeated opportunistic infections who has gradually responded less and less well to treatment for them has a worse outlook than a man who is well except for some KS.

- The second case is that of the person who is visibly close to death because he is not responding to treatment, or he is so weak that he is clearly dying, or he has some untreatable tumour.

If the patient asks, 'Am I dying?' then the answer can only be, 'I think you are'. If the patient doesn't ask then there is no need to make the fact that he is close to death verbally explicit. However, it is important not to treat such a patient as though he will live forever. He will know that he is very ill, he will know that he may well die and he needs to be encouraged to take those steps which he would like to take concerning his death (these issues are covered in more detail below).

*When to discuss death*

Death will naturally be discussed at certain times — at the time of diagnosis and, sometimes, when the patient becomes very ill. However, counsellors often worry about whether they should bring up the issue at other times, particularly in cases where the patient doesn't bring it up. In part this stems from a reaction to anxiety. Counsellors are often anxious about discussing death, they do not wish to evade the issue because of their own anxieties, so they react by going to the other extreme and seeking every opportunity to talk about death. Sometimes this can have interesting results:

> One of us visited a PWA at home late one evening to see how he was getting on. He didn't seem terribly keen on discussing anything very profound so the conversation turned to sport. After a few minutes the PWA suddenly said, 'Thank God you've come round, you're the first person that's come to see me today that hasn't wanted to go on and on about death and AIDS. Can't they talk about anything else? It's so incredibly boring.'
>
> He spoke with considerable good humour. He had had a number of visitors that day from various statutory and voluntary agencies, each one determined not to 'evade the issues', each one unaware of what the others were doing.

The counsellor should aim to take his lead from the patient. If the patient wants to talk about death then the counsellor should be willing to do so. If the issue of death comes up naturally as part of something the counsellor is saying he shouldn't go out of his way to avoid the issue. On the other hand there is no point in forcing a patient to talk about death simply because the counsellor thinks either he or the patient *ought* to talk about it.

### Planning for death

Anyone faced by a possibly life-threatening illness should 'put their affairs in order'. If they don't eventually die they won't have lost anything by doing so. Things which they might do include:

- Making a will.
- Particularly with gay couples where the partner has not got the legal status of next-of-kin (as a wife or husband would have), they may need to take steps to secure the partner's financial future.
- Stating any special request or making special arrangements for the funeral. Sometimes people want special music, or a special oration. Sometimes people go even further. Several PWAs we have seen have made all their own funeral arrangements as far as possible, down to choosing the sort of coffin they want.
- Any religious requirements they may have either at the time of death, or as death approaches, or after death.
- Deciding where they want to die. Some people have a clear wish to die at home if at all possible.
- Anyone they would want to be with them when they are dying.
- Who should be informed when they are dying.
- Putting personal papers together and leaving any special instructions about their affairs.

Once these things have been arranged they can be forgotten and the person can get on with his life. Tackling this sort of issue should be presented as insurance, something which it is wise to do, not as a sign that death is certain (unless it is).

## Clearing up loose ends

For some people there are loose ends in their lives which they want to tie up before they die. These can be of many types — people they have fallen out with who they would like to be reconciled to, things they have not done that they feel it important to do, people they have not seen for a long time that they want to see again.

## Spiritual matters

Some people have deeply held spiritual beliefs, some find such beliefs when they are faced with death, others have none at all. It is helpful for the counsellor to find out about these and to make any necessary arrangements for the person to see a chaplain or rabbi or priest or whoever else can deal with these issues with them.

## Doing things they have always wanted to do

Some people have things they have always wanted to do but have put off. The point where they are facing death is often the point where they want to do these things. Within the limits of the patients' physical abilities it is important to help them as far as possible to achieve what they want to. Sometimes this creates a conflict with clinical issues. Patients may want to travel and there may be a question of whether they will become ill abroad and find themselves in difficulties. As far as is possible, though, they should be helped to travel even at some small risk that things may go wrong.

## Treatment or not

Patients may have strong views about the extent to which they want treatment if they are dying or whether they want to be resuscitated. These views should be respected and followed.

## What happens when you die?

A number of patients want to know about what happens physically to the body when they die. What does the hospital actually do, for instance? In these cases, a full and sensitive explanation should be given.

### Reassuring patients

For many patients fear of death is a less important issue than the fear of dying alone or in pain. They should always be reassured that they will not be allowed to die alone or in pain. Someone will be there with them when they die and adequate medication will always be given to suppress pain.

Sometimes patients ask a similar but distinct question: 'Is it painful to die?.' The answer is that it is not. We know this because some people have died and then been resuscitated and they do not report it as an unpleasant experience. Experiences of seeing other people die peacefully can also be discussed.

### Carers

The person facing death is often not the only one who wants to talk through the issues above. It should be remembered that carers and lovers may also need to go through these issues with the counsellor and they should be given every opportunity to voice anxieties and have them addressed.

## Those left behind: death and the carer

In this context 'carer' means exactly what it says, lovers, wives, husbands, friends, family and anyone else emotionally affected by the death or possible death of the patient.

Carers often need as much support and help as the patient, not infrequently considerably more. There is a particular problem with carers because they are often reluctant to say that they are having problems. There are several reasons for this:

- They feel that they have to be 'strong' so as to be able to help the patient.
- They feel that it is the patient who should be getting all the staff time, not them.
- They feel that their problems are trivial in comparison with those of the patient.

Because carers are so often reluctant to come forward for help they need to be given every possible opportunity to express any difficulties they may be having. Particularly when the patient has come into hospital or is being visited at home, the counsellor will have the opportunity to talk to the carer. It is helpful to actually set aside some time to talk to the carers and to find out how they are getting on. It is surprising how many will say they have difficulties when it comes to the point.

Every effort should be made not to downgrade the importance of the carer. It is easy for carers to think that their usefulness is very limited compared with the 'real experts' of the hospital. As far as possible they need the chance to talk to staff and a point needs to be made of how valuable their contribution to the care of the patient is, being careful not to corner them into a situation where they then can't admit that they are not, in fact, coping.

Sometimes a carer needs to be 'given permission' to withdraw. They simply cannot cope any more and the hospital must say, 'You have done everything it is possible for one person to do, we will take over the physical burden now *but you still have an important role in being there'*.

When a person is approaching death as much as possible should be done to prepare the carer for what is going to happen; if they are going to be there, what the death will be like; and what will be done after the death.

## Tying up 'loose ends'

Carers themselves may have loose ends to tie up with the patient, things they have never said, things that have been difficult between the two of them for years, things they need to discuss for their peace of mind. The carer too has needs and rights. He should be encouraged to sort out things he needs to sort out before the patient dies. Leaving things settled makes dealing with death easier:

A PWA's mother had been taught from her earliest years onwards not to show emotion. She had never been able to tell her son that she loved him. She had shown her disapproval of his being gay and had never been willing for the patient to bring his lover to her house. When she saw that he was dying she began to regret these things. She at last found the strength to tell her son she loved him. She saw how upset the lover was and found she understood that he too loved her son. They talked and got on well, much to the patient's delight. After the death they were able to support each other and became friends, indeed the lover became something of a son himself.

## The carer as patient

It is important to remember that carers are often themselves infected with HIV or have AIDS. They will need, in this case, just as much counselling as, or more than the patient, since they may be facing a double stress.

## Bereavement

The time of a death is a busy one for everyone concerned. It is important that carers should not simply get lost in the overall 'business'. They will continue to have their needs and require support and help through an often extended period.

For people suffering a bereavement the first few days after the death are often a terrible shock. However, there are often sympathetic people around who will share the burden of loss and are willing to talk over the death with the carer.

After a short while, however, carers are expected by the world to 'pull themselves together'. It is considered that they are grieving too long, or 'being morbid'. The friends who flocked around at the time of the death now begin to get on with their own lives again. The amount of support that the carer gets drops off, even though he may feel worse than he did immediately after the death.

There is no 'natural' length of mourning. A person can mourn for days, or weeks or months. Even over many years he may still get pangs of mourning, particularly on anniversaries, or when some favourite piece of music they both shared is played.

There is a difference between mourning and depression, although normal mourning may have days of depression in it, and the counsellor should be careful to pick up the carer who becomes depressed after the death (see Chapter 12).

There are several things the counsellor can do which will help. Some of these are covered below.

### Reassuring the carer

Some bereaved carers feel that they are in some way failing by not coming to terms with the bereavement quickly enough, a message all too often echoed by their friends. They need to be reassured that it is 'all right' to mourn, it is natural. It is also all right to cry sometimes and all right to be depressed from time to time. Above all, they must be reassured that the counsellor has time for them.

Not all carers mourn after a death. They may feel a sense of relief, particularly if the dead person had been very ill before the death or had been suffering from severe dementia. They can feel that they are abnormal in this respect and should be reassured that they are not. There is no evidence for the commonly held view that someone who fails to mourn will come to great psychological harm. What *is* harmful is the carer who is mourning but is not able to express that mourning, usually because of the behaviour of others.

### Discussing the dead person with the carer

Many people who are bereaved want desperately to discuss the dead person with someone. They want to talk about him partly to put things into perspective, partly because talking about him eases the pain. They find sometimes that friends are reluctant to discuss the dead person in case the carer becomes 'upset'. In fact discussion, if the carer wants it, is the best thing.

Talking things over with the carer and listening are the two most important things that the counsellor can do to help.

### Dealing with guilt

Few people who are bereaved escape without at least some guilt. They look back over their lives with their loved ones and see only the things that they regret, arguments, things they feel they prevented the other person from doing, things they failed to do. They need time to talk through these things, but they also need gently to be brought round to thinking of all the good times they have had together. They need to be helped to put the good and bad things into perspective. It is also helpful to reassure them that feelings of guilt are natural.

### Accepting the good and bad parts of the deceased

'Speak no ill of the dead' is an old adage, but not a very sensible one. Few people are saints and carers will have to come to terms with the good and bad aspects of the deceased. At first they may well tend to idealise them; however, as time goes on they will come to take a more realistic and integrated view. For the counsellor the issue to stress is that the deceased was a real flesh-and-blood person with a real person's faults and qualities. If he had not been, would the carer have loved him in the first place?

### Dealing with avoidance

Sometimes carers are reluctant to go to particular places they have been to with the deceased, usually places where they have been happy together. They may be reluctant to go to the grave, not because they do not want to go — which can be a perfectly natural reaction ('there's no point in going, *he's* not there anyway') — but because they are afraid to go. They should be gently encouraged to go; they may feel bad at first, but many people find great comfort from going to places where they have been with the deceased once they get over the initial anxiety. It helps them to feel close to the loved one.

### 'The shrine'

It occasionally happens that, after a death, the carer makes the joint home, or part of it, into a sort of shrine, keeping it exactly as the deceased left it and resisting all attempts to change it. This is rarely helpful, the deceased does not live on in material objects, but in the memories of those left behind.

In this sort of context it is often helpful to gently and gradually encourage the carer to make necessary changes, a little at a time.

### Talking to the dead

Where there are issues which the carer and the deceased have not resolved it sometimes helps to get the carer to actually talk to the deceased. Whether this is in the form of him going to the graveside and talking to the deceased, or setting up an empty chair and talking to that, or simply talking, it can help immensely. He can say all those things he never said when the deceased was alive. A technique we have sometimes used is to get the carer to write a letter to the deceased and then burn it (a sort of way of 'sending' it).

It must be noted that no belief in after-life in the carer is needed to make these things helpful. They are symbolic rather than magical or religious acts. They work because so many bereaved people feel the closeness of someone who is dead.

### Odd experiences

'Odd' experiences after death are very common. The carer may 'see' the deceased, perhaps fleetingly in the street but sometimes in the house. A feeling that the dead person is close, or actually in the room, is very common.

These experiences often distress people greatly. They may think that they are going mad, or they may think that they have seen a ghost. It is only when the subject is touched on by the counsellor that carers will sometimes admit that they have had these experiences.

They should be reassured that they are quite natural and normal experiences. If a carer feels that they are spiritual experiences no attempt should be made to argue with him by a sceptical counsellor. On the other hand it is possible to explain them in terms of normal products of the mind which is mourning, a part of the process of coming to terms with grief and mourning, a benign and helpful process.

## Letting go

After a time the image of the deceased often becomes weaker in the mind of the carer. He may find that he can no longer clearly picture the face or imagine the voice of the deceased. This can cause great distress if, for the carer, the deceased seems to live on only in his memories. He can be reassured about this. The image will often return in the future and can, in any case, be strengthened again through photographs of the deceased.

## Thinking what the deceased would want

One great ally which the counsellor has is the deceased himself. In general, if the deceased had loved the carer, he would want him to have a happy life. Talking through what the deceased would want with the carer and trying to come to some conclusions is often a liberating and pleasing experience.

## References

Kubler-Ross, E. (1970) *On Death and Dying.* London: Tavistock.
Parkes, C.M. (1972) *Bereavement. Studies of Grief in Adult Life.* London: Tavistock.
Cartwright, T.A., Hockey L., and Anderson, J.K. (1973) *Life Before Death.* London: Routledge and Kegan Paul.

# Chapter 15

# Male Homosexual Sexual Behaviour

TOM McMANUS

Since the advent of the AIDS epidemic, there has been more of a realisation among carers that understanding the whole person is an important part of helping people cope with illness. This includes attempting to understand the influence that sexuality has on all our lives, and the impact it may have on the way we cope with adverse circumstances.

HIV, the human immunodeficiency virus, can be spread sexually. The earliest AIDS cases both in the USA and the UK were in homosexual men. Soon it became obvious that a need for more understanding of male homosexual behaviour was necessary, both to mirror the spread of the infection and to help professional and voluntary workers care for individuals with HIV infection.

## Sexual orientation

We know from the investigations of Kinsey *et al.* in 1948 that a person's sexuality may express itself in different ways at different times throughout life. Although the vast majority of men in Kinsey *et al.*'s sample regarded themselves as heterosexual in thought and deed, one in three of their interviewees had had a homosexual experience leading to orgasm between the ages of 16 and 55. There is no evidence to say that this is not true today. In fact, doctors working in genito-urinary medicine clinics are finding that, because of the fear of AIDS, more men are admitting to a bisexual life style.

Society, though, tends to categorise people into either homosexual or heterosexual, recognising that a small percentage of people are bisexual. Bisexual men are thought of as being able or willing to have sexual intercourse with either men or women as the opportunity arises. In dealing with the spread of a virus such as HIV and in counselling men who either know or wish to know if they are carrying HIV, it is essential for health care workers to be aware that men who seem to be obviously heterosexual may well be having or have had sex with other men. They may not regard themselves as homosexual if asked, and may be shy of bringing up the subject unless the counsellor specifically mentions it, and raises it in an obviously comfortable and non-judgemental way.

Many people see homosexuals as only those who lead a so-called 'gay life style'. This means that not only are their sexual partners male but the vast proportion of their social life centres around gay bars and clubs. The danger here is that this misconception may lead to the assumption that the two societies — homosexual and heterosexual — are totally separate.

## Attitudes

Admitting to a homosexual or gay life style is not an easy option. The attitude of most of the general public to gay men is still less than tolerant. The spread of HIV is allowing this intolerance to be expressed more publicly. Therefore covert gay sexual behaviour and an unwillingness among gay men to express their sexual orientation to others is still prevalent today.

Men and women have long recognised that openly admitting to themselves, their family, friends and workmates that they are gay is a difficult option. Admitting publicly to being gay is seen, by many, as a distinct act in their lives, although the process itself may take several years. This process is called 'coming out' and the anxiety which may be associated with 'coming out' can overwhelm some individuals. This is especially true if rejection by their family and/or loved ones occurs. Many who are in the process of coming out require the assistance and advice of friends and often of professional counsellors, even if the 'coming out' is a planned event.

Increasingly men are forced to come out because they find out they are HIV antibody positive or have AIDS. This can lead to an especially stressful course of events and counsellors will need to be aware that their clients will need help not only in adjusting to their antibody status but also in coping with others knowing that they are gay. Rejection by the family, because of homophobia rather than because of the HIV status, is common. Further problems will arise if the man is married or bisexual.

The stresses of coming out and the problems that many gay men face because of the public's attitude towards homosexuality are all issues that need to be addressed when a client is first diagnosed as having HIV infection. The counsellor will gain the confidence of the client if he shows an awareness of these problems and is willing to discuss them in an open, understanding and sympathetic manner.

### Relationships

Relationships within the gay scene are as diverse and complex as in the heterosexual way of life. Since most of us have at least a nodding acquaintance with heterosexual relationships, having been brought up in one, they are often used as role models for the gay scene. But there is a strong belief that gay men are incapable of or unwilling to form long-term relationships.

However, in a recent study using postal questionnaires circulated via gay magazines, around 20 per cent of gay men who responded had had a steady sexual relationship with one other man for more than six months. Many had had one partner for more than five years.

Monogamy is therefore not an unusual state among gay men, although in the 60s and pre-HIV, there was a strong body of opinion among gay men against having just one regular sexual partner. Then there was a need to explore a new-found sexual freedom and a sexual identity and life style recognised as different from that seen in heterosexuals. Included in this was a tolerant attitude to casual sex. Long-term commitments were not sought. Today, however, there is a willingness to work at a relationship with another person and to try to make it last.

Gay men may have one or more regular sexual partners and may also have casual sexual encounters. In an 'open' relationship each partner will know at least some of the other's sexual exploits outside the relationship, and a degree of acceptance will exist. Implicit in this acceptance is the understanding that neither partner will do anything to put the other at risk of catching infections. This type of relationship is often accompanied by unspoken worries and fears. In a 'closed' relationship each partner will be expected to be faithful to the other.

Irrespective of the type of relationship, there is usually an understanding (or hope) that casual sex will be of the safer sex variety to protect the other partner. If an infection such as gonorrhoea appears in a so-called 'closed' relationship, not only is there a feeling of having been let down but also a great fear that HIV infection may be present

in this stable relationship. This may come out during pre-test counselling. The reaction of the individual may be one of despair, anger
and fear. The friendship may break up because of broken trust and the
stress may be greatly increased as a man who thought he was at little
risk of catching HIV suddenly sees himself as vulnerable. The counsellor
then has a marriage guidance role and it may be necessary to see both
partners in an attempt to save or at least define the present state of
affairs.

The sex drive in gay men is as strong as in other men, so there is
still a great temptation for sex with casual acquaintances or with men
who are not well known to the individual. In San Francisco and other
US cities where many men are HIV positive there is strong peer group
pressure to cut down on casual sex or to practise safer sex with
partners whose HIV status is unclear. A similar attitude is developing
in the UK gay scene.

Another change in the development of a new relationship today is
that, early in the friendship, the new friends will broach the subject of
HIV status and each other's state of health. Some will demand that
HIV testing be done and some will want to do it anyway before
starting a new friendship. There should be a respect nowadays not
only for your own health but that of your partner, and a responsible
feeling of not wanting to put others at risk, especially if a new loving
friendship is developing.

Gay men realised early in this epidemic that a responsible attitude
was necessary in their sex lives to prevent both catching and spreading.
Counsellors are already aware of this feeling and of the importance
gay men attach to it.

Gay men also feel that not enough members of the general public
realise how responsible they have been in this area and that they have
seriously attempted to halt as far as they can the spread of HIV
infection. There is no evidence, apart from the occasional and oft
quoted cases, that homosexual men, infected with HIV, are deliberately
and irresponsibly spreading the virus.

## Sexual behaviour

An understanding of male homosexual sexual behaviour is necessary
before a constructive discussion about changing to safer behaviour can
take place. There are general misconceptions and misunderstandings
about gay male sexual behaviour which gay men will spot if the

counsellor is not well informed on this subject. Homosexual sex, apart from occurring between two people of the same sex, differs very little from its better known heterosexual counterpart. There are virtually no gay sex acts which do not occur in the heterosexual or straight scene.

A common belief is that all men who have sex with each other have anal sex. Sodomy has always been closely equated with being male and homosexual. In a recent survey of gay male sexual behaviour (McManus and McEvoy, 1987), less than 50 per cent of almost 1300 respondents said they practised anal sex regularly with either their regular or casual partners.

Another feature of all sexual behaviour is that it often varies with different partners. For example, if a gay man likes being the receptive partner in anal sex he may restrict this practice to his regular partner or partners only. In casual sex, anal sex is very uncommon and if it does feature, condoms are used.

The wishes of the partner are equally important, meaning that a man may have oral sex regularly with one partner but if he changes to another partner this might stop. There is no average gay man and no simple rule book to gay sex.

There are a variety of sexual acts which form the panoply of gay sex. There is no set pattern and it is wise to ask a person what his regular sexual habits are before proselytising that changes should take place. He may already be practising the sort of sex that, as a counsellor, you would encourage.

It may be helpful to work through, in this chapter, some of the sexual practices commonly seen in homosexual sex.

### Masturbation

This is the commonest form of sexual behaviour among men in the UK. With the onset of HIV disease and the worry about casual sex, more emphasis is being placed on thinking up ways of making masturbation more interesting as a regular form of sexual behaviour. Gay videos, books and, in the US especially, 'hot lines' where stimulating talk can be paid for, are all playing a part in revitalising the fantasies which surround solo masturbation.

Mutual masturbation, where two or more men masturbate each other, is obviously thought of as safer sex. Mutual masturbation has always been popular, and again nowadays outside stimulation, such as sexual videos, enhance the enjoyment.

There are common terms for masturbation which are often used by clients. Among these are 'wanking' and 'jacking' or 'beating off'. It is important that in all interviews the counsellor uses words with which the client is comfortable.

## Oral sex

Oral sex comes high up in the list of sexual behaviour common on the gay scene. The so-called sixty-nine (69) position is when two people are sucking each other at the same time.

Seminal fluid is known to contain cells which may carry infections. Although it is recognised by gay men that oral sex, with ejaculation into the partner's mouth, is not as unsafe as the anal counterpart, there is a fear that HIV or the hepatitis B virus might enter the body through cuts in the gums. Therefore while sucking is still popular, most men would not allow their partner to come into their mouth. Occasionally condoms will be used, but interruption before ejaculation is more common.

## Anal sex

The act of inserting or receiving a partner's penis into the rectum used to be a popular form of sexual expression. Many still think it is the commonest sexual practice among gay men. It is not. As stated above, the frequency of anal intercourse varies with sexual partner. While it may be common in a relationship involving a lot of trust, it is becoming less practised in casual affairs.

Lubrication is necessary to facilitate entry of the penis into the rectum. A variety of lubricants have been used during rectal intercourse. These are broadly divided into naturally occurring fluids, oil-based and water-based lubricants. Saliva and seminal fluid can be used as lubrication, the former being more popular; semen is less used now because of the knowledge that it may carry HIV and other viruses. Among the oil-based lubricants the most commonly used are Vaseline, baby oil, Nivea, etc. These are less used now because they are known to irritate the rectal mucosa causing inflammation. They also seriously weaken condoms causing them to rupture during intercourse. Water-based substances, such as KY Jelly, are increasing in popularity, particularly as they can be used with condoms.

Several new lubricants are being introduced to gay men in an effort to find an ideal and safe lubricant. Newly popular creams contain nonoxynol-9, a chemical which is known to have viricidal properties against HIV.

Anal sex both insertive and receptive — also called 'active' and 'passive' respectively — is not so frequently practised now in the UK.

Early in the AIDS epidemic it was realised that seminal fluid could transmit HIV and that the passive partner, especially, was at high risk of catching the infection. One way of knowing that anal sex is less favoured now is the dramatic fall in new cases of rectal gonorrhoea among gay men and, happily, a drop in the numbers of recently acquired HIV infections.

Although there is uncertainty if an entity such as safe sex exists at all, the vast majority of gay men know and accept that anal sex is the least safe form of sexual behaviour, especially with casual partners. Those who like anal sex know that they must learn to use a condom effectively, with satisfactory lubrication. Unprotected anal sex is re- garded as only being safe with a known and trusted long-term partner. This safer sex behaviour needs to be continually encouraged and monitored by health care workers and leaders of the gay community.

As regards anal sex generally, the safest line for health advisers to take is that anal sex is unsafe sex. If the client is absolutely certain of his partner and has known him for more than six months, then it is possible that anal sex would carry little if any risk. All other relation- ships contain a certain element of doubt about the partner's past. Even if the HIV status is known, gay men realise, or should be told, that this offers only slight security: their partner may have seroconverted since he was tested.

Abstinence from anal sex should therefore be encouraged. Condoms are seen as only a safety barrier and not always effective as such in the prevention of infection. We all know that they have not been tested out of laboratory conditions and certainly not under the conditions present during anal sex. Rupture may therefore occur. Gay men may also not be as skilled as their heterosexual counterparts in the use of condoms. Therefore definite instructions on the use of the sheath by counsellors is important.

### Analingus

This is the insertion of the tongue into the anus, or licking the perianal area. This practice is also less popular these days as it is known to spread gut infections, such as *Giardia lamblia* and hepatitis B.

### Other less common sexual practices

Insertion of a finger or of a fist or arm through a dilated anal sphincter – known as 'fisting'; urinating upon the sexual partner – 'watersports'; and handling or smearing faeces as part of the sexual act – 'scat' – have all become less fashionable. They were never as popular in the UK as they were in the metropolitan parts of the USA. We are more aware now that body secretions may carry infection from one person to another. Fisting has the danger of tearing the anal sphincter or rectum present every time, except, perhaps, when it is used by those experienced in this form of sex.

Sadomasochistic acts, bondage, and the insertion of rings or bars through the nipples or genitalia are popular with a minority of gay men.

## Abstinence

One other problem which will be encountered during counselling sessions is that of the gay man who, through fear of catching HIV, has given up sex altogether. He may find it easier to have no sex with others and to stay away from gay venues altogether. While this will certainly ensure a safe life style it may cause loneliness and depression. If he has had sex in the past he may develop an irrational fear of having HIV. This 'AIDS phobia' may be recognised in men not reassured by the HIV test results.

Both the problems of the isolated homosexual and of the AIDS phobic man are challenges for today's HIV counsellor.

## New horizons

There is good evidence that a change in both the sexual practices and the attitudes of gay men to casual sex has taken place. The importance of making sex as safe as possible for both partners was realised early in the HIV epidemic by gay men living in the cities hardest hit by the disease. This change was initially brought by a fear of catching HIV. Gay men were the first group in Europe to see their friends dying prematurely from AIDS. However, they developed a certain maturity about understanding their own sexuality, caring about their partner's needs and wishes, and a willingness to experiment with forms of non-penetrative sex.

Initially in the USA and then in the UK, the facts about AIDS and what to do to prevent catching it spread around the gay communities. Gay newspapers and leaders of the gay community emphasised the need for safer sex. Peer pressure ensured that it became the norm in the mainstream gay scene. It is also recognised that a single campaign is not enough to ensure that safer sex continues. Gay men themselves are responsible for keeping their counterparts informed about the developments in the AIDS field and especially as new information affects their sexual behaviour. Continued community support is seen as essential and has been seen to work in cities such as San Francisco.

'On your partner, not in him,' was an early slogan indicating where it was safe to deposit semen. Consequently, exploration of more interesting forms of masturbation; body rubbing, especially with the penis being massaged by various parts of the partner's body; whole body massage; sexually explicit videos, etc., are now openly talked about, shared and practised in the gay scene.

The rules of safer sex need to be continually disseminated.

All is not rosy, however. It is easy to have a safer, fuller sex life with a regular partner or partners. However, many men can only get or only like to have casual sex. This is where a knowledge of safer sex rules is important and where many gay men need help from others. Enjoying non-penetrative sex may have to be learned, and workshops on the background and mechanism of safer sex may be needed. These are not always available. Therefore both professional and lay counsellors need to spend some time familiarising themselves with the rules of safer sex and become at ease discussing and teaching them to their clients. If we, as health care professionals, do not take this matter seriously, neither will our customers.

## References

Kinsey, A.C., Pomeroy, W.B., and Martin, C.E. (1948) *Sexual Behaviour in the Human Male*. London: WB Saunders Co. Ltd. p.650

McManus, T.J., and McEvoy, M.B. (1987) 'Some aspects of male homosexual behaviour in the United Kingdom' *British Journal of Sexual Medicine*, April, pp. 110–120.

# Chapter 16

# AIDS in the Community

TERRY COTTON

## Introduction

This chapter provides an outline for setting up and developing Community Support Services for people with HIV-related illnesses, based on the experience of one Local Authority in Inner West London.

Hammersmith and Fulham Council have been providing a comprehensive range of services for people with HIV-related illness since 1983. From 1983 to 1985 the numbers of clients were extremely small and there was a perception (with hindsight an incorrect one) that AIDS was not going to be a problem for the council. However, in 1985 two events dramatically changed things.

Firstly, a client in his fifties, who had been supported by six different home helps while at home, died in hospital. His name and cause of death were reported in the local newspaper. The story also reported that the hospital had fumigated his room and the porters had refused to transport his body to the morgue. The reaction from the home helps and their union was to be expected. Staff were frightened and anxious, and very quickly the issue turned into a industrial relations problem. Home helps, Meals on Wheels service, etc., stated they would not work with people who had AIDS.

This prompted the Borough to hold a study day for staff to try to defuse the situation. The study day, although not very successful, managed to raise 139 questions related to AIDS that were causing concern to staff:

'Will I be forced to go in?'
'Can I refuse to go in?'
'Do they really know how you catch AIDS?'
'Can I catch AIDS from a client's money?'

'Why should I look after homosexuals?'
'Will a drug addict bite me?'
    and so on...

These questions highlighted the scale of the problem facing the council. The home helps already working with people with AIDS had been too afraid to admit this as they feared rejection from their colleagues and friends.

The second event was an employee who informed the council that he had AIDS and wished to be redeployed.

The council was forced to look at issues such as health and safety, confidentiality, discrimination, attitudes to gay men and drug users, the needs of a young client group living with a life-threatening condition, and the need for staff support.

The council's response was twofold. Initially a corporate group was established to produce a policy guidance booklet for managers and staff. Secondly, a large training initiative was started. Trade unions have played a crucial part in this process, ensuring management think through the possible industrial relations problems that might arise.


**Policy guidance**

Because of incidents of staff refusal to work with people with HIV the council was prompted to look at their responsibility as employers and the responsibility of staff to their clients. New employees are now informed at interview of the council's non-discrimination policy on HIV/AIDS. For existing staff the policy and practice guidelines state that staff refusing to work with HIV/AIDS clients should not be forced to do so, but should be offered the opportunity to discuss their concerns in confidence with an informed staff member. In our experience to date this has alleviated staff concerns and all have subsequently agreed to work with these clients.

Corporate guidelines were drawn up in consultation with the trade unions and were approved by full council in January 1987. The guidelines sought to ensure that appropriate and sensitive services were provided for people with HIV infection and that no person experienced discrimination in the provision of these services. The guidelines stated that policies, practices and procedures should be regularly reviewed and updated. Included in these guidelines was a clause ensuring confidentiality for any client with HIV infection.

The sheer range of services involved means that there must be planning and co-ordination between Local and Health Authorities in the provision of services. It is clear from Hammersmith and Fulham's experience that supporting people with HIV-related illness has become a community care issue.

In drawing up the council's policies it has been our practice to involve clients with HIV/AIDS to ensure that services are being targeted appropriately.

Since January 1987 several working parties have been established to review policies and to ensure quality of care:

- The Social Services HIV Policy and Practice Group, who consider policy practices and resource issues in the provision of Social Services to people with HIV in the community. Members of the group include home helps, social workers, the Director of Social Services and representatives from local AIDS organisations.
- The HIV Housing Needs Planning Team, who develop policy and practice in respect of housing services for people with HIV illness. They also are responsible for training programmes and support groups for housing staff.
- A task-orientated planning team established with Riverside Health Authority. The team includes representatives from the Health Authority, Local Authority, Community Health Council, Family Practitioner Committee, Housing Associations, local voluntary organisations and AIDS organisations. The aims are to develop consistent policies and practices in the provision of services between agencies and to consider areas of mutual concern, such as confidentiality.

## Training

Discrimination is probably the biggest issue in HIV/AIDS. In the early days staff anxieties about working with people with AIDS were not just caused by fear of infection, but were often about hostility and prejudice to gay men and injecting drug users. These groups were seen as the 'guilty perpetrators' of HIV infection, and haemophiliacs as the 'innocent victims'.

Given that gay men and injecting drug users have been the group most affected by HIV in the UK, it is likely that the majority of people seeking support to remain at home will belong to these two groups. Indeed the majority of people we have supported to date have been gay men. Staff need to examine their own attitudes and feelings about homosexuality and drug users. Training is essential in this area.

There is a compulsory initial training course for all home care staff, with optional further training including a three-day counselling skills course.

Training programmes available cover a wide range of topics, in particular medical issues of HIV/AIDS, infection control, confidentiality, discrimination, sexuality, safer sex, etc. It has been our experience that training has been successful in helping staff overcome their fears.

Staff support is provided in several forms — one-to-one counselling, peer support groups, or built into the training programmes.

### Services available for people with HIV illness

The following list is an outline of the most common services available to people with HIV illness.

- The Hospital Discharge Team provide intensive support for up to eight weeks following discharge from hospital.
- The Area Home Help Services provide practical input to assist daily living.
- The specialist home helps provide support for children and families at risk.
- The Home Care Team provide respite care, overnight care and support to people who have a terminal illness.
- Meals on Wheels provide meals on a daily basis.
- Social workers monitor the physical, emotional and social needs of individuals.
- Area social workers provide a wide range of care including long-term counselling, co-ordinating community services, assisting with welfare benefit and housing problems.
- Visual handicap specialist social workers provide visual handicap loan equipment and assist in rehabilitation at home.
- Occupational therapists assess the client's physical ability and provide loan equipment and adaptations as required.
- The Housing Services Department provides general advice on housing problems. They are responsible for housing the homeless, rehousing people due to ill health or because they are suffering harassment.
- Day care support facilities have traditionally cared for the elderly but are now having to look at a younger population who may require their services.
- Residential care services have not as yet fully addressed the issue of HIV illness but have been involved in assisting a small supported housing project in the south of the Borough.

- Respite care and residential/foster care provide services which include counselling children, young people and their families.
- The Environmental Services Department provide a collection service for clinical waste.
- Advice and Law Centres provide information and advice on legal, financial and social problems, etc.
- The Libraries Division provide health education through leaflets and displays. Campaigns which target the various ethnic communities living within the Borough are being established with the Black Communities AIDS Team.

Under the provision of the Chronically Sick and Disabled Persons Act the council has also provided telephones and travel permits to people with HIV illness.

The sheer range of services involved in the care of those who are affected by HIV, directly or indirectly, means that good planning is at a premium. Without a clear overall plan and mechanisms for co-ordinating care it is impossible to provide the sort of high-quality service necessary.

AIDS dementia is a particularly worrying problem. The council is currently reviewing the provision of day care, residential care and respite care with a view to extending the role of these services to accommodate the specialist care involved in supporting these clients and their carers.

Since 1983, Hammersmith and Fulham Council have provided services to over 200 people with HIV-related illness at a cost in 1987/88 of £600,000. The council has seen a doubling of referrals every ten months.

It has been our experience that specialist teams do not need to be created; rather, existing services should be tailored to meet the needs of people with HIV illness.

Local authorities over the next decade will become increasingly involved in the care of people with HIV infection and AIDS, and therefore it is crucial that planning starts immediately to ensure adequate and appropriate provision of services.

# Chapter 17

# The Role of Voluntary Groups in the Community

JANET GREEN

## Background of the voluntary movement in the UK

Voluntary groups are not a new concept. Prior to 1905 and the emergence of statutory Social Services, voluntary groups were the sole providers of many forms of assistance. Even after the Beveridge Report in 1942, with its recommendations of a comprehensive system of social security, the voluntary sector was still the main provider of basic services.

The late 1950s onwards has seen significant developments in voluntary action. Some existing services have redefined their role in order to differentiate their service from that of statutory organisations. There has been a rapid growth of pressure groups, as well as the emergence of self-help groups. The last 30 years have also seen the growth of co-ordinating bodies at regional and national levels. Both Local and Central Government have encouraged voluntary groups, mainly through financial help.

Traditionally the range of services offered by voluntary organisations was limited. It mainly consisted of giving financial and material assistance or accommodation to the socially deprived. Today, these groups often recognise the need for emotional and social support, as well as financial assistance, whilst pressure groups attempt to treat the cause of the problem, rather than the symptoms, by lobbying Parliament, demonstrating, and monitoring the performances of Local and Central Government.

Voluntary organisations can be seen to have three major purposes: to promote or campaign around a specific issue; to provide a service; to co-ordinate activity. An agency may combine two or more of these aims, or may even change their purpose over time as different, but related, needs become apparent.

Methods of financing voluntary action mainly consist of contributions from individuals and grant-giving bodies, fiscal assistance from Central and Local Government, or returns from their own investments. It may also, of course, be a combination of all of these.

Legislation was passed in 1966 which allowed local authorities to grant money to voluntary organisations, as well as using voluntary groups for statutory functions, and in recent years financial aid from governments to these agencies has risen dramatically.

However, the receipt of public funds can give rise to certain problems. It may be that the voluntary group will be subjected to control by the donor, thus threatening their freedom to respond to new needs; government can threaten to withdraw money if the project does not comply with their demands.

There is also the danger that the project may be used as an extension or cheap substitute for particular services, allowing Parliament to overlook their own responsibilities. Recent cut-backs in social services, together with the rise in grants to voluntary organisations, indicate that the latter are being utilised as alternatives, although it does mean that politicians can be seen to be acting around a particular issue.

The degree of professionalism within a voluntary organisation varies enormously. Some agencies will be staffed by highly qualified personnel, whilst others depend entirely on the efforts of volunteers. Unpaid workers will be interested and concerned about a particular issue, but may have no relevant qualifications, or they may be professionals from various disciplines.

Although not all voluntary groups are charities, it will be to their advantage to seek charitable status. It will affect their finances in terms of reduced payments of income tax and rate relief, as well as adding to their credibility as a worthy cause. However, the main criterion in applying to the Charities Commission is the condition that the group must not be indulging in political activities (although with the current trend towards advice-giving and campaigning the definition of 'political activity' becomes cloudy), nor support any particular political party.

Voluntary groups dealing with HIV infection have developed from the above background. As we consider some of these projects, and their specific areas of interest, we will see how they fit into this framework.

## London Lesbian and Gay Switchboard

Gay Switchboard (as it was originally named) volunteers must have felt at a loss in those early days of the AIDS crisis, trying to counsel

frightened gay men when they, themselves, knew so little of the
nature of the illness. Over the past few years they have had to continu-
ously train their volunteers in how to deal with this category of callers.
During 1986 the Switchboard received 16,000 calls specifically relating
to AIDS. They provide a telephone helpline service to lesbians and
gays from all over the country, and if necessary will refer callers to a
number of specialist voluntary groups.

This 24-hour service is staffed entirely by volunteers and has recently
been granted charitable status. They have been operating for 14 years
and now receive funding from the DHSS, the London Boroughs Scheme,
benefits and donations.


## Body Positive

This project grew out of the first HIV Antibody Positive Support
Group organised by The Terrence Higgins Trust. The people attending
realised that, in coming to terms with their own diagnosis, they could
offer others in the same situation a unique service—help and advice
from people who really understood what it means to be diagnosed
with HIV.

Initially founded as a support and advisory group in 1985, Body
Positive now include an educational function both for those at risk of
being infected with HIV, and for health professionals who treat and
counsel those with the virus or at risk from contracting it.

Having made changes in their own life styles since diagnosis in
order to counter the spread of infection, Body Positive members provide
encouragement to others at risk. As well as providing peer counselling
for those who are antibody positive in groups, by telephone and by
one-to-one attention, the project also organises social events to counter
the isolation felt by many who are found to have the virus.

Body Positive do not receive any funding from Government bodies,
nor do they employ any paid workers. In spite of this, they organise
seminars and classes to encourage a positive and active approach to
protecting health, and work closely with both statutory and voluntary
agencies. They also campaign for the allocation of more resources for
counselling, treatment, health education and research in connection
with HIV infection, through the media and at parliamentary level.

In 1987 Body Positive were granted charitable status and they are
currently preparing to move into their new centre in West London.
The centre will provide a counselling service, as well as a social setting
for its members. This latter function is particularly important as so

many people with HIV have to leave their jobs due, mainly, to their misinformed and frightened employers suspending them.

Since Body Positive is largely, though not exclusively, made up of gay men, an off-shoot has now been introduced for heterosexual men and women who have been diagnosed with HIV. The Beacon Project will have a similar self-help function to Body Positive, and will continue to have close links with the founding organisation.

## The London Lighthouse

PWAs are often physically weak and in compromised financial states. One of the major material problems experienced is the lack of suitable accommodation. There is a great need for a range of housing, so that the PWA can choose between a completely independent living situation, sheltered accommodation, or somewhere to die with dignity. Although moves are now being made to meet these needs, existing hospices have been slow to accept this group of patients. In an effort to address part of this problem, the London Lighthouse have initiated a residential unit for both those who are approaching death and those who require respite care. The emphasis at this unit will be on relieving physical and emotional distress, thereby assisting people to cope better with their lives in these circumstances.

This voluntary group will also offer information, counselling, support and education for the recently diagnosed, as well as a range of health programmes to assist those with HIV to remain healthy, and will include such methods as visualisation and stress management. A domiciliary support scheme is also planned to help people with AIDS remain in their own homes for as long as possible.

## The Haemophilia Society

This voluntary organisation was founded in 1950. Its primary function since that time has been to provide support, friendship, advice and information to people with haemophilia and their carers, as well as to encourage and support research into the condition. Today they face the additional complication of AIDS, which has come to dominate the work of the Society.

A registered charity, the Society has a number of local groups through-out the country, with a Head Office in London. This group publish a number of leaflets, including several specifically relating to HIV and AIDS.

Other services provided by the Society consist of counselling by telephone and in person, together with advice and information on welfare rights and insurance policies. They have a number of holiday caravans and run an annual Adventure Holiday week for young haemophiliacs.

AIDS is now a worrying feature in the lives of all those with haemophilia. This voluntary agency is committed to supporting them and their families, as well as promoting the need for research into the illness.

## The Terrence Higgins Trust

Since the Terrence Higgins Trust was the first voluntary group in the United Kingdom specifically concerned with HIV issues they have, perhaps, had time to develop their services to meet many needs. Since 1984 their work has escalated to keep pace with the growing menace of AIDS.

Health education is one of the prime functions of the Trust, encompassing many forms and responsibilities. As well as producing a wide variety of leaflets, they also provide speakers and trainers for other agencies (both statutory and voluntary) and have a mobile 'Roadshow', travelling around the country so as to be accessible to answer questions and distribute leaflets to the general public. The Drug Education Campaign was set up to cater for the needs of the second largest HIV risk group, as well as to provide advice to other organisations (including prisons) who are dealing with injecting drug users.

The Trust has always attracted a number of volunteers from medical backgrounds. These doctors and nurses advise the Trust on all the medical information published, as well as helping to train our own volunteers, and workers in other agencies. They play a vital role in maintaining the Trust's close links with the medical services.

The organisation also have a group of lawyers giving their services voluntarily to provide legal advice to those who are antibody positive or have AIDS. They, too, are involved in training Trust volunteers, in addition to performing research into the legal problems and various forms of discrimination that people with AIDS and HIV are confronting, so that solutions may be found.

The Trust Inter-faith Group was set up to bring together ministers, rabbis, priests, buddhists and workers in all faiths to advise and help the Trust. This group's main objective is to set up a network of people throughout the country to give pastoral care to PWAs, their friends and family, should they be seeking spiritual guidance. The group are also disseminating accurate information to the religious community, as there have been numerous incidents where such knowledge was obviously lacking.

One of the first functions of The Terrence Higgins Trust was to set up a Helpline—a telephone service to answer the public's many questions about AIDS, as well as to provide a caring counsellor for those affected by the illness. New volunteers for this service are trained and supervised for a total of 30 hours. Their monthly group meetings contain elements of support, Trust business and further training. The calls taken by the Helpline volunteers are enormously varied and range from comforting the distressed newly diagnosed, to reassuring the extremely anxious callers who are at no risk whatsoever.

The Trust runs a 'One-to-One' service, so that individuals who need immediate short-term help can receive counselling. For example, when parents are told that their son has AIDS—and is also gay, their response to the situation is likely to be a mixture of anger, confusion, sadness and guilt. They may (since AIDS is a severely stigmatised condition) have no-one in their informal support system with whom to share their feelings. The One-to-One counselling provides a place for such parents to express themselves freely. The volunteers involved in this work all have extensive experience in counselling.

We live in a culture which has taught us to hide our fears and grief and, therefore, precious time with those we love is often inappropriately spent. When they die, we may be left with unresolved issues. Terrence Higgins Trust Support Groups now exist for the families of those with AIDS; for their partners or lovers; for women who have HIV or AIDS; for those who wish to explore a holistic approach to their illness; for men with HIV and, of course, for PWAs. All of these groups provide a safe, loving environment where individuals can break out of their isolation and share their experiences, thus giving each other support and comfort. All the groups have one or two skilled facilitators to guide its members along a sometimes difficult and painful path. However, it would be a mistake to view the Support Groups as a place purely for tears, useful though this can be. These groups also contain laughter, warmth and a positive approach for their members.

As the number of AIDS cases steadily increases, the need to provide emotional and practical support grows. A diagnosis of AIDS is very frightening. The person diagnosed has many issues to face. While some PWAs and their significant others will have a strong support network, others will not. They may feel very alone, weak and scared. Others may have caring people around them, but feel that they cannot burden their loved ones, who are also coping with the AIDS diagnosis, with their own fears and needs.

The Terrence Higgins Trust Buddy Service can provide a volunteer to visit the PWA at home or in hospital. They may provide counselling, but are just as likely to provide practical help, such as cooking a meal, or doing some shopping, or simply being there. The befriending function of the Buddy will mean developing an on-going relationship with the PWA, which will include accepting the full expression of powerful emotions which the PWA may experience. It will involve advocacy on their behalf, as well as being aware of the needs of their friends and family. At the same time the Buddy is expected to encourage self-determination, and to avoid undermining the PWA's independence.

The Buddy may be one of a number of people involved—friends, relatives, professionals—yet his or her role will fall somewhere between that of professional and that of relative or friend. This latter group will be under emotional strain themselves, and will not necessarily be under any commitment to provide constant comfort. The Buddy is not under the same emotional pressure, and s/he does have a commitment to give consistent support. Professionals tend to have a fairly specific relationship with their client. There is normally some underlying function in terms of provision of resources, services or treatment, whereas the Buddy is much more personally indentified with the PWA.

Buddies come from a variety of backgrounds. Some may incidentally be employed in the caring professions, but many others have quite unrelated occupations. They can offer peer group support, without many of the presumptions and preconceptions which those of us in the professional caring fields may have acquired.

When asking a group of PWAs what they wanted in a Buddy, their response was quite clear: 'A good listener, a sense of humour, and someone to make the chicken soup!' We try to ensure that all would-be Buddies have at least the first of these qualities. However, we also provide relevant training to ensure that they acquire others. A potential Buddy will be required to participate in the Trust's basic training, which all volunteers have to complete. This consists of medical information, along with some input on associated social issues. They will then be asked to complete a Buddy application form, receipt of which is followed by a formal interview. If they are selected as suitable, they then attend an intensive, residential training weekend. At the end of this they are allocated to a small, local support group, where there will be the opportunity for Buddies to share their experiences in complete confidence. In this way burnout, frustration, feelings of sadness or powerlessness can be expressed and support given. There are also regular opportunities for further training.

We have found that the needs of PWAs are as varied as the people themselves. A Buddy can help with emotional and practical problems up to a point, but whilst some of those diagnosed with AIDS or ARC will be able to continue working for some time, others have to give up employment, either because their employers are badly informed and demand that they leave, or because of ill health. For a young person who believed they would continue working for many years, the results can be devastating—not just in term of emotional reactions to being unemployed, but also financially.

In November 1986, the Terrence Higgins Trust set up a fund for those with AIDS or ARC. Requirements for receiving money are simple: the applicant must have been diagnosed with AIDS or ARC and, secondly, the purpose must be to improve their quality of life.

One final Trust group must be mentioned. The Frontliners are, as the name implies, the people who are most affected by AIDS. Made up of those who have been diagnosed with AIDS or ARC, this self-help group has several functions. They visit, befriend and counsel the newly diagnosed. They will act as an intermediary between the PWA and the Buddy service, introducing the Buddy when necessary. The Frontliners are involved in both training Trust volunteers, as well as outside agencies, and in advising the Trust on matters concerning services to PWAs. They have also written a booklet to be given to those who have just been diagnosed with AIDS or ARC, to inform them of the personal experiences of problems which have been confronted and overcome by others in the same situation. Represented on the Steering Committee of the Trust, they supply the voice of the PWA in the decision-making process. They continue to amaze all of us who work closely with the Frontliners by their energy, enthusiasm and positive approach to their illness.

The above voluntary groups represent only a few of the many organisations which now exist around the country. The services offered by these regional projects vary widely. A number of them initially opened with a Helpline, and have gone on to offer befriending or counselling services. Some produce their own literature and are training local statutory and voluntary agencies. As AIDS spreads to include areas outside the major cities, these projects will prove invaluable to both those at risk and the general public who need accurate information.

Most of the voluntary groups dealing with HIV and AIDS are in their infancy, and have grown rapidly in a short time. We hear scattered complaints about their methods, that they are bureaucratic, disorganised or 'a bunch of do-gooders'. It would be foolish to dismiss these criticisms. No doubt mistakes are made and, hopefully, lessons learnt, as one might expect from young organisations.

As most are largely staffed by volunteers, experience of the consumer can depend on chance. Whilst one volunteer may be sweet-natured and extend him or herself, another may be war-weary and a little distant. If, however, a consumer is dissatisfied with the service he is receiving, he should make this clear to the project organisers, and give the agency a second, or even a third, chance. Bad practice can be reprimanded, and incompatible befrienders or counsellors can be changed.

Voluntary AIDS groups can offer a special response to those with HIV or AIDS. They avoid judgements and criticisms, respect confidentiality, provide support, affection and caring, are committed to the dissemination of accurate and clear facts and to the campaigning for better resources for all those on the 'frontline'.

## The future

There is a danger that statutory services may use voluntary groups as an extension or substitute for particular services, and may overlook their own responsibilities in meeting needs. Voluntary organisations can provide a cheap or easy alternative. If local authority Home Helps refuse to attend to a client, or ambulance workers will not transport a patient, statutory agencies often call upon voluntary groups to provide such services, instead of educating their own workers and thus dispelling much of the fear and misinformation which surrounds AIDS.

However, the very fact that voluntary groups were amongst the first to respond to the AIDS crisis, in all manner of ways, illustrates that such groups can identify and meet needs that local and health authorities cannot, or will not, acknowledge. Certainly, the worried well, who have proved to be an enormous drain on health service resources, would have completely overwhelmed medical staff without these projects dealing with thousands of callers who simply needed reassurance, and would have otherwise attended hospital clinics.

Perhaps, too, voluntary agencies are able to be more flexible and innovative. They can provide a quick, possibly experimental, reaction to new needs, whilst statutory legislation tends to be safe and slow. The Terrence Higgins Trust, for example, were distributing leaflets several years before the Government's campaign against AIDS. There can be no doubt that, in spite of some criticisms from some quarters about the basic language used, the Trust literature has had an effect in restricting the spread of HIV infection.

Many of those diagnosed with HIV or AIDS may be suspicious of statutory agencies. Welfare services tend to exclude the gay community: they are planned around the notion of the heterosexual nuclear family. Gays are discriminated against in various ways – in housing, in being accepted as next of kin, in fostering, and so on. Consequently, it may be difficult to receive help from these services, or even think of them as applicable to the gay community.

It is also difficult to receive such services from professionals who continue to communicate hostility, hesitancy or inappropriate interest. For instance, we have come across professional workers who have told us how much they enjoy working with gay men because 'they all have such a good sense of humour'. It is not useful in working with gay men with AIDS to persist in identifying them as stereotypical images.

Injecting drug users and those perceived as 'promiscuous' have also experienced judgemental attitudes from professional carers. Little wonder, then, that some will find it difficult to ask for help from statutory services. Voluntary organisations provide a choice in the provision of help.

Voluntary groups also act as a watchdog on Central Government, pressing for new legislation, more resources, and drawing attention to areas of need which may have been overlooked.

All the existing groups working around the issues of HIV infection liaise as much as possible. There is a strong feeling of co-operation, arising from the concern which we share. Both volunteers and paid workers in these organisations are committed to enabling PWAs to maintain their independence, thus attaining a higher quality of life.

None of the groups works in isolation, and they have constant contact with other unrelated organisations such as Citizens Advice Bureaux, the Samaritans, the Alzheimers Disease Society, housing and advice projects, Social Services, hospitals, and Social Security, to mention just a few. Together, we can *all* work towards providing a continuum of care, from giving reassurance for the worried well, to acknowledging the need for pre- and post-test counselling, to supporting those with HIV, ARC or AIDS, and helping people with AIDS both to live with their illness, and to die with dignity and compassion.

We can continue to exchange ideas and challenge each other, reach out to those who need us and those we need, and discuss our concerns frankly. Let us continue to build a solid community willing to challenge our weaknesses, exciting by our strengths and energy, and proud of our accomplishments.

# Chapter 18

# Counselling in Developing Countries

JOHN GREEN

## Background

The model of counselling used in Western countries is, inevitably, a response to local conditions. As such it has certain characteristics:

(1) Counselling tends to be carried out by specialist counsellors who are either committed to HIV/AIDS counselling or take it on as part of their work in sexually transmitted disease counselling or in infectious diseases. Counselling and primary medical care tend to be carried out by separate individuals.

(2) There are well-established voluntary groups, often with telephone helplines, aimed at those who are particularly at risk or know themselves to be infected.

(3) Most patients are aware when they are at high risk because most cases of infection continue to be amongst gay men, intravenous drug users and haemophiliacs.

(4) As a result of (3) most individuals who receive counselling come forward for it themselves. They have ready access to medical and counselling facilities on demand. Counselling can, therefore, be concentrated on a few sites.

(5) A lot of counselling work centres around individuals who come forward for the test or who have been diagnosed as having AIDS.

The situation in many developing countries is different. A successful counselling model needs to take these differences into account. Key differences include:

(1) Many patients are not close to hospitals or sexually transmitted disease clinics. They may find it difficult to reach them, particularly

in rural areas. In the West most people are readily able to travel quite long distances because of the availability of relatively cheap public transport and personal vehicles. In much of the developing world patients simply do not have these services available. Either counselling has to be available locally, or the counsellor has to come to them.

(2) The provision of counselling through the creation of specialist counsellors alone is unlikely to meet the demand in those developing countries with high rates of infection.

This is most easily seen through an example. Assuming that a specialist counsellor might provide input into 500 cases per year, a country of 3 million people would need 60 counsellors if the infection rate was 1 per cent. It would need 180 if the infection rate was 3 per cent.

In practice it is only likely that a counsellor would reach this sort of case load if the patients were coming to see him in a hospital or clinic. In a rural area where the counsellor had to go out and see patients, probably travelling long distances, the number of cases seen might drop to 100 or 150 per year. This would increase the number of counsellors needed by 3–5 times.

Many developing countries would find it very difficult to obtain or pay for such large numbers of specialist counsellors.

(3) Patients may not be able to identify whether they are at risk or not. Although health education campaigns play an important role in raising general awareness of AIDS, and are thus of crucial importance in any AIDS strategy, there is little evidence that, in themselves, they have a great deal of impact on sexual behaviour. There is also little evidence that, in themselves, they make it possible for people accurately to assess their personal level of risk.

(4) In Western countries the impetus for self-help and community counselling agencies came in most cases from gay men. It is difficult to imagine a self-help group based purely on heterosexuality or on high levels of sexual activity. Ready access to transport and telephones has meant that self-help groups have been able to cover much larger geographical areas than would be possible in most developing countries.

(5) Where medical resources in the broadest sense are scarce, particularly in rural areas of developing countries, it is doubtful if it makes sense to separate primary medical care from counselling about HIV and AIDs. Primary care is where patients at risk or ill are likely to be identified and cared for. Sending them to a central facility would, in most cases, be impossible.

(6) Not only is it difficult for patients to assess their personal risk of infection, it can also be difficult for medical personnel to do so.

(7) Resources in terms of money, materials and, crucially, manpower are likely to be in extremely short supply in many developing countries.

(8) In contrast to developed countries which have well-resourced voluntary blood donation systems, many developing countries rely for a substantial proportion of blood supplies on donations by relatives and friends. Under these circumstances it is difficult to deter high-risk donors. Thus detection of positives through donations is likely to be higher than in Western countries.

(9) In most Western countries there is a fairly uniform culture across the country. In many developing countries there are marked differences within countries, because national boundaries often fail to reflect tribal or religious boundaries. Differences within countries between rural and urban areas are often far more marked than in Western countries. This means that the specialist counsellor may have to be familiar with a wide range of different cultures.

Similar considerations apply to language. Few geographical areas in the West have more than two major language groups and, where these exist, it is common for people to be at least partially bi-lingual. In many developing countries there are many languages, of which a patient may speak only one or two. Counselling through an interpreter makes things doubly difficult — if a suitable interpreter is available at all.

## Developing an appropriate model of counselling for local circumstances

It is clear from the above that simply taking what has been done in many Western countries and applying it to developing countries will not provide the best possible service.

The scarcity of resources, both economic and human, means that a successful system is likely to have to make the optimal use of existing resources, particularly in terms of trained health professionals, but also in terms of making the best use of what systems already exist for delivering health care. Because patients are less likely to present with worries about HIV, since they cannot necessarily identify themselves as at high risk, health staff will have to be much more active in identifying those at risk in other settings. Where specialist health care staff are used for counselling, particularly in rural settings, they may also have to undertake non-counselling aspects of health care. Since the setting up of self-help organisations and groups is less likely to occur spontaneously, existing groups in the community will need to be used to carry out health education and provide support or the counsellors will have to try to set something up themselves.

A successful counselling system in a developing country is likely to be a truly local system — that is, it is likely to be the result of applying certain general principles to a local situation and coming up with a plan of action which is suited to that area and the resources available. However, even with quite scarce resources it is possible to produce an effective model.

Taking as an example a rural health district with a hospital, a health centre and a dispensary, a model which would take these issues into account might be:

(1) To use existing health contacts, including hospital admissions, family planning programmes, maternity services and vaccination programmes to provide face-to-face health education and health education materials.

(2) To train staff in hospital, dispensary and health centre as well as community staff to ask the necessary questions to find out who is at high risk and to provide basic counselling on the prevention of infection.

(3) To aim for a limited number of specialist HIV/AIDS counsellors to provide back-up, advice and training to workers and assistance with particularly difficult cases on a referral-on basis. If the hospital offers testing-on-request at a single centre they would also provide the services in that clinic.

(4) Where resources permit, to train community staff who will both provide counselling and support to PWAs and their families and also provide a range of simple medical assistance, for instance advice on infection control, anti-diarrhoea medications and pain-killers.

(5) To ask simple questions of relatives who may be going to give blood in order to identify those at high risk so as to avoid donations occurring during the 'window' period between infection and seroconversion.

(6) To use existing groups in the community, for instance women's groups, church groups or other local and national groups, to provide health education and support.

(7) To make a local assessment as to who is at high risk currently. This assessment is likely to be imperfect but will still allow better

concentration of scarce resources than if such an assessment has not been made. The idea that in an area of heterosexual spread almost everyone is at risk, while strictly correct, is unhelpful since in all areas of the world there are gradations of risk.

The model suggested above might also be appropriate in an urban area. However in urban areas patient access to health facilities is generally better than in rural areas because of better transport. In a large city it might be appropriate to aim for more specialist HIV/AIDS counsellors, if resources were available, on the basis that it would be easier for other health care staff to refer them on to specialist counsellors. This would not remove the need for other staff to be trained in the issues since they would still have to be able to recognise who was at risk. It is unlikely in most developing countries that, even in a large city, sufficient resources would be available to provide all HIV/AIDS counselling through specialists. Again, it is a matter of balancing what needs to be done against what is available, and coming up with a sensible system.

### Assessing risk

In any area it is helpful to try to make some assessment of who is at greatest risk of infection. This is of greatest importance where infection rates are low or moderate but is still of value even in areas where infection rates are high. There are good reasons for this:

- It makes it easier to focus a health education campaign when resources are limited and to match the content to the specific needs of those at risk.
- If a busy health professional can spot those at most risk they can target them for discussion and education about HIV.
- It helps in diagnosis and in deciding which samples or patients to send to a hospital.
- High-risk donors can be discouraged from giving blood.

Because in most developing countries HIV is a heterosexually spread infection it is not possible to predict who will be infected with anything like the accuracy that is possible in the West, where high rates of infection are still found mainly in particular risk groups. However it is possible to produce worthwhile *local* predictions based on local conditions. These will need periodic up-dating.

The starting point for such a prediction is to try to assess how common infection is in a particular area. There are several possible sources for this information:

- One can look at positives detected through testing facilities or blood donor screening. When using such data allowance has to be made for the fact that identified positives may not be an entirely fair representation of those who are positive in a particular area.
- Where seroprevalence data is available this can be used to make predictions.
- It is possible to gather some useful information by looking at cases of frank disease, although this tends to be relatively crude data since the appearance of cases of AIDS tends to lag by some years behind the spread of infection.
- Where no data is available it is usually possible to make some intelligent guesses by looking at other comparable, geographical areas where such data is available.

At the same time as information is gathered on how common infection is, information should be gathered on the possible risk factors of those found to be infected, through, say, testing facilities. This will give important clues as to which untested people are likely to turn out to be infected. As Chapter 3, on pre-test counselling, made clear, assessing risk in those coming for the test is an important part of counselling. Test facilities should always keep records of the risk factors of those found to be infected as pooled non-identifiable data so that the spread of the infection and any change in the pattern of risk factors in an area can be charted.

Often data on people infected will be sketchy or non-existent. Or it may be available but suspect in some sort of way. However, it is possible by knowing, or guessing, whether the prevalence in an area is high, medium or low to make some intelligent predictions about who is likely to be at risk.

Obviously the chances of anyone catching any sexually transmitted disease is related to two factors: how many partners they have unprotected sex with, and the rate of infection amongst potential partners.

### Low incidence areas

In a low incidence area those *most* at risk are likely to be:

(1) Those who travel to areas where the incidence of infection is high, for instance truck drivers or businessmen. Where prevalence varies within a country between rural and urban areas, as is

usually the case, those who travel to the cities to work, particularly single men leaving their families or married men separated for long periods, are also likely to be at risk.

(2)   Those who have sex with travellers. This will include their wives or lovers but will also include 'barmaids' and prostitutes who have sex with travellers.

### Medium incidence areas

(3)   As HIV infection spreads in an area the next group to be at high risk will be those who have a very high number of sexual partners, because they increase their risk of meeting someone in group 2 above, i.e. in effect of coming into *indirect* contact with a traveller. Those at risk in low incidence areas will, of course, continue to be at risk.

### High incidence areas

As the infection spreads so people with fewer sexual partners start to be at risk. For instance, if the rate of infection in an area is 1 per cent then a man with five partners per year has a one in twenty chance of having sex with someone infected. If the rate rises to 5 per cent he has a one in four chance. As the local rate rises travellers of one sort or another have less and less importance as agents of general spread. However, while rates remain higher outside the rural area than inside it, individuals in groups 1, 2 and 3 still remain at most risk.

In an area of medium to high infection it is not just the number of partners an individual has that matters, it is also the number of sexual partners that the individual's sexual partners have. So a man may have only one sexual partner but if that partner is a prostitute he may still be at relatively high risk. Similarly a woman whose husband has many sexual partners may be at high risk.

In an area of medium to high incidence placing someone in a higher or lower risk category for the purposes of counselling according to the number of partners they have is likely to be rather arbitrary. It will depend on how much is available in the way of resources for counselling.

### Specific risk factors

Besides the general considerations above, certain groups of people are particularly worth thinking about when assessing risk or drawing up a list of risk factors to look for in, say, a testing clinic. Some of them have already been mentioned above. Because of the key role that they can play in spreading infection it is worth considering these groups in more detail.

(1) *Prostitutes* In any country with significant rates of heterosexual infection prostitutes are likely to be a high risk group, unless they act to reduce their risk of infection by consistently using condoms.

There is clearly a spectrum of prostitutes in terms of their clients, how much they earn and where they operate. Not all prostitutes in a country are likely to be at equal risk. However, which group will be most at risk will vary according to local factors.

In a country where levels of infection are low it is likely to be prostitutes who cater to travellers who are most at risk early in an epidemic. This includes the prostitutes who service clients in hotels, even though they may have fewer clients than street prostitutes or 'barmaids'. However, street prostitutes who service truck drivers and other travellers are also at very high risk if the people they are servicing come from high risk areas.

On the fringes of prostitution are those women who occasionally engage in prostitution or who have sexual relationships with relatively few men in order to gain money or food or other services. They are likely to be much more difficult to identify and to reach, firstly because they may be reluctant to admit to prostitution or may not consider that what they are doing is prostitution, and secondly because they are less likely to be locatable in particular places. In most large cities there are areas where prostitutes congregate, particular streets or hotels or bars, and therefore they are relatively easy to locate for a health education drive. This is likely to be much more difficult with the casual or occasional prostitute.

(2) *Travellers* In Africa truck drivers who may travel large distances are particularly at risk because they pass through areas of high prevalence and may have sex there. Not only are they at risk themselves but so are their sexual partners and, as noted earlier, they may act as a major route by which the virus is spread across a country. Truck drivers are not the only travellers; those working on railways or airlines may also be at high risk.

One should not only think in terms of travel to other countries; travel *within* a country may be equally important. With HIV it is usually the case throughout the world that cities are much worse affected than rural areas. Spread is limited by the lack of contact of people in rural areas with those in the cities. However, where men or women leave their homes and travel to the cities to work for periods and then return home, they tend to travel from low to high prevalence areas. On their return they may bring back HIV to their own area. Again, their sexual partners are at risk.

(3) *Those cut off from normal social restraints* In general every society to some extent tends to act to regulate the sexual behaviour of its members, whether by explicit rules or by social approval and disapproval. Families often also act as powerful restraining influences on sexual behaviour (although they can, of course, have the opposite effects sometimes). When people are freed from the social constraints of their society and family they are free to act in ways which would otherwise be unacceptable. In this respect the key group are probably those who move away from their families into cities, either permanently or for extended periods. Not only are they out of sight of those who might influence them but also in cities opportunity for sexual licence is increased and the anonymity of the city means that no-one in their new setting is likely to worry much what they are doing.

(4) *Prisoners* Even in areas where homosexual behaviour is unusual it tends to be common in prisons and other all-male institutions where access to women is denied. This is of particular importance because prisons have been used frequently as reliable sources of blood donations.

(5) *Those in other all-male institutions* Wherever men are taken away from their families and from normal access to the opposite sex they are *potentially* at higher risk. People in the army, navy or air-force are one example, men living away from their families in mining camps are another. In general, such men are more likely to seek casual sexual contacts and to make extensive use of prostitutes, although of course by no means all will.

(6) *Recipients of frequent transfusions before the introduction of screening of blood* This might include some haemophiliacs and those receiving transfusions for sickle-cell anaemia as well as those who have had major surgery.

(7) *Babies of HIV infected mothers.*

(8) *Those who have received repeated injections with poor sterile technique in areas of high HIV prevalence.*

(9) *Sexual partners of those who are known to have HIV or who are the widows or widowers of those with HIV* Also the sexual partners of anyone in the above groups.

In addition to the main groups considered above there is a question mark over those who have had skin piercing or ritual scarification under non-sterile conditions.

Although it is becoming less common throughout most of Africa, circumcision under non-sterile conditions of men, and less commonly of women, still occurs. For HIV to be transmitted in this way it is necessary for at least some of those being circumcised to be already infected with the virus. Where circumcision is carried out before puberty or before those being circumcised are sexually active the risk is likely to be fairly low. Only if one or more of those being circumcised have been infected through transfusions or through materno-foetal transmission is there likely to be a clear if unquantifiable risk. At the moment there is no reason to suppose that circumcision is a major route of spread of HIV although there is, clearly, a risk.

Ritual scarification for cosmetic or for traditional healing purposes in adults is a potential transmission risk if unsterilised instruments are being used on more than one person. The difficulty for the counsellor is in trying to assess whether an individual who has had ritual scarification or skin cutting or piercing is at risk of HIV infection. The situation is complicated by difficulties in assessing the risk of transmission from contaminated 'surgical' instruments. This will vary according to:

- the amount of blood transmitted.
- the time elapsing between the instruments being used on one person and being used on the next.
- the rate of infection of individuals on whom such instruments are being used.

It is worth bearing in mind that where skin cutting is being used for traditional healing the people involved are more likely to be ill and therefore may have a higher rate of infection with HIV than the normal population. Given these factors, whether those who have had scarification or skin piercing in recent years are at increased risk of HIV infection is something which can only be decided at a local level and even then estimations of risk are likely to be little better than crude guesswork.

## Drawing up a list of risk factors

Once some assessment of who is at risk locally has been made this can be used in a variety of ways:

(1)  Specific health education campaigns aimed at specific target groups

might be started; for instance prostitutes might be targeted. A plan might include:

- Identifying prostitutes in sexually transmitted disease clinics and other settings and spending extra time informing them about the risks of HIV.
- Getting a worker, perhaps even an ex-prostitute, to go to bars, hotels and onto the streets to talk to prostitutes about the risks and to hand out information, either written or in the form of comic strips.
- Handing out condoms to prostitutes through clinics and outreach work.
- Forming groups of prostitutes to spread information and disseminate condoms.

Prostitutes are only one example of what can be done in terms of health education. Health education drives aimed at single men living in hostels or at young single women working in cities are possible. The advantage of selecting specific target groups is that the health education message can be tailored directly to the needs of that particular group and put in such a way that it seems to address their own personal way of life.

(2)   Identifying those at high risk for the purposes of offering counselling, face-to-face health education, and to aid diagnosis.

In a sample rural area of low prevalence a list of high risk individuals might be drawn up with the following reasoning (obviously this is only an example of what might be done):

- *At high risk* will be those travelling to the city to work and their sexual partners; prostitutes because they cater to travellers of various sorts; also, for the purposes of offering counselling on risk reduction; those with more than ten sexual partners a year, because the rate of infection is not expected to be more than 0.5 per cent locally and this gives a one-in-twenty chance of that person having sex with someone with HIV infection in a year. For the purposes of aiding differential diagnosis where testing is not readily available, individuals rated as high risk, given that they already have some symptoms which might be HIV associated, might be set at a lower number of partners.
- *At relatively little risk* will be those who have had repeated blood transfusions in the past because all blood used was collected locally and prior to the last couple of years infection rates were low. Similarly, babies born before this year are unlikely to be infected because of low infection rates except where the mother was the sexual partner of

someone who travelled, or was a prostitute. Since there is no mining and no prison neither of these need a great deal of attention. Since HIV infection is relatively low individuals who have been circumcised or have had cosmetic scarification are at low risk. So are those who have had traditional healing skin cutting up to this year since infection was low in the past and AIDS cases which might be dealt with by a healer are low at the moment.

On the basis of this sort of list, staff in hospitals and rural clinics might be encouraged to ask patients about travel, sexual contact with travellers and number of sexual partners their patients have. This could be a part of routine history taking for patients coming to see them.

### Who is at low risk of HIV?

In the same way as high risk can be estimated, so low risk can be estimated?

(1) Anyone who is celibate and has been during the period when HIV has been prevalent in an area. This is likely to include the obviously celibate like nuns and priests but also older children, before puberty but too old to have caught the virus through materno-foetal transmission. There will be others who have been celibate in most societies, perhaps widows or widowers.

   As noted above, some people such as prisoners who might be expected to be celibate turn out not to be so.

(2) Individuals who are monogamous or who are in 'closed' poly-gamous relationships, in which no member of the relationship has sex outside that relationship. One of the difficulties with this group is that, unlike celibates who *know* that they have been celibate, few people can be absolutely certain that their partner has been faithful to them.

(3) Young people very early in their sexual careers in some societies. If young people tend to have sex only with others in their own age-group, particularly if they restrict their sexual activity to those in their own locality, they are at relatively low risk. If no-one in that age-group starts out with HIV they are not going to spread it amongst themselves. As time passes HIV will get into an age-group because some members of it will catch the virus from those older than themselves or by travelling.

   In a culture where older people tend to have sex with those younger than themselves on a large scale, this assumption tends to break down.

(4)  In low prevalence areas, those who have very few sexual partners are at relatively low risk.
(5)  Those who have consistently used condoms during sex.

### What can estimates of low risk be used for?

Estimates of low risk can be used as part of a plan to assemble low-risk donors for a 'pool' blood donation drive. They can also be used to check test results. An individual who tests positive in groups 1 and 2 and sometimes in the other groups merits some checking to make sure a mistake hasn't been made. Wherever in the world a blood test is carried out it is important for the clinician to apply common sense to the result. Mistakes happen ven in the best laboratories and to wrongly tell someone they are infected on the basis of a mix-up is a true tragedy.

## Organising a counselling service

On the basis of considerations of who is at high risk it should be possible to go on to plan how services will run, who will carry out the counselling, who needs to be trained and what sort of information and skills they will need.

There are several different aspects to the provision of a comprehensive counselling service and it is helpful to look at each of these in turn.

### Testing on request

Where possible the provision of testing on request is usually very helpful, for reasons which the rest of this book makes clear. However, it is not always easy to work out exactly how testing on request can be best provided. There are two possible models with a range of possibilities in between.

#### Single centre model
A single testing clinic can be set up to which anyone coming forward and requesting the test can go or be sent. There are several advantages to this approach:

• The clinic can advertise itself effectively and it is likely that patients will come forward more readily to a specially set up centre.
• It is possible within such a setting for workers to build up a great deal of expertise rapidly, because of the numbers of patients they

are dealing with. This helps in ensuring that a small number of counsellors can rapidly become adept at counselling. This means that a nucleus of experienced staff can be formed to advise others, to provide training and to provide a centre for referral-on by other workers.

- It is easier to collect information on risk factors on a limited number of sites so that information can be built up on the pattern of spread in an area. Where sera comes in from distant sites it is usually difficult to assemble information on who was tested and what their risk factors were.
- It is possible to concentrate other resources on the same site — a laboratory carrying out HIV testing, facilities for investigating HIV-related problems, medical facilities, etc.

There are, however, disadvantages in concentrating testing-on-request on a single centre:

- Where communications are bad, individuals who want to be tested may be unable to reach a test site. At the very least they may be deterred from coming forward for testing.
- The professional taking on the counselling of a patient may be different from the professional looking after his physical health, and communications between the two may be a problem.

*The testing-at-multiple-sites model*
In this model any health professional is encouraged to counsel and take blood on request from the patient and then send that blood for testing and give the patient the results of the test.

There are several advantages to this approach, and several disadvantages. Since these are the exact opposites of the advantages and disadvantages of a single-site model they will not be repeated.

Which model is adopted will depend in part on the situation. Having a single centre may be workable in an urban area but may be quite inappropriate in a rural area simply because most patients are unable to reach it.

In most areas, outside big cities, a middle path is likely to be chosen initially: testing is likely to be offered on more than one site but not at every point where it could, in theory, be offered. As more and more health care staff begin to develop expertise in the area more and more will be able to offer the test. However, as the number of people offering the test increases it is important to ensure that the information they are collecting about spread is not lost. It is also important to ensure that they have a source of specialist expertise to refer to when they are in difficulties and that they are able to meet with others carrying out testing to discuss the problems they are meeting and possible solutions. It is also vital that anyone offering the test should keep up-to-date on progress in the understanding of HIV infection and AIDS. In practice this means that they will need continued training input.

If testing-on-request is to be offered at a limited number of sites, the question of who should carry out the counselling is then important. Can the existing staff at these sites carry out the extra work? If they can then the only need is for extra training. Suppose they can't, who should be recruited? The key question here is whether to bring in staff specifically designated to carry out only HIV work or whether to bring in extra staff to increase the numbers of existing staff so that everyone can carry out the work.

Which of these options is taken is likely to be the result of local considerations. Partly it depends on how well the existing staff can be expected to do the work after training, partly it's a matter of getting the best results from limited resources. Sometimes it is best to try to expand the existing staff and get everyone to do the work.

### Others being offered the test

There are other settings in which it might be desirable to actually offer the test to patients. For instance it might be thought desirable in a high prevalence area to offer the test to pregnant women.

Again, the system which is arrived at is likely to be dependent on local conditions. However, it is clear that if antenatal staff are to be involved in the issue of testing then they need to be able to offer counselling to go with the test. The issues here are covered in more detail elsewhere in the book.

### Blood transfusion counselling

In the West most blood donations are acquired at mass donor sessions or through 'panels' of donors with rare blood types. This type of donation can be called 'pool' donations.

Pool blood is not sufficient to meet the need in many developing countries. Additional blood has to be obtained from relatives and friends of those going in to hospital — 'relative blood'. Most relatives think their blood is going direct to the patient. In fact in most cases it goes to swell the overall blood supply.

In the West the blood supply is protected by two mechanisms. All blood is screened. Also, donors at high risk of HIV infection are vigorously discouraged from donating. This reduces the number of positives the blood transfusion services have to deal with to a handful. It also reduces the risk of an infected donation from someone who has not yet seroconverted slipping through the net. Discouraging high-risk donors is easy in the West where most of those infected have clear risk factors. It is more difficult in developing countries.

Counselling positive would-be donors is irretrievably mixed in with overall policy towards blood collection. There are at least three elements to this policy: trying to reduce the number of donations from high risk donors, trying to maximise donations from low risk donors, and getting a system for the recall and counselling of those who are infected.

Discouraging high-risk donors has the advantages noted above. Where for any reason testing of blood is not available, discouraging high-risk donors becomes crucial. However, it can cause problems:

> The medical officer in an African rural district hospital in an area of low seropositivity decided to try to discourage those who had had multiple sexual partners in the city from donating blood. She put up posters in the hospital and handed out leaflets to potential donors as well as having a member of staff mention the issue to would-be donors, in case they were illiterate. The result was a fall in the number of individuals giving blood. Some of those who did not give blood seemed to be at low risk.

Here two possible approaches to the problem might help to screen out those genuinely at risk without discouraging low-risk donors. The problem seemed to be that people coming to donate blood had enough information to make them concerned and reluctant to give blood but not enough information to make them realise that they were at low risk. There would seem to be two possible solutions to this sort of situation.

- The hospital might have put much more time into educating potential donors, and this would include employing someone who would have time to go into the issues with potential donors. This would be a good time investment with regular donors.
- Rather than trying to educate the donors in advance it might have been possible to use a short series of questions to identify possible high-risk donors and to use this to screen out those at high risk rather than encouraging donors to self-select.

With relative blood the situation can be more difficult. It is not so easy to sort out a set time for them to arrive to give blood and they may not be very happy at finding themselves treated to a lecture on

AIDS. As with pool blood, asking potential donors a few simple questions will significantly reduce the numbers of positive donations.

Getting more low-risk donors is an issue that was addressed under 'Who is at low risk of HIV?'.

Where HIV-positive blood is identified it is likely to be necessary to bring in the donor for counselling. This means keeping good records. It also means having someone attached to the department collecting blood following them up. Particularly with relative blood they may have to travel to track down infected donors.

It is particularly important to get a second sample from an infected donor for confirmation: making a clerical error and telling the wrong person they are positive can be catastrophic.


## Those showing symptoms of HIV infection or AIDS

One of the difficulties with AIDS is that it has such a wide range of manifestations that people with HIV infection-related problems can appear at just about any part of the health services of an area. Surgeons, physicians, psychiatrists, midwives, health visitors, staff in family planning clinics and a whole range of other staff are likely suddenly to be presented with patients showing signs of HIV infection or AIDS. Patients will present at hospitals, at clinics, at health centres and at dispensaries, and community staff, if they are in an area with high prevalence and they have their wits about them, are likely to turn up further cases.

The first step in being able to provide a service for those with AIDS or HIV-related problems is to be able to recognise them in the first place. There is often a problem in detecting who has AIDS in developing countries. Most of the infectious diseases and tumours seen in Western AIDS patients are usually uncommon in adults. This is not always the case in Africa; tuberculosis is common in both those with AIDS and those without AIDS. Where problems such as pneumonia are caused by unusual organisms like *pneumocystis carinii* lack of laboratory facilities may make identification difficult.

However, given the very real difficulties it is clear that everyone in contact with patients needs to know how to detect which problems are particularly likely to be seen in AIDS. All staff must be aware of the need to ask patients about possible risk factors, and what questions they should be asking. As was noted above, assessment of risk can play an important part in forming a preliminary diagnosis in an untested patient.

It is relatively easy to set up a counselling service for those with AIDS-related problems in a district hospital. Provided such patients can be recognised by staff it is possible for them to pass on the counselling aspects of the work to one or more staff who take a particular interest in the area.

In a rural area the situation is likely to be very different. It is important that whoever is dealing with the patient should be aware of the basic issues surrounding counselling and be able to provide at least basic support and counselling. For this to be possible it is important to have staff with greater experience − specialist or semi-specialist staff to provide back-up advice and help, even if they have to travel out from the district hospital on an occasional basis.

Arranging follow-up for someone with AIDS after discharge from a district hospital is also likely to be a problem. If the patient is too far from the hospital to travel to it regularly, or too sick to travel, then either care will have to be organised through local health centres or dispensaries or the counsellor from the hospital will have to go out and see the patient. Either way there is a need to double up the purely psychological aspects of care with simple physical home-care measures.

Teaching relatives looking after a patient about good hygiene and how to use simple medications to control pain and, where it is a major problem for carers, diarrhoea, are all parts of counselling in this sort of situation.

In any counselling system, as in any medical system, the point where a patient is transferred from the care of one professional to the care of another is when the system is most likely to break down. It is vital to provide whoever is taking over care with as much information as possible, to ensure that the patient knows who he will be dealing with in the future and to ensure that whoever is taking over care knows who has been looking after the patient so far and feels able to get in contact if anything is unclear.

## Counselling those at high risk of HIV infection

Locating and counselling those at high risk of HIV infection is likely to be a key problem in any country. For the reasons discussed earlier it is likely to be even more of a problem in a developing country simply because so few people will identify themselves as at high risk. It is worth considering that, while it may be time-consuming to identify someone at risk and to counsel him, it is likely to be a good deal less time-consuming than treating him for AIDS.

In an area where HIV infection is common it is likely to be helpful to train every health professional in at least the basics of identifying those at risk and the sorts of advice which they need to give to reduce that risk. It should be a part of routine history-taking to ask questions about risk factors. Asking about sexual behaviour does not always come easily to health staff and they may need help and encouragement to ask the right questions. However, asking those questions is vitally important.

Making condoms readily available wherever possible is just as much a part of counselling as talking through the issues with patients. Provided condoms are available to health staff to distribute, it is important to make it as easy as possible for them to be handed out and for the patients to be able to get more supplies. Where men are unwilling to collect them in person it may be possible to get women to collect them.

It is also important that, where condoms are being distributed, staff spend some time explaining how to use them properly. Condoms are reliable if they are properly used, much less so if they are misused. The instructions which come with condoms are often less than helpful, and, if the user is illiterate, totally useless. Clearly staff need to stress using each condom only once, only putting them on when full erection has been attained, not withdrawing and then re-entering during sex (because this increases the breakage rate), and holding on to the base of the condom during withdrawal after ejaculation. While these measures may appear self-evident they are far from self-evident to someone who has never used a condom.

## Using every opportunity for health education

While there is no substitute for specific, face-to-face counselling in terms of changing behaviour it is important to use every opportunity to provide health education.

Most societies already have groups of various sorts – everything from women's groups to local church groups; these gatherings can be used to get across basic information about HIV infection and ways of avoiding it. By building up relationships with these groups health professionals can also develop a valuable resource for assisting in the care of those with AIDS and HIV infection. Where a patient has no family, or where the family is sick, it is important to try to use whatever resources are available in the local community for providing basic care. People are only likely to provide such care if they understand about AIDS and understand about the transmission of HIV — and how it *cannot* be transmitted.

Sometimes it may be helpful to try to start up self-help groups from scratch. There are, as was noted earlier, many problems in doing this. But at least in the case of some people at risk it may be possible. The example of prostitutes was used earlier but there may be other groups which can be formed.

Often in an area there will be local health education initiatives in existence already. There may be campaigns aimed at other diseases, or immunisation programmes or even family planning programmes. Successful campaigns in other health areas can be useful, not only in terms of the information they will have gathered about the best way to get health messages across, but also because a certain amount of health education about HIV can often be delivered at the same time.

There are sometimes problems with this approach, of course. Mixing HIV education and family planning, for instance, has to be handled carefully. Where family planning programmes are having difficulties there is a danger that promoting the use of condoms for prophylaxis may appear as just another way to introduce an unpopular restriction on family size. Conversely, the association of contraceptives with HIV may make it more difficult to promote family planning. However, there is at least the possibility that each campaign may benefit from the other.

Besides attempts to influence groups there is also a need to try to influence opinion leaders, whether local politicians, religious leaders, teachers, local officials or village elders, anyone who might help to get across the message of what people need to do to protect themselves against AIDS.

## Should patients be told that they are infected?

The above model assumes that people will always, where possible, be told if they have HIV or if they have AIDS. However, for those setting up a service for the first time this is not necessarily a 'cut and dried' issue. One element in the uncertainty is the fear that those who are told that they are infected may decide that they are going to go out and infect as many other people as possible. There are frequent news-paper reports in many areas of the world of individuals deliberately infecting others, often coupled with urging from the newspaper that 'something should be done' to prevent this happening. People seem often to know someone who knows someone who had a patient who did just this. However, it is rare to find someone who actually *had* a patient who behaved like this.

All the evidence is that this sort of reaction is likely to be very, very rare. It appears to be more frequent in newspaper reports than in real life. It is certainly likely to be such a rare event that it should not deter a health worker from informing patients that they are infected with the virus or that they have AIDS.

Of course the individual who deliberately goes out and infects others must be distinguished from the patient who knows that he or she is infected but simply does not change his or her behaviour. This is a more common response, although still surprisingly uncommon. However the fact that people may not change is not a reason for not telling, rather it is a reason for good counselling of such individuals.

Against the theoretical risk of someone deciding to infect others deliberately must be set the advantages in telling the infected person. Firstly, many counsellors would argue that it is the right of an individual to know information about his own health. Secondly, there are many practical reasons for telling someone of his HIV status once this is known:

- A person who knows that he is infected is able to take steps to protect his current partner and possible future partners.
- He is able to plan for the possibility that he may become ill in the future and make some provision for the support of his family if he should die.
- He is able to inform his sexual partner or partners that they too may be infected with the virus.
- He is able to take steps to protect his own health, for instance by avoiding catching other sexually transmitted diseases and by trying as far as possible to maintain good health in the ways outlined in Chapter 4.

These considerations provide compelling reasons why, under all but the most extraordinary circumstances, it is best to tell individuals that they are infected with HIV or that they have AIDS.

## Special problems

The general process of counselling in developing countries is not different from that found in Western countries. The reactions of people to the news that they are infected with HIV or have AIDS are much the same in Africa as they are in Budapest or London. The steps which people must take to protect their health are much the same also.

There are, however, some differences. These are the result of cultural differences which, while they do not affect the aims or methods of counselling, mean that the counsellor may be faced with a slightly different balance of problems in trying to help people to change their risk behaviours.

### Informing sexual partners

This issue is covered in detail in Chapter 4. However it is worth summarising some of the issues here in order to look at some of the specific problems in developing countries.

Someone who is infected with the HIV virus should tell his current sexual partner and immediate past partners if they have been put at risk of infection. It is important that they too should have access to counselling and, if they want it, testing.

Where a patient is going to inform a sexual partner it is important to rehearse with the patient what he is going to say to make sure that it is factually correct. It is also important to get him to bring in the sexual partner as soon as possible after telling him so that counselling can take place.

One difficulty with immediate past partners is to know how far back a patient should go in contacting them. A patient will seldom know for sure when he was infected. However there is little point in patients chasing after, and unnecessarily alarming, partners they may have had five years ago in an area where HIV infection was rare up until two years ago. How far back to go is a matter for common sense but in areas where HIV is common it is rarely going to be beneficial to go back beyond very immediate past partners.

With current partners the patient sometimes wishes them to be told but feels unable to do so. The issue then becomes one of who will tell the partner. One possibility is to get the patient to bring in the partner and the counsellor can tell him. However it is always worth considering alternatives with the patient. Sometimes an intermediary in the family may be able to do the telling and, because of their social relationship with the partner, handle the situation better than the counsellor could.

Particularly in extended families there may be an elder member of the family, an 'auntie' or 'godfather', who fulfils a general advisory role for the family; sometimes such roles are informal, in some societies they are socially recognised. Otherwise a sister, a brother or other relative might be brought in to break the news. Such messengers need to be chosen with care and need to be discreet: it would be a mistake to choose a messenger who then told a whole village about the situation. On the other hand where resources are scarce and a patient comes a long way from the counsellor's base sometimes it may not be practical for the counsellor to go out himself:

> A man came to a district hospital and was diagnosed as having AIDS. His wife did not believe that he was very sick and would not come to the hospital. He did not want to tell her himself because she was a woman with a sharp tongue and he did not feel he could cope. The counsellor identified an 'auntie' − a distant relative who acted as a sort of general advisor to the women in the family. The 'auntie' then informed the wife, who came to the hospital for advice.

Suppose a patient will not tell his current sexual partner, say his wife, and will not give permission for anyone else to do so. Clearly this is a situation where the counsellor needs to apply all possible persuasion. However, if the patient still refuses, what then? The temptation for the counsellor to tell the wife is strong; however, to do so might create difficulties of its own. If people think that if they have a blood test for HIV other people will be told about the result without their consent then they will not come forward in the first place. If they don't come forward then there is no way that they can be persuaded to inform their sexual partners. In the end it is this sort of consideration that suggests that, even in a difficult situation, it is best to maintain confidentiality.

Some counsellors will feel that they are morally obliged to inform a sexual partner if the patient will not do it himself. This is an understandable view and clearly an acceptable one, provided they make their position clear to the patients before they take them on. If such a situation is not acceptable to the patient then the case should be passed on to another counsellor.

Although confidentiality is important there can be no obligation for the hospital to actually lie to a partner about what is wrong with a living patient. If a wife asks what is wrong with her husband and he does not wish the hospital to tell her the only thing the hospital can do is to tell the wife that it is only the patient who can say what is wrong with him. It is then between the two of them to sort it out; there is a limit to what the hospital can do to protect a confidence.

Maintaining confidentiality can occasionally present unexpected difficulties:

> A woman whose husband was dying of AIDS came to see the hospital. She said that since he had become sick some of his relatives suspected her of poisoning him or of engaging in witchcraft.

In some societies it is important that the partner should be able to explain why the patient has died, or even, as in this case, why he is sick. It must be stressed to the patient that confidentiality, where sexual partners are concerned, does not extend beyond the grave. Once someone is dead there is a clear primary duty to look after the living and, whatever the patient wants, the wife will need to be told. In the meanwhile the wife needs to be given at least enough information to allow her to avoid unjust accusations. She can be assured that he is genuinely sick and the relatives, if they can be contacted, can be told the same thing.

Another set of problems comes up with the patient who is being cared for at home by relatives:

> A man with AIDS was being cared for by relatives. He had profuse diarrhoea and open sores. He believed that, if his relatives were told he had AIDS, they would abandon him because of their great fear.

Here the most important thing is that the relatives should take elementary hygiene measures, not that they should know exactly what is wrong with the man. There are two alternatives: either the patient can be persuaded to let the hospital tell the relatives and spend time with them reassuring them and educating them about AIDS; or the relatives can be told that the patient has an infection and be told how to carry out the necessary hygienic precautions without the word 'AIDS', or the local equivalent, being used. Which course is taken depends very much on how far education about AIDS is thought likely to succeed and on other factors in the situation which can only be judged at the time.

## What happens when a patient dies?

Standard advice surrounding death is to place those who have died of AIDS in a leak-proof cadaver bag. This tends to raise a number of problems. The argument in favour is that the body may leak and so put people at risk. On the other hand nursing staff and relatives who have been looking after a patient who leaked when alive tend to reason that if a man was safe to look after when he was alive why is he so dangerous when he is dead? Moreover there tends to be rather a shortage of leak-proof cadaver bags in most developing countries.

The problems surrounding death tend to be most acute when they cut across local death customs:

> After a man's death it was the local custom to engage in feasting around the body in the man's house. This became a particular problem for the local medical officer during a cholera epidemic.

Interfering in the usual practices surrounding death may not only be very difficult, it may also leave the relatives with extra grief and in those cases where death rites have religious significance it may leave them frantic because of fears of what may happen to the man's spirit.

Again, it is a matter of finding out about local death rites, trying to talk through what is to happen to a man's body after death and trying to talk through with relatives ways of ensuring that there is no risk while at the same time ensuring that the minimum interference possible takes place in the normal mourning process.

## Problems in changing behaviour

An effective counsellor tries to change the behaviour of those he is counselling in order to achieve certain objectives. *Amongst* these objectives are:

- Getting those at risk to change their behaviour so as not to get infected.
- Getting those infected to change their behaviour so as not to put others at risk.
- Getting those infected to change their behaviour so as to reduce as much as possible their own risk of going on to get AIDS.

In order to achieve these objectives it is crucial to understand what forces act to make people behave in particular ways and what forces act to prevent them from changing their behaviour. This section looks at some typical difficulties.

### Sexual behaviour

Many countries have laws enforcing monogamy, in the sense of only allowing one legal wife, or, where polygamy is legal, restricting the number of wives a man may have. The laws concerning divorce vary from country to country, in some countries it is easy to obtain a divorce, in others more difficult. However legislation does not necessarily alter behaviour, especially where other social forces act counter to it.

In some parts of the world, there are societies which remain essentially polygamous whatever the law says. A man may have a legal wife or wives, but he may also maintain a relationship with a number of other women, some of whom will be married, others of whom will be single. These relationships may be long-standing or they may be brief episodes. The way in which they tend to differ from the case of the man in a non-polygamous society who has a mistress (if they differ at all), is that the arrangement tends to a greater or lesser extent to be socially acceptable, even sometimes socially approved or encouraged.

Having other partners outside marriage is not always the sole prerogative of the male. It may also be the societal norm that a woman has more than one liaison at a time, whether she is married or single.

The counsellor may thus be faced with a problem of attitude in that monogamy or celibacy may be less acceptable options in some places than in others.

Throughout the world relationships between men and women often fulfil a financial as well as a sexual role. Where the ability of women to support themselves financially is limited, a single woman who cannot rely on her family may have to have a man in order to obtain the basic necessities of life. So a woman who is widowed or divorced may more or less be obliged to form a liaison with one or more men. Clearly if the husband has died of AIDS there is a large risk that infection will be passed on to a new partner. Under these circumstances 'safer sex' is not just a restriction on the range of sexual behaviours available to an individual, it may also be a restriction on her ability to form a new liaison and hence to obtain the basic necessities of life.

The financial element is also a major factor in the existence of what are called 'sugar-daddies' in some areas of the world, for example in parts of West Africa. These are older men, often married, who take on a younger woman as a mistress. It is important to note, of course, that there is nothing uniquely West African about this. It is common in many parts of the world and is, of course, far from unknown in London or Paris. However, it is likely to be particularly common wherever women find themselves financially disadvantaged.

For the man the advantages are a relationship with a young, attractive woman, and also status in the eyes of his peers. For the woman the advantages may be emotional and status-linked, but there is often also a financial element. The woman is usually living in a city, unmarried, and often on a low salary. The man can provide many extras and allow her to live in a style she could not manage otherwise. If he is generous she may be able to save something for the future, towards a house, or more often towards a business.

The financially dependent role of many women in many developing countries also has implications in terms of a woman's relationship with her family. Customs relating to the behaviour of widows show wide variation from place to place. In some African societies it is customary for a husband's brother to take on the husband's responsibilities if he dies, including responsibility for his wife, both financial and, in some places, sexual. In other societies the wife may have to move back to her own family's village and may be expected to remarry there. In countries where there is no social security and very few people have life insurance — which is most countries in the world — the pressures on a single woman whose partner has died of AIDS to form a new sexual liaison may be almost overwhelming.

Particularly in the case of women, then, the counsellor may be faced with the fact that the scope for change in behaviour may be severely restricted by the simple need to survive.

For the man there are also likely to be pressures in terms of forming multiple relationships. It may give him status in the eyes of his peers. It may be the expected social norm. Sometimes it may have financial advantages. There may also be specific reasons why he may form more than one relationship.

In many societies men marry late, often because they must achieve a certain financial or social status before being able to do so. They may form liaisons with married women or, in those societies where pre-marital sex for women is acceptable, with a number of young women, either serially or at the same time. Late marriage may also increase the use of prostitutes, as it did in Victorian England. There are often taboos against sex for a period after childbirth, either in terms of a number of months or years, or during the period when the woman is breast-feeding. This also can create the occasion for men to look outside their marriage for sexual relationships.

Again, this is partly a matter of attitude, particularly where individuals in a society feel that having sex is essential to physical well-being, and partly a matter of social forces acting on individuals to encourage them to have many partners in order not to 'lose face' with their friends and peers.

In many societies there is a strong emphasis on the bearing of children, both for men and women. In particular there is often a strong emphasis on the bearing of male children, both from the point of view of ensuring support in old age and from the point of view of status in the eyes of others. Consequently if a couple are unable to produce children the man may divorce his wife and re-marry or the wife may seek sexual relations outside the marriage. The difficulties this raises when advising one partner to use condoms or advising a woman not to get pregnant are obvious.

The first step for a counsellor in any culture is to think carefully about the prevailing social and sexual norms and to try to identify the pressures which operate to make people behave as they do. Where a counsellor is operating in an area where there are many different cultures it will be necessary to seek, through questioning of patients and others who understand those cultures, to build up a picture of what are the forces operating in each culture. When helping a patient to change his behaviour the prevailing culture sets up the framework within which problems have to be solved. Not to understand that framework is to risk helping the patient to solutions that he is simply not going to be able to put into practice.

## Conclusion

There is no such thing as a 'typical' developing country. Every country has different problems and different needs. Models of counselling which work very well in Paris or New York cannot simply be transplanted wholesale and unchanged to a different culture and a different country. Local workers have to develop their own models and methods of counselling appropriate to local circumstances. This is already happening in many parts of the world. Some of the work going on in developing countries has strongly influenced my own work in London. It is a trend I expect to continue.

# Chapter 19

# Training Models

ALANA McCREANER

## Training in HIV/AIDS

With the rapidly increasing incidence of HIV/AIDS in the population, the health service finds itself having to meet a growing demand for information not only from the public but from within its own ranks. For example a growing number of staff find themselves having to counsel HIV positive patients, those considering taking the test, and worried or bereaved friends and relatives. Other staff may feel the need for information on health and safety and infection control procedures and how best to implement them. Others still may find themselves in less direct contact with HIV/AIDS by having to deal with general but concerned enquiries. This has led to an urgent demand for training courses, some highly specialised, others of a more general nature, and an energetic pursuit of experts in such fields as pre- and post-test counselling, bereavement, sexuality, health and safety, epidemiology, immunology, and virology.

In meeting this need health care managers can look to established training bodies such as the National AIDS Counselling Training Unit (NACTU), funded by the DHSS, or to their own 'in-house' expertise, or perhaps to both. Practised trainers in HIV/AIDS — or, indeed, any other field — will take care to assess in advance the needs of those seeking training and to establish their own requirements in terms of organisation and facilities. However, for those with the necessary medical experience but little or no experience in training, a request to organise a course can be daunting. At first sight, it may appear that the answer to everyone's problems would be an all-purpose 'trainer's handbook', the basic elements of which could be neatly rearranged to meet every training contingency. However, this 'lecture-Lego' approach, although it may have the initial appeal of reassurance for newcomers, would inevitably frustrate their own spontaneity and flexibility. On a more practical level, it may assume access to teaching aids, facilities and even a certain kind of audience which are simply not there.

The outline which follows, therefore, is not a prescriptive account of HIV/AIDS training, but rather a descriptive one of how trainers work and some of the possibilities open to them. Hopefully, it will provide a basis for discussion for new trainers and managers when planning courses.

## Preliminary assessment

Trainers should first take stock of which aspects of HIV/AIDS they feel competent to deal with personally, and at what level. A pool of specialist speakers should be established and called upon where necessary to reinforce the quality of the course content.

A simple preliminary exercise which can assist trainers in identifying possible problem areas while highlighting the potential for success is to list strengths, weaknesses, and opportunities. Naturally, this list will be highly personal but it may contain such items as the following:

| | |
|---|---|
| *Strengths*: | Strong personal commitment |
| | Ability to recruit participants |
| | Sound practical experience and expertise in the following areas... |
| *Weaknesses*: | Lack of suitable venue |
| | Pressure of waiting list |
| | Staleness through repetition |
| *Opportunities*: | Possibility of well-resources venue |
| | Growing need for information and training |

## Identifying training needs

Training will have to be provided at various levels and with differing emphases to meet the needs of all groups of health workers. Within a hospital, for example, the following groups may require training: medical, nursing, social work, ambulance, physiotherapy, auxiliary, clerical and management. Non-hospital based health workers in contact with HIV/AIDS can include GPs, dentists, home helps, drug workers, etc.

The aim should be to achieve consistency and quality of information across the board. Interviewing staff and their managers can help to highlight not only acknowledged areas of training needs, but also those where a particular aspect of HIV/AIDS may have been mistakenly dismissed as irrelevant to a particular group. For example, the need for information about infection control is widely seen as essential for home helps: less obvious may be the benefit of an understanding of the emotional and social stresses which their HIV positive clients are undergoing. Social workers, on the other hand, may see little need for information about infection control until they stop to consider not only their own safety — for example, in an emergency involving blood spillage — but also the possibility of questions about domestic contact from anxious clients, friends and relatives. Irretrievable damage can be done where health care workers in the same locality give out conflicting advice or appear to be unaware of information given out by colleagues.

Trainers should familiarise themselves thoroughly with any organisational, departmental or professional guidelines covering HIV/AIDS and should incorporate these into training programmes. However, where these are found to be misleading or inaccurate in any way, trainers should discuss the failing at the relevant manager level before commencing the course.

Having established the spectrum of training required, trainers can then move on to consider the most appropriate and cost-effective method of training. It should be borne in mind that some sections of staff may need to attend more than one course (or may even need a special series of courses designed specifically for them). GPs, for example, may want a specialist medical update programme as well as training in counselling techniques.

## Course models

Various models have proved effective in HIV/AIDS training. A comprehensive discussion of these is not possible in the space available, but hopefully those sketched below will provide a useful indication of the nature of choices available.

### Hourly sessions

These can be 'one-off' or a series covering different aspects of HIV/AIDS. They are most suited to groups which require minimal and straightforward input, for example, clerical staff with general questions about health and safety, or a group of workers requiring updates on particular aspects of procedure or policy.

Presentation can be in lecture format with time for questions at the end; questions and answers throughout; or, with topics of a more controversial nature, opposing views from the floor can be taken and discussed. An example of the latter may be a session on the compulsory testing of pregnant women as part of a course for midwives.

To allow for full but informal participation in questions, a recommended maximum for such sessions is 30 participants.

## Specialist seminars

These can last from half a day to two days depending on need, and are appropriate for groups such as doctors and nurses who need intensive updating. This is most effectively done through lectures given by expert speakers with time for questions and discussion. A chairperson is useful to ensure that the programme runs to schedule.

It is possible to incorporate workshop sessions into seminars. If this is done it is important to ensure that the venue has enough rooms to house the workshop groups and that there is a facilitator available to lead each group. Unless workshops are offered, the restriction on numbers will be dictated by the size of the main lecture theatre.

## Experiential workshops

These can be tailored to meet the needs of particular health workers, e.g. home helps, social workers, doctors, etc., or they can be structured around topics to be explored by a multidisciplinary group. Training in HIV/AIDS counselling is particularly suited to experiential workshops.

Numbers must be limited. Twenty-four is ideal: less may circumscribe the scope of the group, more may inhibit group cohesion. Venue is of particular importance here as the sessions are intensive and tiring and can last for anything up to five days or more. Comfortable seating is essential and there should be enough room to accommodate syndicates (i.e. small groups). For example, a group of 24 may split into three syndicates; therefore a minimum requirement is one room capable of housing 24 and two more capable of housing eight. Trainers should also ensure that there are facilities for making tea and coffee and secure storage space to hold equipment overnight.

Experiential workshops require detailed preparation. Syndicate tasks must be well researched. Clear instructions and objectives, preferably written, should be given for role-plays and exercises. Equipment for syndicates must be readily available and in the right quantity. As the workshops involve an intrusion behind the personal and professional security of the participants the creation of a 'safe environment' is of paramount importance, and all participants should be asked to enter a confidential contract at the outset.

One of the most valuable features of experiential workshops is the opportunity they provide for workers from different branches of health care to gain insight into each other's priorities, methods and problems, and to explore new ways of working together to improve health care. For example, managers and policy makers may gain from such a workshop a fuller understanding of HIV/AIDS patients and the objectives of those who care for them, hopefully taking one step on the road to the development of more vital policies.

### Follow-up courses

These have been shown to be most beneficial for the 'frontline' and key managerial participants via experiential workshops. The format of follow-up courses can be flexible but should provide participants with the opportunity to discuss case studies and problems which they should prepare in advance for presentation. Ideally, the same people should meet again in the follow-up sessions. Information update can be included but experience to date suggests strongly that the greatest benefit is gained from the mutual support in the exchange of experiences. Follow-up courses should last from two to three days, depending on need.

### Designing course content

Having interviewed staff and decided on the kind of course which would be most appropriate, trainers should then make a careful list of the needs which they have identified. From these, they should proceed to crystalise course objectives and detail course content.

The following lists of needs and objectives were drawn up in the course of planning a multidisciplinary experiential workshop in HIV/AIDS counselling. They are offered by way of illustration only and are in no way intended to be comprehensive or prescriptive: different trainers will identify different needs in prospective groups, but the discipline of identifying these and of building a course around them is essential to a successful workshop. Staleness quickly creeps in if one fails to look at each group afresh.

## Needs

(1)  Basic facts and information
(2)  Safe environment for personal exploration (e.g. as preparation for training in sexual counselling)
(3)  Improvement and practice of communication skills
(4)  Developing an awareness of patients' rights
(5)  Improvement of teamwork and co-ordinated care
(6)  Demystification of AIDS and counselling
(7)  Review of professional practice
(8)  Instilling a sense of what it is like to actually counsel and encouraging and directing personal initiative.
(9)  Breaking through professional roles to create greater responsiveness and responsibility
(10)  Attitude change and behaviour change.

## Objectives

From the above needs the following course objectives were formed:

(1)  To enable participants to communicate complex and technical information in a way that patients will understand
(2)  To raise awareness of social, legal and ethical aspects and implications of HIV and AIDS
(3)  To enable participants to recognise the options open to patients
(4)  To review counselling practice
(5)  To explore personal attitudes, beliefs and fears about sexuality, sex practices, death and bereavement.

Bearing these summaries in mind a programme can be designed to fit the time available. Trainers will naturally try to cover fully all the points which have arisen in their list of needs and objectives, but it is perhaps worth stating that it is not necessarily a mark of failure if there is still ground left uncovered at the end. A training course is not the 3.30 from Cheltenham. It is far more satisfying for participants to have covered a few major aspects of HIV/AIDS and come away feeling that they have really learned something which they can carry confidently into practice, than to arrive breathless at the end of several days' training having galloped through every topic but in fact having assimilated and consolidated very little.

**Written materials and presentation aids**

A printed summary of factual information is always welcome. However, where lecture material is concerned views among trainers differ as to when it is most usefully distributed. Some feel it is counter-productive to distribute it in advance of the lecture as this encourage inattention. Others prefer to do so, arguing that it reduces automatic and thoughtless note-taking.

Basic factual information on such matters as virology, drug therapy, infection control, etc., may be usefully distributed in advance of experiential workshops to ensure that participants in syndicates are working from the same baseline. If this is done, however, it is advisable to ensure that extra copies are available at the workshop as all too frequently participants forget to bring it. Case studies for discussion and role-play in experiential groups should be clearly presented with full instructions.

Trainers should be thoroughly familiar with any equipment they plan to use in their presentation, and in particular be able to correct basic malfunctions. The following is a list of the most commonly used equipment, but in considering their possible use, trainers should bear in mind matters of cost and transport and, when invited into an unfamiliar venue, should always check in advance whether or not there are facilities to use their equipment.

| | |
|---|---|
| White or black board: | Always try to ensure that a room has one of these, especially where groups are being asked to 'brainstorm' |
| Flipcharts: | One should be available for each syndicate to record results and facilitate presentation to the group |
| Tape recorders: | With the advent of video, these have become less important for role-play, but participants often find it useful to make their own relaxation tapes to increase their understanding of relaxation techniques |
| Video camera and playback facility: | Mainly used for recording role-plays to give participants the opportunity to criticise their own counselling techniques |
| Pre-recorded videos: | 'In-house' videos can be made of good and bad counselling techniques for discussion<br>Recent TV programmes are also useful for discussion |

Overhead projectors: These are particularly useful for displaying statistical information, which is constantly changing and therefore too costly to be put on slide

Always check that a screen or a clear wall is available for projection

Slide projector: These can be used either as a lecture prompt for the trainer or as a clear and easily preserved record of relatively static key information, which is repeatedly presented

Photographic information can also be kept on slide to illustrate clinical symptoms

## Evaluation

Ongoing evaluation of courses is necessary to ensure that they are keeping abreast of new developments and that trainers are using the most effective methods and are targeting their audience accurately. Evaluation can be done internally or externally. The latter is ideal as it reduces the chance of bias in interpretation of results, but the cost can be prohibitive.

In-house evaluation can be valid provided that checks are built in to the procedure to ensure objectivity. The following is only one suggestion as to how this might be achieved. Before the course starts, participants are invited to complete a questionnaire which aims to ascertain their present level of knowledge about HIV/AIDS. The results can then be compared with a second questionnaire to be completed at the end of the course, asking basically the same questions. A comparison of the two should give some indication of the degree to which information has been effectively conveyed and learning has taken place. The second questionnaire may also contain questions inviting participants' comments on the course and suggestions for improvement. An enjoyable course can prove to be the most difficult to assess as there is a danger that participants will score the second questionnaire highly on a pure 'liveliness' factor rather than on hard content. One remedy — perhaps not the one that springs immediately to mind — is to contact participants for a third evaluation after about six months, when they will have had the opportunity to put what they have learned into practice and be in a position to gauge the contribution the course has made to improving their technique.

Even the best prepared and most professionally presented of courses become stale with repetition and dated by new developments. Honest evaluation will give advance warning of the need for a change of direction.

# Chapter 20

# Legal Aspects

DIANA KLOSS

There is very little legislation about medical problems in the United Kingdom: it is the common law as enunciated by the judiciary which determines the legality of most forms of medical intervention. This has advantages over the long term since it means that the law can be developed in the context of changing social mores, but it makes it very difficult in the short term for a lawyer to advise a medical practitioner exactly where the boundaries are set. However, lest the reader turn away from this chapter in despair, he should be made aware of two important trends in the courts over the last decade.

The first is the judicial awareness of the dangers of defensive medicine as practised in the United States, and a clear resolve that our law shall be steered away from the worst aspects of the system. English judges are clearly determined that health care professionals should be liable in the courts only for failures of care which members of their own profession would also condemn. The standard is that of the reasonable member of the relevant profession, as explained by an expert in that speciality.

The second is an underlying realisation that advances in medical science have created a new world which demands that the common law develops realistic responses to the new state of affairs, as in the prosecution of a man accused of murder whose main defence was that it was not he who had killed the victim, but rather the doctor who had switched off the life-support machine on which the victim had been placed after the attack.[1] The court rejected the defence, holding that the victim had 'died' before the machine was switched off.

It is necessary to make these preliminary points, because the spread of HIV has given rise to many legal problems about which so far there has been no time for the courts to give specific guidance. What follows is an attempt to give answers in the context of what has gone before and taking into account recent judicial attitudes. It may be that future governments will decide that legislation is necessary to supplement the common law, but so far the attitude of the UK Government has been to concentrate on information, counselling and research, rather than the introduction of statutory regulation.

### The criminal law

Suppose that a man (or woman) is told that he is HIV positive. Embittered by this news, he decides that he will revenge himself on humanity by having unprotected sexual intercourse with as many partners as possible, hoping that he will thereby infect others with the virus. He is successful in infecting five other people, and within five years one of these has died. Is he guilty of any crime? (A similar case involving an American convicted in West Germany of attempting grievous bodily harm was recently reported in the Press.)

In 1888 Charles Clarence was charged with unlawfully and maliciously inflicting grievous bodily harm contrary to s.20 Offences Against the Person Act 1861 on his wife, or in the alternative, assaulting her occasioning actual bodily harm, contrary to s.47 of the same statute. The accused knew that he was suffering from gonorrhoea. His wife did not know, and if she had known would not have consented to the sexual intercourse which infected her with the disease. On appeal, the accused's conviction was quashed (by a majority of nine judges to four).[2]

The main justification given by the court for their decision was that both the offences charged required that the act of the defendant constituted a battery in law. A battery is any touching of another *without that other's consent*. Mrs Clarence had consented to have intercourse with her husband and thus the basic element of the crime was absent.

The main argument of those who dissented was as follows. Mrs Clarence only consented to intercourse because she thought that her husband was free of disease: this was false, so her consent had been obtained by a fraudulent misrepresentation and was therefore no consent. A battery had been committed. If the parties had not been married but merely cohabiting, such an argument, if accepted, might have led to the conclusion that Clarence was guilty of rape (men cannot rape their wives in English law).

The reason for rejecting this argument was that Mrs Clarence was not deceived as to the nature of the act of intercourse, merely as to its consequences. If, as in R. v. *Williams*,[3] she had been totally ignorant of sexual matters and had believed that intercourse was a form of medical treatment administered by her singing master to improve her voice, her apparent consent would have been void, but this was not the case. 'The only cases in which fraud indisputably vitiates consent in these matters are cases of fraud as to the nature of the act done.'[4]

However, the legal position is not as clear-cut as this for the following reasons:

- Subsequent courts have held that the offence of inflicting grievous bodily harm contrary to s.20 does not necessarily require proof of a battery — you can inflict harm without touching someone, as in the case of the defendant who so terrified his wife that she jumped out of a window to escape him and broke her leg.[5] These developments may throw doubt on the authority of R. v. *Clarence*.

- There are other possible criminal offences with which a defendant might be charged. In the case where the person infected contracts the full AIDS condition and dies, it would be virtually impossible to convict the infecting agent of murder or manslaughter for, apart from the difficulty of proving that the infection was transmitted by the defendant and not from some other source, at common law death must ensue within a year and a day for an unlawful homicide to be committed.

  However, it has been suggested[6] that another possibility is a prosecution under s.23 Offences Against the Person Act 1861. It is an offence unlawfully and maliciously to administer 'any poison or other destructive or noxious thing'. (Liability under this section was not discussed in the case of *Clarence*.) Is HIV a 'noxious thing' within the meaning of the section? Again, it would be difficult to prove beyond a reasonable doubt either that the infection of the victim had been caused by the defendant or that he either intended to bring about that result or recklessly had unprotected intercourse knowing that his partner might become infected with the virus.[7] Will the publicity given to the AIDS threat perhaps influence the judiciary in the direction of imposing criminal liability on those who deliberately threaten the lives of others? As Hawkins J., one of the dissenting judges in *Clarence*, said: '...I can picture to myself a state of things in which a kiss or shake of the hand given by a diseased person, maliciously and with a view to communicate his disorder, might well form the subject of criminal proceedings.'[8]

Where the commission of crimes like rape, unlawful sexual intercourse with a girl under 16 or homosexual acts with a man under 21, also carries the risk of infecting the victim with HIV, some judges increased the sentence imposed on convicted criminals for that reason, but this has now been discouraged by the Court of Appeal, unless there is evidence that the victim has been infected.

## Identification of carriers of HIV

There are basically three groups who need to be able to identify a carrier. The first is composed of public authorities who wish to be able to compile statistics, and possibly to introduce controls, like the refusal of entry to the UK. The second is individuals who fear that they are infected and the third is individuals who wish to avoid contact with a carrier.

There is no power in English law, even in a judge in a court of law, forcibly to compel any person to give a sample of blood, semen, saliva, urine or other intimate samples. Even where an individual is suspected of a serious crime he may refuse to give a sample, though his refusal may then be admissible against him as evidence of guilt.[9]

In civil cases, no court has power to order adults to undergo a blood test.[10]

On the other hand, though there may be no power to insist that any person undergo a blood test, it may be possible for an individual to be faced with an 'either-or' situation: 'Either you submit to a blood test or you don't get the job', for example.

There are few legal controls over this kind of ultimatum. The prospective employer is in law free to ask more or less any question of an applicant for a job and to refuse him the post if no satisfactory answer in forthcoming. (The situation is more complex where the employee is already established in the job (see below).)

There are no laws in the UK which prohibit discrimination against homosexuals of either sex, but there are laws which make discrimination on grounds of sex or race unlawful (Sex Discrimination Acts 1975 and 1986 and Race Relations Act 1976). Discrimination against male homosexuals, but not against female homosexuals, is a form of sex discrimination. If it can be shown that in practice most carriers of HIV at the present time are male (as would seem to be the case in the UK in 1988),[11] the exclusion of HIV carriers from employment is an act of indirect discrimination against men and therefore unlawful unless the employer can show that the exclusion is 'justifiable', because the nature of the employment is such that HIV carriers would constitute a risk to the public or other employees. Since this is rarely the case, the demand for blood tests from prospective employees with the purpose of excluding HIV carriers is probably unlawful at the present time.

The Equal Opportunities Commission recently was able to persuade the airline Dan Air that its policy of excluding male cabin staff was unlawful sex discrimination and must be abandoned; the attempt to justify the exclusion on the ground that those applying for jobs as male cabin staff were likely to be homosexual HIV carriers was not legal justification for the policy, since even if it were true they would not constitute any health risk to passengers. On the other hand, British Airways' new policy of testing applicants for jobs as pilots for HIV may be upheld if it can be demonstrated that there is a potential risk of associated brain disease which may create a hazard to the safety of aircraft and passengers.

Controls on immigration have been held to be outside the sex discrimination legislation[12] and by definition are exceptions to the Race Relations Act. If the UK Government wished to insist on blood tests as a condition of entry to the UK of persons who have no right of entry, it would be free to do so. Even in the case of nationals of Member States within the European Community, it could be argued that the protection of public health justified the imposition of such controls,[13] though the European Court interprets such defences narrowly, and a 1964 EEC Directive lists diseases justifying refusal of entry, but does not, of course, mention AIDS.

Some insurance companies now demand evidence that an applicant for life assurance is HIV negative, at least in the case of some applicants like single men over 35 or two young men who jointly apply for a mortgage. Although this is discriminatory against men, it is not contrary to the Sex Discrimination Act, because it can be scientifically proven that carriers of the virus have a greatly increased risk of premature death and is therefore justified on actuarial grounds.[14]

It is therefore clear that no-one is compelled to undergo a test for HIV, but that in some cases adverse inferences may be drawn from a refusal.

If the individual is an adult, conscious and of sound mind, and is told that he is being asked to give a sample of blood for the purpose of testing it for evidence of HIV, either with his name attached, or in the form of an anonymous sample, his consent will give complete authority to the medical and nursing staff who carry out the procedure. It is not in law necessary for such a consent to be given in writing, but it is always advisable to have written evidence in case disputes subsequently arise.

The courts have frequently emphasised in recent decisions that consent to medical procedures must be 'informed' — that is, that the patient must be told of the broad nature of the treatment proposed and of any substantial risks involved.[15] The information which must be given is that which a reasonable doctor or nurse would have given to the patient in question; the courts accept that details may be withheld from an exceptionally nervous patient which should be given to one who is more stoic in his attitude.[16]

However, all the informed consent cases concern information about the essential nature of the procedure itself, or about the likely risks or probable outcome of the treatment, not about what is to be done with any intimate samples thereby obtained. As with a criminal battery (discussed above), as long as the patient knows of the broad nature of what is to be done he gives a valid consent and no civil liability for battery will arise, even though facts may be concealed from him (like a 1 per cent risk of paralysis) which might have led to a refusal of consent had he known of them. Only if a reasonable member of the medical or nursing profession following the general practice of the profession would have given further information will he be able to sue for damages, and the cause of action will be for negligence, not battery, which means that he will have to prove a failure to take reasonable care and that he would have been likely to have refused the treatment had he been properly informed.

If we apply this to a blood test, the consent of an individual to the taking of blood will prevent it from being a battery, even if he is unaware that the blood is to be tested for HIV. He may be told that it is to be tested for alcohol or drugs or the effects of lead or ionising radiation, or that it is a routine procedure commonly administered. The fact remains that he knows the *nature* of the process, the taking of a sample of blood, though not the true reason behind it. Unless the courts were willing to invent a new doctrine — that consent to the taking of blood for a declared purpose is conditional on it being used for that purpose only — there is no action for a civil battery in this type of case. However, if the consent is obtained by fraud, that is that the doctor pretended that the test was for one purpose, when it was in reality for another, at least one judge has said that the consent will be vitiated.

As to negligence, as there is at present no treatment for HIV carriers, and the discovery that an individual is infected with the virus can lead to severe consequences, both financial and emotional, it is probably true that a doctor's duty of care to his patient demands that he only administers a blood test after he has warned the patient of the unpleasant consequences if he discovers that he is HIV positive. A doctor who knows that the patient is HIV positive may be compelled to disclose that fact to an insurance company at a later date or, if he is also the doctor of the patient's spouse, to pass on the information to protect his other patient. Since a test on a patient's blood without the patient's knowledge would exclude the possibility of this pre-test counselling, it is possible that it would be held negligent not to inform the patient that he was being tested for HIV and to ask for his consent. Even if the doctor did not give the patient the result of the test (there is, in general, no legal obligation to disclose medical records or information to the patient himself,[17] unless he needs to know in order to undergo treatment, e.g. a woman found by a cervical smear test to be in a pre-cancerous state), the doctor would have knowledge which he might later have to disclose to the patient's detriment.

The testing of anonymous samples, such that the donor cannot be made aware of the result because the tester does not know his identity (as proposed by the Chief Medical Officer to the Government, Dr Acheson) would avoid this, but is thought by many in the medical profession to be unethical, because it deprives the patient of information about his condition.

Testing of pregnant women in antenatal clinics should only be undertaken with their consent and after counselling that if the mother is found to be infected she may wish to consider an abortion.

Where a patient is unconscious and therefore unable to give or refuse consent, necessary medical procedures may be undertaken without consent. It would be for the medical profession to justify a blood test for HIV as necessary in the circumstances of the case. The consent of a relative of the unconscious person is not required, nor would it justify the performance of any treatment which was not a real necessity.

Tests can as a general rule only lawfully be performed on children under 16 with the consent of a parent, or, if a child under 18 has been made a ward of court, with the consent of the court. If a child under 16 is intelligent and mature enough to understand the nature and implications of the test he can give consent on his own behalf.[18]

The mentally ill and adult mentally handicapped can only be tested with their consent, as the Mental Health Act 1983 does not cover treatment for physical, as opposed to mental illness. The same applies to prisoners in the care of Her Majesty.[19]

## Confidentiality

The Hippocratic Oath includes a promise that the doctor will not divulge confidential information about his patient to third parties, but this duty can never be absolute, because sometimes the public interest or the protection of others must take precedence over the rights of the individual. The General Medical Council lists eight circumstances in which confidentiality may be breached, including the sharing of information with other health professionals participating in the care of the patient, disclosure of information by order of a court of law or in pursuance of a statutory requirement, and disclosure in the public interest, for example investigation by the police of a very serious crime, or in cases of suspected child abuse.

AIDS is not a notifiable disease under the Public Health (Control of Disease) Act 1984, though certain provisions of that Act have been extended to AIDS by statutory regulation.[20] There is at present no obligation on doctors to report cases to the local authority.[21] The AIDS (Control) Act 1987 obliges health authorities to compile regular statistics of those diagnosed as suffering from AIDS and those who have died from the disease. It also requires health authorities to report on facilities and services provided for treating, counselling and caring for AIDS sufferers and people infected with HIV, and on action taken to educate the public about the disease.

There are special regulations relating to sexually transmitted diseases: the NHS (Venereal Diseases) Regulations 1974.[22] These provide (Reg. 2) that every health authority shall take all necessary steps to secure that any information capable of identifying an individual obtained with respect to persons examined or treated for any sexually transmitted disease shall not be disclosed *except for the purpose of communicating the information to a doctor or someone working under his direction in connection with the treatment of persons suffering from the disease or the prevention of its spread.*

It is assumed that these regulations apply to AIDS and HIV, though arguably neither is in itself a disease, merely a loss of capacity to resist other diseases, and HIV may be transmitted other than through sexual intercourse.

It would seem that a health authority is obliged by the regulations to order STD clinics not to disclose to any person other than the patient's doctor the fact that an individual is HIV positive, even to that person's husband or wife. But the regulations do not control the extent to which the STD clinics may report the situation to the patient's own doctor, nor how far the patient's GP can disclose the information to third parties. If the clinic told a GP that a child of eight was suffering from a disease inflicted on her by her father by means of criminal sexual intercourse (an actual case reported to the author), no law of confidence would prevent the GP from revealing the facts to social workers or the police.

What if a GP who has both a husband and wife on his list is told by the clinic that the husband is HIV positive: should he tell the wife? It is probably the law that his duty to protect the wife's health justifies, indeed obliges, him to disclose the facts to her, especially as the health of a future child of the couple may also be at risk. Where the GP of the HIV positive patient is not also the doctor of that patient's spouse or sexual partner there is probably no positive duty in law to make disclosure, but if the GP knows that his patient is sexually active and is ignoring advice to take precautions it is probably justifiable to break confidence in the general public interest of restricting the spread of the virus (especially if the courts are willing to hold that this kind of conduct by the patient is criminal).

Medical personnel caring for the patient may be themselves put at risk if precautions are not taken. The same may apply to laboratory workers dealing with blood samples and domestic staff dealing with soiled clothes or bandages. It is argued that these workers must be told of the condition of the patient to be able to protect themselves. Pressure has been brought to bear on administrators to make disclosure to all kinds of ancillary staff like catering and portering staff in hospitals and home helps and 'meals on wheels' helpers in the community, to whom the risk, if there is any, is small. In consequence, AIDS sufferers have been subjected to threats and have even had their homes attacked because so many precautions were taken by overzealous health authority employees that the community was alerted to their condition.

It is difficult to find any legal justification for such wide disclosure. Ancillary workers are rarely at risk and could usually be protected by general hygiene precautions which could be applied to all patients, whatever their condition. The ill-informed belief of employees that they are at risk is no justification in law for their employer's breach of confidence, especially when the outcome may be as threatening to the patient and his property as the virus itself.

If a local authority holds a case conference to discuss an AIDS patient it should confine it to those who need to know of his condition, either because they are giving him counselling or medical treatment or because they need to take special precautions. If the patient wishes others to know he should have the right to decide for himself.

Where an employee wrongly discloses confidential information to a third party, the employer is vicariously liable even if he has given strict instructions that information must be kept secret. A receptionist who, as in a recent incident, announced to a crowded surgery: 'Oh my God, it's the man with AIDS', would make both herself and her employer liable to pay damages. Where the fault was all on the employee's side, her employer could both dismiss her and claim reimbursement of any damages paid to the patient (the latter course of action would only be worthwhile where the employee was insured against professional liability — for example, if she was a member of the Royal College of Nursing).

Cases have arisen of mothers who are HIV positive giving birth to a child and asking for it to be taken for adoption. Such a baby has a 25/35 chance of infection (through transmission in the womb), but it is not possible for technical reasons to test the child. The adoption procedure under the Adoption Agencies Regulations 1983[23] requires the adoption agency (either the local authority or an approved adoption society) to provide a prospective adopter with written information about the child, his personal history and background and his health history and current state of health (Reg. 12). In the course of its pre-adoption investigations it has to enquire into the family health history of the mother, including details of any present illness, and any other relevant information (Reg. 7 and Schedule, Part IV). If the mother has been diagnosed as HIV positive, it would seem clear that the prospective adopters are entitled to know this, though if the mother refuses to be tested for HIV there is more of a dilemma. Although there is no power to force the mother to undergo a test (the agency must do that which is reasonably practicable to persuade her to do so), the courts would probably hold that the agency was entitled to tell the prospective adopters that the mother was in a high risk group and had refused to be tested, and probably that it had a duty to do so, even though it led to the rejection of the child.

The DHSS Circular LAC (84) 3 advises that health information on the natural parents should be sought from a doctor who knows the parents and has access to the relevant records, who will usually be the GP. It states that the prospective adopters must be advised about any health problem. 'If the placement of a baby direct from hospital is proposed, the medical adviser should ensure that it is carefully explained to the prospective adopters that only preliminary health screening and assessment has so far been possible; he should also ensure that the implications of any particular risk factors are explained. It is essential for the prospective adopters to receive these explanations, so that they can decide whether they wish to go ahead with the placement, and so that any risk of their undertaking more than they feel they can manage is minimised.'

If the mother's doctor, either her GP or the hospital doctor, knows that she is HIV positive and wants her child adopted, should he tell the adoption agency? As the Adoption Agencies Regulations require the agency to obtain medical reports on the child and, so far as is reasonably practicable, his natural mother 'with the results of any tests carried out during or immediately after pregnancy' (Schedule, Part IV), even a doctor who at the mother's behest *refused* to disclose medical records would in practice probably prevent the child from going forward for adoption, because the necessary documentation would not be available.

The courts have held that confidence may be broken in the public interest.[24] Unless medical personnel and adoption agencies are able and willing to reveal all the relevant facts, even in breach of the mother's confidence, prospective adopters and foster parents will be deterred from coming forward through fear that they will not be told the whole truth. This cannot be in the public interest, nor in the long-term interest of the child.

Of course, the court, which must eventually approve the adoption, has power to order the disclosure of medical records and to order that the child's blood be tested,[25] though not that of the mother. Finally, once the adoption is complete the child becomes the responsibility of his new family who cannot send him back if he is later diagnosed as HIV positive.

### The isolation of HIV-infected persons

Where a patient has developed the full blown clinical condition of AIDS, legal powers exist to confine him compulsorily in hospital if this is necessary to protect others. The Public Health (Infectious Diseases) Regulations 1985 have extended certain provisions of the Public Health (Control of Disease) Act 1984 to AIDS, including the magistrates' power on the application of a local authority to make an order for detention in a hospital of an AIDS sufferer if he would not take proper precautions to prevent the spread of disease if allowed to go free.

What if a member of the caring professions discovers that a patient is HIV positive or suffering from AIDS? May he lawfully for that reason refuse to treat him? Where he has already undertaken the care of a patient, as in the case of a GP who has the patient on his list, he will have a duty to take reasonable care of that patient. If the GP fails in his duty by refusing to treat him the patient will be able to sue for damages for negligence if he thereby suffers injury. Also, although the NHS regulations governing the doctors' contracts with the Family Practitioner Committee provide that a doctor may refuse to accept a patient or may ask for a patient already on his list to be removed, they do not allow him to act unilaterally without following the proper procedures, so that the Family Practitioner Committee which investigates failures by GPs to comply with their terms of service might take proceedings against him.

If the patient is not registered with a doctor there is no legal obligation to act as a Good Samaritan and come to the aid of a stranger, other than emergency cases arising in the GP's own district.[26]

A hospital doctor or consultant might also be liable for negligence if a patient in the hospital is denied essential treatment because he is HIV positive and thereby suffers injury. The only legal justification for such a refusal is self-defence, that the situation is so dangerous because of a lack of proper precautions that the doctor is being asked to undergo an unreasonable risk. What if a surgeon refuses to perform a non-essential operation like a hip replacement on an HIV positive patient? The patient will suffer extra pain and distress through the surgeon's refusal and would be able to sue for that, but in addition the surgeon's employer, the health authority, could take disciplinary action, and, of course, the General Medical Council might decide that any doctor who refused to treat his patient was guilty of professional misconduct and unfit to be a doctor.[27] Much would depend in such a case on how the profession as a whole viewed the reasonableness or otherwise of the doctor's conduct. The General Medical Council has warned that it is unethical for a doctor to refuse to treat a patient because of personal risk to the doctor, or moral judgement on the patient's life style.

What about the common situation where an employee is suspected by his employer and fellow-employees of being an HIV carrier? Often, workers put pressure on the employer to sack such a person. First, there is no power to force an employee in employment to undergo a blood test or any medical examination on pain of losing his job if he refuses, unless there is a term in the contract of employment which obliges the employee to submit to such examination. Secondly, if an employee is found to be HIV positive and the employer is informed, it will be unfair dismissal to sack him for that reason unless the employer can show that the presence of the virus or the development of symptoms renders the employee unfit to do the job (only full-time employees [employed for 16 or more hours a week or eight or more hours a week for five or more years] who have worked for the employer for at least two years at the date of dismissal are able to complain to an industrial tribunal that they have been unfairly dismissed). It is no defence to a claim for unfair dismissal that the employer was under pressure from other employees, who were either threatening industrial action or actually striking, to dismiss the infected person.[28]

Where a dismissal is an act of sex or race discrimination no qualifying period of employment is required. As has been argued before, inferior treatment given to HIV carriers is indirectly discriminatory against men, so that an employer whose policy was to dismiss those who were diagnosed as HIV positive would be acting contrary to the sex discrimination legislation, unless he could prove that for reasons of safety it was necessary to exclude such persons.

## The legal obligations of the patient and others

Once an individual is given the news that he is HIV positive he is faced with a continuing dilemma: to tell or not to tell.

If he subsequently wishes to take out life assurance he is likely these days to be asked whether he has had a blood test. It is pointless to lie, because even if he obtains a policy by suppressing the truth the contract will not be binding and the insurance company may eventually refuse to pay. Even if he is not asked the question, there is a duty in an insurance contract to reveal material facts known to the proposer, so that the insurance company may refuse to pay if it is later discovered that he knew that he was HIV positive at the time he applied for insurance and did not reveal it. This deters some people in high risk groups from having the blood test: it is financially better to be ignorant.

There is no obligation on an employee to inform his employer that he is HIV positive, nor if he is applying for a new job to reveal the fact to his prospective employer. As a general rule, and subject to the laws against discrimination (see above), when an employer is choosing employees he can ask applicants about their health and refuse to employ them if the answers are unsatisfactory. If an applicant lies in answer to such a question, it has been held that this may justify his dismissal when the truth is eventually discovered, but only where the illness or disability actually makes the employee unsuitable to do the job, which is rarely the case with HIV.[29]

What of the individual who knows or fears that he is HIV positive and realises that he may constitute a danger to others? There may be liability for negligence − a failure to take reasonable care. For instance − a surgeon believes that because of his life style he may be infected and that, if so, there is a slight risk to his patients. The surgeon's duty of care means that he must take all reasonable precautions to protect others against possible infection, but it does not necessarily require him to have a blood test or give up surgery. The same rule applies if he knows that he is infected − he must take reasonable care, which does not require him to tell his employer or his patients.[30] A patient would be entitled to refuse to allow him to operate if the surgeon was unable or unwilling to give an assurance that he was free of infection, but only because it is always the case that a patient may refuse to be treated by any individual member of the medical profession, for a good reason or for no reason at all.

If a man donates blood to the transfusion service knowing that he is in a high risk group and may be infected, he could in legal theory be sued for negligence if it could be proved that his blood had infected a patient. His belief that the fact that the blood is tested would exclude infection (when there is a chance that he could be infected but tested negative) would be a defence unless he had been specifically warned when he gave blood that this was not the case.

An individual who has unprotected sexual intercourse or who allows another to use his drug needle when he knows or has reasonable cause to suspect that he is HIV positive could be sued for damages for negligence by anyone whom he infects, but in all these cases it would be for the victim to prove that the HIV infection came from that source, which might be difficult if he or she had had several sexual partners, for instance.

One AIDS sufferer is reported to be suing the UK Government after he contracted the virus through a contaminated supply of factor VIII, purchased by the UK Government in the United States and given to haemophiliacs. He is presumably arguing that the Government was negligent in applying insufficient tests to the American product. Similar cases brought in the US have all been unsuccessful and the Haemophilia Society has advised AIDS sufferers not to pursue action through the courts, because of the difficulty of proof. The Consumer Protection Act 1987 is now in force: it is possible that those infected by tainted blood will be able to rely on 'product liability' (liability of the producer without the need to prove negligence), but this will not be retrospective.

## Conclusion

As has been seen, there are many situations in this area of medical and social work practice where the law has yet to be clarified. On the other hand, counsellors who adhere to the following principles are likely to avoid condemnation in the law courts:

* You have a duty to patients and clients to take reasonable care. If you follow the practice and principles of most of your professional colleagues this will in law in the majority of cases constitute reasonable care.
* Your duty to your patients and clients requires that you keep their

confidence *unless* there is a real danger to others or the public interest demands disclosure.

- It may be a serious disadvantage to an individual to discover that he is HIV positive, because there is no treatment for the condition and the knowledge may prevent him from obtaining insurance and could be passed on by his doctor to his wife. No-one should be tested without his consent, and the possible implications of a positive result should be explained before the consent is obtained[31]. Anonymous testing is probably lawful, whatever the ethical objections may be.

# References

1. *R.* v. *Malcherek* [1981] 2 All ER 422.
2. *R.* v. *Clarence* (1988) 22 QBD 23.
3. [1923] 1 KB 340.
4. Stephen J. at p.43.
5. *R.* v. *Halliday* (1889) 61 LT 701; *R.* v. *Wilson* [1983] 1 All ER 993.
6. Fortin and Wauchope (1987) *Law Society's Gazette*, March 25, p.884.
7. *R.* v. *Cunningham* [1957] 2 QB 396.
8. (1888) 22 QBD at p.52.
9. s.62(10) Police and Criminal Evidence Act 1984; s.7 Road Traffic Act 1972.
10. *W.* v. *W.* [1963] 2 All ER 841. A statutory exception is a case where the paternity of a child is in dispute: Family Law Reform Act 1969.
11. Official DHSS figures up to the end of 1986 show that of those who have contracted AIDS, the majority are homosexual men.
12. *R.* v. *Entry Clearance Officer*, ex parte *Amin* [1983] 2 All ER 864.
13. Art 48 Treaty of Rome; Directive 64/221.
14. s.45 Sex Discrimination Act 1975. The EOC advocates the repeal of this section: *Legislating for Change? A Consultative Document* (1986).
15. *Sidaway* v. *Board of Governors of the Bethlem Royal and the Maudsley Hospital* [1985] 2 WLR 480.
16. *Bolam* v. *Friern H.M.C.* [1957] 1 WLR 582. 16 A *Bristow J. in Chatterton* v. *Gerson* [1981] Q.B., 432.
17. The Data Protection Act 1984 contains provision for subject access to medical records held on computer, but it is likely that regulations will modify this obligation which only came into force in November 1987.
18. *Gillick* v. *W. Norfolk and Wisbech H.A.* [1985] 3 All ER 402.
19. *Freeman* v. *Home Office* [1984] 2 WLR 802. See *Re B. (a minor)*, [1987] 2 All ER 206 (Sterilisation of mentally handicapped girl).
20. Public Health (Infectious Diseases) Regs, SI 1985/434.
21. The voluntary system of reporting cases without the identification of individual details to the Communicable Diseases Surveillance Centre is not a breach of confidence, since the information is anonymous.

22. SI 1974/29.
23. SI 1983/1964.
24. *Lion Laboratories* v. *Evans* [1984] 2 All ER 417.
25. *S.* v. *S.* [1970] 3 All ER 107.
26. See Brazier: *Medicine, Patients and the Law* (1987) Harmondsworth: Penguin Books, Chapter 15; SI 1974/160.
27. In the case of a nurse, the matter could be reported to the UK Central Council.
28. s.63 Employment Protection (Consolidation) Act 1978; AIDS and Employment, D of E and HSE Advisory Document (1986).
29. *O'Brien* v. *Prudential Assurance Co. Ltd*, [1979] IRLR 140, where the employee who had a history of mental illness lied in an application for a job as an insurance salesman visiting clients in their homes. When the truth was discovered he was held to have been fairly dismissed.
30. The advice of the GMC is that it is unethical for a doctor who knows or suspects that he has AIDS or is HIV positive to continue working without medical advice. Other doctors are instructed that they should inform health authorities if they suspect a colleague of having the virus, but not following advice.
31. The BMA has now received similar legal advice. *BMJ* Vol **295** p.911 (1987).

# Chapter 21

# Ethical Questions

REVEREND DR KENNETH BOYD

AIDS and HIV infection raise a variety of ethical questions for counsellors, their clients and society. Ethical questions normally arise when there is doubt or conflict about what ought to be done for the best, and when the problem cannot be resolved by an appeal to the facts. Indeed, to describe questions as 'ethical' (or 'moral' − the terms are interchangeable for most purposes) is to suggest that there are good moral arguments on both sides of the case, and that, in practice, a fallible human judgement has to be made between them. The most we can expect from discussing or studying ethics is greater clarity, and possibly wider agreement, about the strengths and weaknesses of the relevant moral arguments. Beyond this point, moral choice is a matter for the individual conscience or for collective judgements concerning professional ethics and the law.

The ethical issues raised by AIDS and HIV infection are not essentially different from others related to medical and health care ethics generally. Some of the questions encountered most commonly in the present context in fact are those with which medical ethics traditionally has been most concerned. In the context of AIDS and HIV infection however, many of these questions are being raised more acutely and urgently than hitherto. This chapter will discuss five of them: consent, confidentiality, professional responsibility, euthanasia and suicide, and sexuality.

Before discussing these specific topics, it may be worth noting a degree of agreement which has already been achieved in some studies of the ethics of health care. From the examination of various ethical codes and declarations, it seems clear that many moral problems in health care can be analysed helpfully in terms of three major moral principles which are widely commended − those of beneficence and

non-maleficence, of respect for autonomy, and of justice.[1] These principles indicate what ought to be done for the best in most of the moral
problems and dilemmas encountered by professionals. The principle
of beneficence and non-maleficence requires that good should be done
and harm avoided to patients or clients. The principle of respect for
autonomy (or self-determination) requires that the wishes as well as
the interests of the client or patient should be respected. The principle
of justice requires that the competing interests and wishes of different
individuals should be judged fairly. Ideally, all of these principles
should be satisfied. The professional, that is, should do good and
avoid harm to the patient or client, in a way which is in accordance
with the latter's wishes, and also is agreed to be fair to and by
everyone else involved. If all of these conditions were satisfied, indeed,
there would no longer be a moral problem. The problem, of course, is
that very often it is not possible to satisfy all of these principles on the
same occasion.

**Consent**

Consent to treatment is a moral as well as a legal requirement. It is
required most obviously by the principle of respect for autonomy. We
may not have a duty to provide one another with everything which
the other believes he has a right to: the resources to provide this may
not be available, or others with greater needs may be claiming them.
But the least we owe one another is respect for the liberty not to be
interfered with in making choices, about our own lives, which do not
interfere with the liberties of others. In most cases, the liberty to refuse
medical treatment does not interfere with the liberties of other people.

   In ethics, this moral requirement is now commonly referred to as
that of 'informed consent'. In practice, this means that consent must be
given voluntarily, under neither coercion nor undue pressure. It means
also that the patient or client must be given adequate information, in a
manner which enables him to understand what is involved in the
proposed procedure.[2] The difficulty with these requirements, obviously,
is that they are subject to different interpretations. Undue pressure, if
not coercion, may be exerted in subtle if unintended ways; degrees of
understanding may be affected not only by the patient's mental state,
but also by how, where and when information is given; and what
constitutes 'adequate' information is very much a matter of judgement.
In the United States, the relevant judgement is normally seen as that of
the 'prudent patient', in Britain as that of the 'reasonable doctor'. What

the British reasonable doctor (not wishing to alarm his patient with information about every conceivable risk) may consider adequate information may well differ from what the American prudent patient believes that he has a right to know.

Matters of judgement are involved also in arguments about consent based on the principle of beneficence and non-maleficence. On the one hand this principle can provide arguments for requiring consent. In other words, to treat someone against his wishes may harm more fundamental interests than those it serves: heroic attempts to prolong the life of someone who is dying and no longer wishes to live, can be an example of this. On the other hand, treating without consent a minor, or someone who is mentally disturbed, or someone who is unconscious, may well be in their best interests. In this area, clearly, the most difficult questions are those in which the individual's mental state or the benefits of treatment to the individual are matters of borderline judgements.

The strongest arguments for treating someone without their consent, or against their wishes, derive from the principle of justice. Failure to treat or restrain a known and dangerous psychopath would not be fair to the interests and wishes of others at risk. A similar case might be made for compulsory hospital admission of a mildly confused elderly person, living in a block of flats, who repeatedly forgot to turn off the taps of her gas cooker. In this example however, the problem equally might be solved without compulsion — perhaps by installing an electric cooker, or by finding alternative accommodation, or by voluntary admission to hospital. In judgements of this kind, the details of the case obviously influence how the relevant moral principles should be applied.

In the case of HIV infection, the question of informed consent has arisen primarily in relation to antibody testing and screening. Here too, the details of the case will affect how the moral principles should be applied. Considering the question first with reference to the principle of beneficence and non-maleficence, it is not immediately clear whether the interests of someone who may be at risk will best be served by having a blood test. It depends both on the result of the test, and on what the result means to the person concerned. The obvious benefit of a negative result, for most people, would be peace of mind. In the case of a positive result however, much depends on how the particular individual views this. For some people, the relief of knowing may be more bearable than the uncertainty of not knowing; and the knowledge may be crucial for choices they wish to make about the future. But for others, ignorance or uncertainty may be preferable to the knowledge that they have an ineradicable infection which may (or may not) develop into an incurable and fatal disease. A preference for ignorance may be strengthened, moreover, by an awareness of the potential material and financial disadvantages of being identified as infected. Someone at risk, with a family to provide for, may well have altruistic reasons for preferring ignorance: he may, after all, not be infected, or if infected, not go on to develop AIDS, or be killed in an accident in the meantime; and again, he may be aware that some partners of those who are HIV positive have not themselves become infected,[3] or he may opt for 'safe sex' or even cease to be sexually active.

Considerations of this kind, of course, would carry less conviction if there was an effective treatment for AIDS: testing then would be more likely, in general, to be in the interest of those at risk. In that event also, it might be morally justifiable to test, in their own interest, at-risk individuals who were mentally incapable of giving consent because of psychiatric illness, or who were unconscious. Without an effective treatment however, it is difficult to argue that testing, in general, is in the interest of those at risk. In terms of doing good and avoiding harm to the individual therefore, there would seem to be no argument for testing without consent. This suggests, in other words, that it would be unethical to test unconsultable individuals and that those who were consultable would have to make the choice for themselves. For counsellors, this inevitably involves a heavy burden of responsibility for ensuring that, before deciding whether or not to give consent, the patient or client is fully informed of the possible consequences. Although the law in Britain does not demand that the relevant information should be that which a 'prudent patient' might wish, the counsellor's moral duty of beneficence, non-maleficence and respect for autonomy suggests that such a criterion should be adopted, not least because many of those at risk are young and intelligent, and because the potentially serious consequences of a positive result are already matters of widespread public discussion.

These arguments against testing without consent have not taken account, so far, of the principle of justice. If HIV, with all its consequences, was air-borne for example, and highly infectious, the unfair risk to other people might well tilt the balance of the argument in favour of testing without consent. To reach this conclusion however, one would need to be reasonably sure that the considerable practical difficulties of testing without consent could be overcome, and that more infected individuals were likely to be detected in this way than by voluntary testing. It is difficult to see how this could be achieved in practice, other than by screening the entire population. To screen only sections of the population (for example, those who are sexually active, or homosexuals, or intravenous drug abusers) whose membership is not immediately obvious not only would be ineffective, but also would be highly unjust, in principle and in practice.

Such draconian measures of doubtful efficacy clearly are not demanded by what is known about HIV infection and its transmission. The interest of the public health, of course, might be served if accurate epidemiological data could be gained about the prevalence and spread of the infection; and to this end it has been argued that anonymised screening might be employed – i.e. unidentifiable samples of blood taken for other purposes might be tested for HIV. As the House of Commons Social Services Committee has noted[4] however, the epidemiological usefulness of anonymised screening is limited, precisely because its anonymity precludes identification of the prevalence and rate of spread in high-risk groups. The most to be expected from anonymised screening might be some information of possible future relevance for health planning. But this limited benefit would scarcely justify offending against the normal requirement of consent, particularly if, as has been argued persuasively,[5] 'adequate consent' to voluntary anonymised testing 'seems relatively easy to obtain'.

Testing without consent also might be argued for in cases where identification of an infected individual could protect others in direct contact with him. The other people involved here might be either health workers or sexual partners. In the case of health care workers however, the argument against the normal requirement of consent is greatly weakened not only by evidence[6] of the minimal occupational health risk of working with AIDS patients, but also by the traditional expectation that health workers voluntarily accept some exposure to such risks in their choice of profession. Sexual intercourse too is normally a voluntary activity, in which individuals choose their partners. If an unsuspecting partner is infected by an unidentified carrier, this may well be regarded as unfair. But the unfairness of such cases does not necessarily justify the unfairness of compelling possible carriers to be tested against their wishes.

Compulsory medical examination and detention of patients with AIDS is provided for by the Public Health (Infectious Diseases) Regulations 1985. The general principles and examples discussed above however would seem to support the conclusion of the House of Commons Social Services Committee, when it noted[7], 'To our knowledge the Regulations have been used only once, and the implications they raise for civil liberties make us doubt if they should ever be used again'.

## Confidentiality

Confidentiality is a traditional requirement of professional and particularly, medical ethics. In the case of sexually transmitted disease, it is also a legal requirement under the National Health Service (Venereal Disease) Regulations 1974. The most obvious reason for maintaining medical confidentiality is that if patients do not trust doctors to keep their secrets, they are unlikely to provide the full information necessary for optimal care. Similar considerations apply to counselling, and can be seen as required by the principle of beneficence and non-maleficence. The principle of respect for autonomy also supports confidentiality. Some degree of privacy is necessary, if people are to make choices about their own lives free of undue external pressures; and self-determination implies that individuals should be able to choose, as far as possible, which of their intimate secrets to share, when and with whom. In such vulnerable areas as illness and sexuality, confidentiality protects autonomy.

These arguments for confidentiality support the recommendation of the House of Commons Social Services Committee, that 'there are no grounds for disclosing a patient's antibody status without their consent, except to safeguard another from infection'.[8] This imposes a moral duty of confidentiality on everyone with access to confidential information and, in practice, as the Committee suggests,[9] 'a very strict "need to know" policy': those 'involved in the direct care of a person must be told, but there is no need for everyone involved in care to be told the exact diagnosis'. As the Committee points out, a 'need to know' is likely to exist not so much to protect carers or other patients from the minimal risks of HIV infection, as to protect the health of those infected.

The major argument against maintaining confidentiality — 'to safeguard another from infection' — derives from the principle of justice. An obvious example would be if someone known to be HIV positive refused to inform his wife or sexual partner. In this case, an STD clinic doctor presumably would be required by the 1974 regulations to maintain confidentiality. His legal obligations might be supported moreover by the moral argument that his professional role made his special duty to respect his patient's autonomy outweigh any general moral duties to the patient's spouse or partner who was not his patient. These general moral duties (which we all owe to one another) would be sufficiently weighty however to oblige the STD clinic doctor or counsellor to use every effort to persuade his patient to honour his own moral obligations (albeit making the case in less formal terms). If the doctor involved was a general practitioner with both the patient and his spouse or partner on his list, a much sharper moral dilemma clearly would be involved. The moral pressures for and against breaking confidentiality in this case are so finely balanced indeed, that it is not possible to suggest any general rule about what should be done. On the other hand, the effect of breaking confidentiality on the doctor-patient relationship, not only in this case but generally, would be sufficiently damaging to make it morally permissible only as a last resort, adopted as a rare exception after every effort of persuasion had been made.

In relation to HIV infection and AIDS, it is important to maintain confidentiality in order to 'protect patients and clients from the reactions of the ignorant and the intrusions of the press'.[10] In this context however, it is no less important to emphasise that the main reason for confidentiality, as in any other serious diagnosis, is respect for autonomy. Confidentiality, in other words, should not become the kind of secrecy which implies that the condition is shameful or those affected blame-worthy. These connotations perhaps may fade as the condition becomes more common, and affects friends or members of the families of those who might otherwise condemn. In these circumstances, as in the case of other terminal illnesses, some people with AIDS may wish to talk more publicly about their experience, in order to help others. The initiative here, however, should always be that of the individual concerned.

## Professional responsibility

The health professional's primary responsibility, it has been suggested above, is towards his patient or client. But clearly professionals have other responsibilities − to their families and colleagues, to other patients and society, and to themselves. These responsibilities, it might be argued, could be cited in defence of doctors and other health care workers who have refused to treat people with HIV or AIDS. In other areas of health care, after all, they have a right to decline to treat certain patients: the 1970 World Medical Association Declaration of Oslo,[11] for example, allows a doctor, on conscientious grounds, not to advise or perform an abortion.

The analogy with abortion, however, does not really hold: conscientious objection to abortion is to the procedure, not the patient, to taking life rather than preserving it; and even in the case of abortion, the doctor may withdraw only 'while ensuring the continuity of (medical) care by a qualified colleague'.[12] The case of HIV infection and AIDS, by contrast, involves only normal professional duties, however demanding. The objection here, moreover, seems to be based either on fear or disapproval, neither of which justifies refusal to treat. Disapproval of patients with illnesses attributable to activities of which the doctor disapproves was not unknown, of course, before AIDS — drivers who drink, smokers, and attempted suicides were all examples. But as has been observed,[13] the unacceptability of not treating such patients can be illustrated by inverting the example.

> Suppose, for example, a surgeon who reserves 'the right to decline to operate' contracts syphilis and in the venereal disease clinic encounters a bigoted gay doctor who disapproves of heterosexual intercourse. Would the latter be justified in withholding medical treatment for syphilis on the grounds that it resulted from a voluntary activity of which he or she disapproved

Refusal to treat on the grounds of fear of infection, as already noted, is a disproportionate reaction to the minimal occupational health risks involved. But occupational risk, of course, cannot entirely be eliminated from work in health care, and it would be irresponsible (if not inhuman) if a surgeon operating regularly on AIDS patients did not give some serious consideration to his responsibilities toward his young family. The surgeon's choice here, however, would not be one which allowed picking and choosing among his patients, but whether or not to continue in a profession whose high status in part derives from its historical willingness to accept some degree of exposure to fatal infections.

In the case of doctors, the General Medical Council now has stated[14] that those who refuse to care for HIV or AIDS patients could be charged with serious professional misconduct. In general as well as professional ethical terms, the case against refusing to treat ultimately derives from the unique role in society of doctors and other health care personnel. In human society, there are very few people whom vulnerable individuals (potentially, any of us) can trust with their secrets and look to for non-judgemental advice, help and care. When people are at their most vulnerable, the support and protection offered by health care workers is important not only to the individuals concerned, but also for the future existence of a civilised society.

## Euthanasia and suicide

Euthanasia is a subject on which opinion is divided and strong views are held. Any request from a patient to be put to death painlessly when his suffering becomes too great, is likely to be met by very mixed feelings on the doctor's or other carer's part. In the past, such requests commonly have been associated with the fear of uncontrollable pain or of senile dementia. In response, many doctors have deflected the request by offering reassurance. Modern methods of pain control, they have argued, are highly effective, and the relief of suffering, even at the incidental cost of shortening life, is the main aim of good terminal care. In the case of dementia, insight is lost and those affected are not necessarily unhappy — sometimes quite the reverse. To put them to death in order to relieve other people's distress, moreover, if it were known that this happened, would undermine the confidence of other elderly people in their doctors. The only cases in which it might just be ethically justifiable (although still not legal) to put a patient to death, at his own request, are those involving someone who, after serious rational consideration, wishes above all to die now, but is physically unable to commit suicide — an example of the kind portrayed in the play, *Whose Life Is It Anyway?*. But these hard cases are so extremely rare that the exception does not justify breaking the rule.

In the case of people with AIDS, arguments of these kinds may still be advanced. But many of those suffering from the condition are young, intelligent and educated, and many have already made independent choices about their lives which do not always conform to social conventions. If these patients request to be put to death therefore, the case has moved much closer to what traditionally has been regarded as the rare exception. In these cases, it may be argued, there is still often the option of suicide. But successful suicide may not be easy, and some of those facing the prospect of a terminal condition may well feel justified in requesting death sooner rather than later.

In such circumstances, it is difficult to see how the demands of all the basic ethical principles mentioned earlier can be satisfied. Respect for the patient's autonomy would seem to imply granting his request, but in this case the doctor's autonomy also has to be respected; and legal considerations apart, many doctors will be unwilling to step across the boundary from 'allowing to die' ('passive euthanasia', or just good terminal care) to killing by request ('active voluntary euthanasia'). To do this, they may argue, cannot be construed as doing good or avoiding harm to the patient, and it is not in the general interest, demanded by justice, for doctors to be seen as ministers of death. Nor, they may argue, is this necessary, if the appropriate treatment and relief of pain are administered. To resort too soon to killing, moreover, will decrease the incentive to provide optimal care and treatment in the individual patient's case and more generally.

Arguments against voluntary euthanasia appear to be more strongly held among doctors (who would have to carry it out) than among the general public (who lack the medical knowledge to kill themselves, as some say, 'with dignity').[15] All that can be said about what doctors actually do when confronted with such requests is that no-one knows, but that since most people die in hospital, where some staff at least are very opposed to euthanasia, the opportunity of acceding to a request for euthanasia is very limited. The ethics of counselling someone who wishes to die clearly must take this into account, and must assist the client towards a realistic appreciation of the inevitable conflict of interests and wishes which this question raises.

The ethics of counselling someone who wishes to take his own life are not easier. Obviously, clinical assessment is necessary in such cases to ensure that the individual's understanding of his own condition is realistic and that his judgement is not affected by a treatable mental condition. In the case of someone who has all the information available to a 'prudent patient', and rationally wishes to die, the counsellor (it may be argued) should still maintain a presumption in favour of life, expressed not simply in words, but most of all in ways which help the individual feel valued as himself. The decision thereafter must be that of the individual. As has been argued,[16] our unwillingness to condemn someone who has committed suicide:

> '...both reflects compassion for the conditions which led to the act and an ambivalence that mirrors the moral ambiguity inherent in the act itself. Suicide is always a tragic choice; it is sometimes a misguided choice. But it can be...a conscientious choice.'

## Sexuality

HIV infection and AIDS clearly raise ethical questions about sexuality, and these in turn are related to questions about the place of values in counselling. In schools, for example, it is 'the legal position that sex education must be conducted within the context of a moral framework, emphasising the importance of family life'.[17] In health care counselling, by contrast, a moral framework with this emphasis overtly or detectably present might well deter many potential clients. The values emphasised here, by contrast, are those of life and health; and with this in mind, the counsellor is likely to adopt an approach in other respects as value-free and non-judgemental as possible. On the other hand, there clearly are limits to how value-free even the most non-judgemental counsellor can be. As already suggested, for example, the counsellor has a responsibility to try to persuade the HIV positive client not to hide this fact from any potential sexual partner; and this implies a moral framework in which the values of honesty, and respect for the autonomy of third parties, play an important part.

Values are implied also by the counsellor who decides to provide information about 'safe sex'. This decision may be justifiably regarded as implicitly choosing one moral framework among others; and those who criticise it are correct to argue that, cumulatively, such decisions by those who are perceived as authorities may well undermine so-called 'traditional sexual morality'. In the area of sexuality therefore, it has to be recognised that an entirely 'value-free' approach to counselling is not possible. The situation created by AIDS, however, presents a significant opportunity to re-examine the moral framework in which much discussion of human sexuality has been conducted. In this context, it can be argued that reciprocal care and honesty in sexual relationships are better guides to morality than externally imposed rules of engagement; and that sexual relationships characterised by reciprocal care and honesty can be significant forces for good in the human world, even when they do not conform to the dictates of 'traditional sexual morality'.

Sexuality, of course, also has a social dimension which extends beyond relationships between individuals. In any society, the quality of family life is of the greatest importance, particularly as it affects the need of children for both security and stimulation. Attitudes engendered in caring families, moreover, may well make for a more caring society. In this connection, 'traditional sexual morality' commonly has regarded the needs of family life as frequently in conflict with the desire of adults for mutually fulfilling sexual relationships; and because of this, it has emphasised the rules of celibacy before and (technical) fidelity within marriage, as well as disapproving of homosexual relationships. These rules, however, have always proved difficult for some or many people to adhere to; and those who have broken them often feel not only guilty, but also that there are now no moral guidelines applicable to their situation. These consequences of breaking the traditional rules clearly do not provide the best preconditions for responsible sexual behaviour.

Against this background, it may now be necessary to question the assumption that 'traditional sexual morality' provides the only moral framework which supports the values of family life. A moral framework emphasising the importance of reciprocal care and honesty in sexual relationships, and accepting that different people express their sexuality in different ways, would not always conform to the rules of 'traditional sexual morality'. On the other hand, its emphasis on inner intention, if heeded, might help to make many sexual relationships (outside or within the traditional rules) more responsible and caring. In view of the difficulty many people have with the traditional rules, such a moral framework — outwardly more relaxed, but inwardly more demanding — might make more sense and might have more positive consequences, not only for family life, but also for attempts to limit the spread of HIV infection. Whether or not this is a real possibility, of course, depends on whether society is sufficiently mature to respond to the challenge of a complex rather than a simplistic sexual morality. If society is not mature enough, then only fear may work. But by the time fear does work (when AIDS has actually killed individuals known to others at risk), it may be too late.

## References

1. The best general introduction using this approach is: Gillon, R., (1986). *Philosophical Medical Ethics* Chichester: John Wiley & Sons.
2. See: National Commission for the Protection of Human Subjects of Biomedical and Behavioural Research (1978) *The Belmont Report* Washington DC: DHEW Publication No (OS) 78–0012, pp.10–14.
3. House of Commons Social Services Committee (1987) *Problems Associated With AIDS* London: House of Commons (13 May) p.9 (para.7).
4. *Ibid* pp.12–14 (paras 13–15).
5. Gillon, R. (1987) 'Testing for HIV without permission' *British Medical Journal*, **294**:823.
6. See reference 3, p.75 (para.126).
7. *Ibid* p.100 (para.172).
8. *Ibid* p.102 (para.174).
9. *Ibid* p.103 (para.176).
10. *Ibid*.
11. Declaration of Oslo In: *The Handbook of Medical Ethics* (1984) London: British Medical Association, p.77.
12. *Ibid*.

13. Gillon, R. (1987) 'Refusal to treat AIDS and HIV positive patients' *British Medical Journal*, **294**:1333.
14. Anon (1987) 'GMC advises doctors on duty to AIDS patients' *British Medical Journal*, **294**:1436.
15. Dawson, J. (1986) 'Easeful death' *British Medical Journal*, **293**:1188.
16. Gustafson, J.M. (1984) *Ethics from a Theocentric Perspective, Vol 2* London: University of Chicago Press, p.215.
17. See reference 3, p.60 (para.99).

# Appendix A

# Relaxation

AGNES KOCSIS

If relaxation were easy we would all do it. Ironically, the more stressed one is, the harder it is to relax. It is therefore pointless simply to tell a stressed person to go away and relax. While it is possible simply to give them a relaxation tape and tell them to play it, a large proportion of people will fail to gain benefit from it without further preparation. If someone is often, or has become, chronically tense, that is no accident — he has learned to be that way. Often tension is perceived as a necessary survival tactic, as summed up in the plea, 'Don't tell me to relax — it's my tension that's holding me together'. Teaching someone to relax therefore requires several stages.

## The value of relaxation

It is helpful to review with patients why relaxation is valuable:

- By reducing anxiety and counteracting stress it improves subjective well-being.
- It has direct beneficial effects on bodily functioning by relieving the physical effects of anxiety and stress; for instance it can reduce blood pressure.
- Stress in itself can result in lowering of immune system responses and therefore counteracting it is likely to be very beneficial.

## 1. Preparing the ground

### The objections

While accepting that relaxation is a good idea in principle individuals often give reasons as to why they cannot practise it. They may say that they do not have time, or that those around them would not approve if they were 'not active', or that relaxation is 'self-indulgent'. Or they may feel that their anxiety 'keeps them together'.

Some people get more reward from their stress or busy-ness than they imagine. Being stressed and always 'busy' may fit in with their ideal image of themselves whereas taking time to relax may not. Therefore the counsellor who is preparing a stressed person for relaxation has to start with the basics if the client is to comply with the programme. Things which prevent the person taking up relaxation need to be discussed and confronted. Some issues that can be explored include:

- *Priorities*: The choices between health or stress, work or personal well-being.
- *Giving oneself permission* to look after oneself and one's health.
- *Others* would probably prefer a person who takes time to relax but is well rather than someone who is perpetually stretched.
- *Being realistic*: real efficiency and productivity usually comes with a calm mind and is not necessarily produced by a busy body.

The aim is to establish that the client will give himself *permission* to relax and that he can identify times and places during the day when it will be possible to do so.

### Defining stress

It is important for the counsellor and the client to come to a joint agreement about what is stressful for the client. Things which are stressful for some people are not stressful for others. They also need to explore how the client *recognises* that he is stressed. Different people recognise when they are under stress in different ways. A list can be drawn up jointly of what these are for a particular client. It may be increased irritability, or making more mistakes, or showing symptoms of anxiety, or simply feeling unable to cope, or some other set of symptoms.

The next step is to identify times of day and situations when the symptoms of stress are worst for the client. This can be done by going back over the past few days, recalling and writing down the situations together with the level of tension experienced and rating the tension on a scale from 1 to 5, where 1 is no tension and 5 is very high tension. (See also Chapter 12 on anxiety and depression, for diary-keeping.)

## 2.   Building on what is there

Most people will already have ways of relaxing in their lives and these can be built upon first before suggesting new ways of relaxing. The counsellor must beware of deciding *for* the client what is going to be relaxing, just because it comes under that heading for the counsellor. Violent exercise, hang-gliding, washing floors or watching flowers grow can all be relaxing occupations for different people. Progress will be much easier if you work with these first, before suggesting other kinds of relaxation to try.

It is important to identify with clients the ways in which they relax. There are various general categories to explore:

- *Active physical activities*: e.g. squash, jogging, swimming, dancing, going for a walk, doing the housework, tidying up.
- *Sensuous physical activities*: e.g. having a bath, going for a sauna, having a massage, sex, playing a musical instrument, preparing a special meal, eating and drinking, yoga.
- *Stimulating mental activities*: e.g. watching television, listening to the radio, going to the theatre or cinema, listening to music, reading, conversing, doing the crossword.
- *Mental activities which reduce stimulation*: e.g. locking oneself away in bathroom or home, taking the phone off the hook, day-dreaming, dozing.

These are all constructive ways of relaxing. However, individuals may have ways of relaxing which, in the long term, can cause more problems than they solve: for instance, excessive use of alcohol or drugs. These too need to be elicited and talked through.

When you have a list of ways in which the client can relax it will help you and the client decide whether he tends to relax more through muscular activity or through mental processes. This is of value later.

The next step is to discuss how he is currently using these relaxing activities in his life and to find ways in which he can enhance them or incorporate them more frequently and consciously.

When people are relatively cheerful and coping, they will partake in relaxation often without labelling it as such. They will also spontaneously *use* activities to cheer themselves up and to unwind at the end of the day. Unfortunately when people get anxious and depressed, instead of stepping up the amount of relaxing activities they engage in, they may often not bother about relaxation or put it low on their list of priorities and spend all their time worrying or feeling low. It needs a conscious decision then not only to remember that the enjoyable parts of life still exist, but that incorporating them into everyday life is a sensible way of coping — not meaningless self-indulgence.

### 3. Preparing a relaxation tape

The use of a relaxation tape can be a very helpful adjunct in helping someone to relax. Finding out about the client's preferred forms of relaxation will have given an indication of whether the client has a preference for physical or mental relaxation, or whether perhaps both are enjoyed. This preference will affect the preparation of the tape.

There are many commercially available relaxation tapes. These vary in quality, but the main problem is that they tend to be too general and not to take individual variation into account. There are two advantages in the counsellor and the client working on developing a tailor-made relaxation tape together:

- The client will end up with a tape to suit him individually.
- During preparation, the client will have had to consider, experiment and choose what he does find relaxing, in the process becoming more aware of relaxation as an important activity.

It will probably be most reassuring for the client if, when the content of the tape has been agreed, the counsellor records the instructions onto the tape himself. Occasionally the patient may prefer to ask a friend to do it, or even record his own voice. In the instructions given below, pauses will be required. The counsellor will have to use judgement as to the length of time to pause for.

There are several possible components for a relaxation tape and the balance of these and which are included and which left out will vary with individual client preference.

### Breathing exercises

Control of breathing is a crucial skill for anyone who experiences anxiety with physical symptoms. There are several ways to learn to control breathing. Two methods are given below. Try each of these out with the client in the session and send him away to practise. When he has chosen what suits him best, you can record instructions for that exercise on his tape.

### 1. Hands on stomach

This method is useful in social situations because you can quite com-

fortably keep your hands folded on your stomach without anybody
noticing you are practising relaxation!

### Example instructions

Place your hands flat and touching with fingers laced on the lower part
of your stomach, just above your pelvis. Spend a few moments noticing
how your stomach is moving as you breathe. Now exaggerate the
movement slightly, so that you can really feel your stomach move
upwards as you breathe in and downwards as you breathe out. Now
imagine something slow and peaceful and comfortable. You are strolling
down a country lane on a sunny day and you are listening out for the
distant sound of the sea. You can just hear the regular comforting
sound of the waves breaking on the shore. There is no wind and the
waves make a slow, infinitely regular sound. Breathe in time with the
waves.

This image can be adapted according to the client's preference. If he
cannot easily visualise, he could think of a slow piece of music, or, if
necessary, count. The disadvantage of counting is that when people
are anxious it is difficult for them to count slowly. An alternative is to
say a phrase when breathing in, and another when breathing out:
'Now − be calm' (breathe in); 'Relaxation is a balm' (breathe out), is
an example.

### 2.   Breathing out and up

### Example instructions

This is best done lying flat. Lie down in a warm convenient spot and
make your body comfortable. Place your hands with fingers splayed
on your ribcage, just under your nipples or breasts. Now half breathe
in by pushing your chest up to the ceiling and then finish the breath
by pulling your ribcage towards your head. Hold the breath for a
moment. And let go. Do this just three times. (Pause.) Then breathe
normally and feel the pleasant lightness in your head. Let yourself
float.

### Muscular relaxation

There are two ways of relaxing muscles which can be done while
basically lying still. Both involve going over the body systematically
and relaxing each muscle or group of muscles in turn. It is usual to

start at one end of the body and work towards the other, but this is not essential. Some people like to start with, say, their back, because that is such a nerve-packed area.

The first method is especially valuable for those who have never really thought about relaxing and do not have much awareness of how tense or relaxed their body might be at a given time. It involves, paradoxically, tensing each muscle even more — and then letting go. This method means that everyone can achieve the sensation of letting go some of the tension, even if just a little. It is helpful to synchronise each muscle relaxation exercise with breathing in and out. Instructions are given below for the upper torso. Each muscle group is repeated twice. The instructions should be extended by simply replacing the parts of the body referred to with the muscles of the lower back, the upper thighs, the knees, the calves, the ankles and the toes. The instructions should be read at a slow, comfortable pace, attempting to impose a rhythm on the exercises.

*Example instructions*
Start with your hands. Focus on your hands. Feel the tension in your hands. Now start to breathe in and curl your fingers up into a fist. Tense them three-quarters tense; tense, but not too tense. Prepare to breathe out and let go the tension. Hold — and let go. And again. Start to breathe in. Curl your fingers into a fist. Tense them hard; tense, but not too tense. Prepare to breathe out and let go the tension. Feel the tension move out of your hands. Now your arms. Prepare to breathe in. Now tense your arms and breathe in. Tense, tense up, but not too tense. Hold — prepare to breathe out — and let go. Say goodbye to the tension. And your arms again. Prepare to breathe in. Tense — feel the tension. And prepare to breathe out. Let go the tension. Now your shoulders. Prepare to breathe in. Now move your shoulders back as far as they will go. Push them back under you. Hold — prepare to breathe out — and let go. Now the shoulders again. Prepare to breathe in. Now push the shoulders back, push them against one another. Hold — prepare to let go — and breathe out.

The second method of muscle relaxation is for those who have a sense of their muscle tension and already know how to manipulate it. This can be done lying in any comfortable position, whether on the front or the back. The body must feel well supported. A high pillow is not helpful for most people. Unless very uncomfortable it is probably best to lie quite flat.

*Example instructions*
I want you now to make a journey through your body. You are journeying to the different parts of your body to relax them. As your journey goes on, more and more of your body will feel comfortable. Start at your head. Make your head go heavy. Let it sink into the floor. You do not have to support any part of your head. The floor is there to support it for you. Give your head to the floor to support. Now your arms. Stop holding your arms. Let them go. Let the floor support your arms for the moment. Feel now that you have no responsibility for your arms. Now your upper body. Let your upper body go completely. Let it sink into the floor. Your body is sinking deeper and deeper, is being held by the floor.

The instructions can be extended for the legs and the feet.

## Sensuous imagery

For those individuals identified early on as enjoying mental stimulation and day-dreaming, imagery and visualisation can be a very potent form of relaxation. The essence is to discover images which the client finds very soothing and pleasurable. The images should be texturally rich and detailed, with colour, shape, sound, touch and even smell if this can be achieved. People vary enormously in their ability to visualise scenes or sensations to themselves, and not everyone will find this pleasurable or possible. It is of course vital to explore which images will be pleasant. Some people for example hate lying on a beach and listening to the seagulls; others are allergic to the countryside!

*Example instructions*
It is a warm day in early summer and you are waiting for a friend in the midst of the countryside. You are anticipating having a most happy day together. You are lying waiting on some new grass, close to a willow tree. There is a stream alongside you and you can sense the coolness of the water as it runs past to a small waterfall. As you lie there with your eyes closed and the sun warming your eyelids, you can hear the soft whisper of the waterfall. The water makes you feel thirsty. You take an orange from your bag and run your fingers over its cool skin. It is a beautiful vibrant colour. You peel it slowly with your fingers, feeling the moistness of its thick flesh and smelling the oil as it spurts onto your fingers. You part the orange segments and feel their silky surface. You can anticipate the sweetness of the juice you are about to taste, the coolness and the sweetness.

## Memories of happiness

Along similar lines to the above you can discuss a moment in your client's life when he remembers being particularly happy. This can either be described in detail on the tape, or else, if he prefers to remember it privately, he can be prompted to do this for a few minutes.

## Incorporating music or sounds

Moods are generally very responsive to music and even particular sounds. Clients can be encouraged to identify music which they associate with happiness or relaxation and to incorporate this onto the tape. Flutes, pan-pipes and harps are often used to create a soothing ambience, but again this is idiosyncratic. It can be quite interesting to try to identify your most soothing piece of music.

## Poems, uplifting words

Those who like poetry may wish to record particularly meaningful pieces. Those with HIV are sometimes interested in 'talking to the virus' in their body. Any statements that they wish to use could also be incorporated here. Alternatively, the following statements could be used:

I am becoming a more relaxed person.
I am enjoying taking control of my body, and my life.

## Preparing to use the tape – setting the scene

When the tape has been prepared, discuss with the client when he is likely to use it – and where. It should be used daily if at all possible. Sometimes clients pose difficulties – 'My flatmate is there, I can't disturb her'; 'I'm too busy to listen to the tape every day', etc. These excuses have to be confronted. It is a question of priorities. Friends are usually fascinated by relaxation tapes and if anything, want to join in!

## 4.   Dealing with panic attacks

If the client experiences panic attacks with overbreathing and is planning to try to return to the situations he fears most (see Chapters 12 and 13, on anxiety, depression and problem solving), it is helpful to discuss the strategies he is going to use. Most helpful are likely to be the breathing and to some extent the muscle relaxation. The example is of someone who tends to panic in the supermarket.

*Example instructions*

On your way there I want you to prepare your body. You are preparing your breathing and your muscles. You are going to keep relaxing the muscles of your neck, your shoulders and your chest — your upper chest and your lower chest. You are going to walk out, feeling the strength in your body. You are going to walk confidently and with suppleness. Keep checking your breathing and your muscles. Think of the exercises. Now you are taking control. Do not take any notice of your heart beating or any of your body's fear responses. You are going to go into the supermarket and you are going to beat your anxiety. It is not a dangerous place. If you feel your anxiety rising, practise your breathing. Breathe as much as you need, but remember the rhythm of your breathing. Aim for a natural, smooth rhythm. Remember the rhythm of the waves, beating on the shore.

Although it is usual to listen to the tape when in a private place and lying comfortably, some people have used their tapes in a personal stereo while on the street or in the underground. This can be very helpful for people who are worried about experiencing panic attacks or who are practising getting back into their feared situations. Additional comforting thoughts can be pre-recorded. Examples are:

'I'm not alone in this. My counsellor is going to be really pleased that I've done this. *I'm* going to be really pleased that I've done it.'
'Even if I panic, it's only my body playing up. I've got to reassure my body. There's no real danger. There are no lions in this supermarket.'
'My heart's beating very fast, but it's not doing me any harm. Physically I am quite all right. This just shows my body knows how to react to danger if it has to. But here it doesn't have to.'

## 5.  Tape, diary and programme

The whole relaxation programme therefore comprises two, or possibly, depending on the individual, three parts:

- The incorporation of relaxation into everyday life.
- Preparation and use of the relaxation tape.
- Preparing to deal with a panic attack.

In order for the client and counsellor to monitor how the programme is going, it may be helpful to keep a daily diary. This can be in the form of a check-list, incorporating the relaxing activities discussed, to be filled in every day:

| MONDAY | | |
| --- | --- | --- |
| | **Time** | **How Relaxed (1–5)** |
| Tape | 11 pm | 5 |
| Jogging | 8 pm | 3 |
| Bath | | |
| Listened to music | | |
| Spent time with friends | 6–8 pm | 2 |

Alternatively, if someone's anxiety varies a great deal during the day and he wishes to practise incorporating relaxation as much as possible, a fear 'thermometer' chart can be used for each day, marking shifts in state of relaxation (Fig. A.1).

### Modifying and perfecting the programme

As the client becomes increasingly skilled at relaxing using the relaxation tape, some of the exercises will become second nature and he will be able to do without the tape. This applies particularly to the muscles exercises. He may then prefer to use the tape only for imagery, or music. He may wish to prepare another tape.

The diary-keeping should not be continued if it is a chore. Sometimes it is better to keep a diary, say, every third week.

### General points to remember

During the whole of the relaxation work with the client, it is important to emphasise monitoring of tension.

'The more tense you are to start with, the harder it is to relax. It is therefore important to get into the habit of monitoring your level of tension, so as to be able to intervene early enough. This may mean checking and relaxing as often as every minute in some situations, every few hours in others. Relaxation must become an integral part of life.'

People who have been anxious for many years, prior even to HIV infection, rather than just in response to becoming seropositive or being diagnosed as having AIDS, may find relaxation itself quite

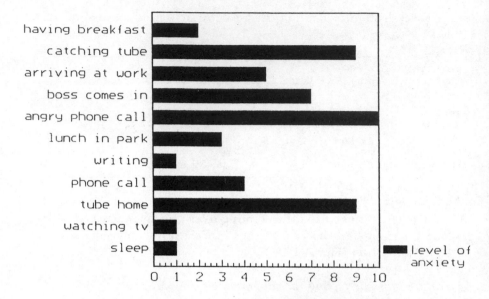

*Fig. A.1* Illustration of a way of keeping a 'fear thermometer' —
linking events in the day with anxiety levels. Hourly checks on anxiety
levels can be made.

anxiety-provoking at first. It should be pointed out to them that this is
not surprising, since they have been using anxiety to cope, as a sort of
attempt at survival. The trouble is that the attempt was counter-
productive. Now they will be learning a more effective survival method.
But for a while they will feel anxious about letting the old one go. This
is normal and they should just practise regularly. The anxiety will fade
quickly.

However carefully counsellor and client prepare, it is *crucial* to emphasise that relaxation takes time. All the exercises have to be learnt
and practised regularly. At first it will very probably feel laborious and
clumsy, like the initial awkwardness of learning to drive a car. This is
inevitable and clients will only feel disappointed and discouraged if
they are allowed to expect an immediate, heady sense of relaxation. It
will certainly come. But daily practise with the tape, as well as the
active incorporation of the relaxing pastimes and activities identified
at the beginning of the sessions, will be necessary. The aim is to allow
relaxation to permeate their life style — not simply to be added on top
of an existing life style.

# Appendix B

# Suggested Reading List

SIMON VEARNALS

## Journals

Included below are some of the main scientific journals which might be of use to you, and which cover various aspects of HIV/AIDS work. Topics covered vary considerably from journal to journal so it might be useful to read a few back copies to see if they are relevant to your area of work.

*British Medical Journal (BMJ)* weekly
Very informative up-to-date material of a scientific nature. Other issues covered include social, legal and ethical problems like HIV testing without consent, screening and counselling.

*The Lancet* weekly
Very similar to the *BMJ* in scientific information and social dilemmas. Very good for preliminary research reports.

*New Scientist* weekly
Popular scientific weekly with a section called the 'AIDS monitor' which covers worldwide issues relating to HIV/AIDS.

*Nature* weekly
General information relating to HIV/AIDS.

*AIDS* an International Bimonthly Journal
Covering scientific research from around the world on HIV/AIDS. Also includes the latest World Health Organisation's statistics on HIV/AIDS.

*New England Journal of Medicine* weekly
Includes some of the larger longitudinal studies in the USA on subjects

such as progression of HIV in patients, behaviour trends and drug trials.

*Journal of the American Medical Association* weekly
Covers a much wider range of issues regarding HIV/AIDS. Also has a section on the CDC's morbidity and mortality weekly report (MMWR).

## Books

The following list of books are just our selection from the many which have been written on the subject of HIV/AIDS.

*The Management of AIDS Patients*
Macmillan Press (1986)
D. Miller, J. Weber, J. Green
A very comprehensive book written by experienced HIV/AIDS workers. An invaluable source of information for any HIV/AIDS worker.

*Living With AIDS (A Guide to Survival by People with AIDS)*
Frontliners (1987)
Written by PWAs for PWAs, a useful book with chapters dealing with most aspects of HIV infection like 'Preparing for the future', 'Going into hospital'.

*AIDS, A Self Care Manual*
IBS Press (1987)
AIDS project Los Angeles
A step-by-step manual for health care workers and people with HIV infection.

*AIDS, A Strategy For Nursing Care*
Arnold (1986)
R. Pratt
An excellent book covering the major areas of caring for people with HIV infection. A very useful book for both nurses and other health care workers.

*AIDS Nursing Guidelines*
Royal College of Nursing (1987)
RCN AIDS working party
Gives a good outline of areas which may be causing concern for nursing staff regarding HIV/AIDS. Covers infection control, support and community care.

*AIDS and Employment Law*
Financial Training Publications (1988)
C. Southam, Gillian Howard
A comprehensive textbook covering the issues around UK employ-
ment law, confidentiality and discrimination. A useful book for lawyers,
trade union workers and for people with HIV infection.

*Living With AIDS and HIV*
Macmillan Press (1987)
D. Miller
A step-by-step manual for people with HIV infection and health care
workers. It covers some of the major psychological and practical areas
which people with HIV infection and health care workers may
encounter.

*Women and the AIDS Crisis*
Pandora Press (1987)
D. Richardson
An interesting book dealing with aspects of HIV infection with a
particular emphasis on problems that women may encounter.

*The Complete Guide to Safe Sex*
Specific Press (1987)
The Institute for Advanced Study of Human Sexuality
Useful introduction to facts and information on safe sex counselling
and education.

*Sexuality Nursing and Health*
John Wiley and Sons (1985)
C. Webb

*Dying*
Penguin (1984)
J. Hinton

*On Death and Dying*
Tavistock Publications (1970)
E. Kubler-Ross

*ABC of AIDS*
British Medical Association (1987)
Edited by M.W. Adler

# Index

Adoption, 164–5
  Adoption Agencies Regulations 1983, 294
Advantages of the test, 25
AIDS Related Complex (ARC), 5, 6
Anal intercourse, 48, 229–30
Analingus, 48, 230
Antenatal screening, 158
Antibodies, 4, 5, 6
Antibody testing, 135–6
  legal issues, 289
Antigens, 4, 5
Anxiety
  check list, 101
  management, 80–81
Assessing risk, 22, 252–3
AZT, 11

Behaviour change, 26
Body fluids
  breast milk, 36
  faeces, 36
  saliva, 36
  tears, 36
  urine, 37
  vaginal and cervical secretions, 36
Body Positive, 240–41
Body rubbing, 49
Blood and blood products, 36
  Factor VIII, 101–12

Factor IX, 36, 101–12
Blood transfusion counselling, 262–4
Breaking the news, 28, 29, 30, 31
Buddies, 244–5

Carers, 65, 99–100
CD–4 antigen, 2
Co-factors, 9
Cognitive impairment, 92–4
Community care, 136–7
  services available, 236–7
Confidentiality, 21–2
  ethical question, 306–307
  legal issues, 291–5
Consent, 302–306
Consumer Protection Act 1987, 298
Counselling significant others, 83–4
Criminal law, 286–8

Day and foster care, 163–4
Death and dying, 76, 118–19
  death and the carer, 218–219
  discussing death, 214–15
Dentist, 59–60
Depression
  check list, 101–102
  combatting, 81–2
Discussing the test, 23
DNA, 3

Drug treatments
    anxiety, 181-2

Emotional reactions, 70-3
Encephalopathy, 8
Epidemiology, 10, 11
Euthanasia and suicide, 309-10

Family, 86
Fisting, 48
Flushing, 122
Friends, 87
Frontliners, 245

General Practitioners, 24, 59-60

Health boosting, 62-3
Health education, 266-7
Haemophiliacs
    adolescence, 115-16
    adult, 116-17
    schoolboy, 115
Haemophilia Society, 241-2
Heterosexuals, 64
HIV-1, 1, 2, 3
HIV-1 antibody tests, 13
    confirmatory tests, 15
    screening tests, 15
HIV-2 virus, 2
HIV education in schools, 165-6
HIV seropositive women, 159-60
Hypochondriacs, 168

Immunisation, 162-3
Informing sexual partners, 52-5,
    269-71
Injecting drug use
    management of the drug problem,
        128-9
    outreach work, 133-4
    self-help, 131-2
    treatment services, 131-4
Insurance, 24
Interviewing
    getting the discussion going, 31
    infection control, 35

IV drug related, 124-5
    relationships, 42-6
    transmission, 35-9
Isolation of the HIV infected person,
    295-7

Keeping well, 60-3

Legal obligations of the patient and
    others, 297-8
Legal repercussions, 24
Lesbian and Gay Switchboard, 239-40
London Lighthouse, 241
Lovers, 42, 46, 99-100

Mental Health Act 1983, 291
Mass screening, 145
Masturbation, 49, 228-9

NHS (Venereal Diseases) Regulations
    1974, 292
Neurological involvement, 100-101
Neuropsychological tests, 94-7

Obessional behaviour, 194-6
Obessional thoughts, 196-7
Offences Against The Person Act 1861,
    286, 287, 289
Opportunistic infections
    Candidiasis, 7
    Cryprococcal meningitis, 7
    Cryptosporidiosis, 7
    Cytomegalovirus, 7
    Herpes simplex, 7
    Pneumocystis carinii pneumonia, 7
    Toxoplasmosis, 7
    Tuberculosis, 7
Opportunistic tumours
    Ano-rectal carcinoma, 8
    Kaposis sarcoma, 8-9
    Non-Hodgkin lymphomas, 8
Oral sex, 48, 229
Organising a counselling service, 260-2

Panic attacks
    dealing with, 321-2

Persistent Generalised Lymphadenopathy (PGL), 5
Planning for death, 216–18
Planning pregnancy, 152–5
Practical help, 65–6
Pre-test counselling in pregnancy, 146–8
Professional responsibility, 302–309
Prognostic tests, 16
  antigen testing, 16
  core (p24) antibody testing, 17
Prostitutes, 255
Public Health (Control of Disease) Act 1984, 294, 295

Race Relations Act 1976, 288–9
Recreational drugs
  reducing use of, 63
Reducing risk, 26–7
  intravenous drug use, 125–6
  personal risk, 39
  sexual risk, 39–42
Relaxation, 63
  preparing a tape, 317
Risk to child, 142–3
Risk to mother, 141–2
RNA, 2, 3

Seroconversion, 14
Sex
  dealing with sexual issues, 127–8
  safer sex, 39–42, 47–52
  sexual difficulties, 83

sexual behaviour, 127, 272–5
Sex Discrimination Acts 1975 and 1986, 288
Sex toys, 48
Sexuality
  ethical questions, 310–12
Shooting galleries, 122
Staff support, 119–20
Stress
  defining, 315
  reduction, 63
Suicidal thoughts and actions, 188–9
Support, 57–60, 73, 79

Telling others, 52–5, 75
Termination of pregnancy
  counselling for, 148–9
  effects of, 143–4
  post termination counselling, 150–51
The Terrence Higgins Trust, 242–5
T-helper cells, 1, 2
Training, 235–6
Transmission, 35, 36
  tissue and organ transplants, 36
Travel, 24
Travellers, 255–6

Vaginal intercourse, 48
Virus culture, 13

Water sports, 48
Who to tell, 25